3

PREGNANT WOMEN AT WORK

PREGNANT WOMEN
AT
WORK

Edited by

GEOFFREY CHAMBERLAIN

Professor of Obstetrics and Gynaecology
St George's Hospital Medical School
Cranmer Terrace, London SW17 0RE

Published jointly by
The Royal Society of Medicine
and
The Macmillan Press Ltd

First published jointly in 1984 by
THE ROYAL SOCIETY OF MEDICINE
1 Wimpole St, London WIM 8AE

and

The Scientific and Medical Division
THE MACMILLAN PRESS LTD
London and Basingstoke
Companies and representatives throughout the world

British Library Cataloguing in Publication Data
Chamberlain, Geoffrey
Pregnant women at work.
1. Pregnant women — Great Britain
2. Women — Employment — Great Britain
I. Title
331.4'3'0941   RG 525

ISBN 0-333-36881-9
ISBN 0-333-37117-8 Pbk

Printed in Hong Kong

Contents

The Contributors

Prof Raja W. Abdul-Karim
Dept of Obstetrics and Gynecology
College of Medicine
State University of New York
Upstate Medical Center
750 East Adams St
Syracuse, NY 13210
USA

Nicholas A. Ashford
Center for Policy Alternatives
Massachusetts Institute of Technology
Cambridge
Mass 02139
USA

Ms Frances J. T. Baker
Senior Nursing Officer
Scottish Gas
Granton House
4 Marine Drive
Edinburgh EH5 1YB

Prof N. R. Butler
Dept of Child Health
Royal Hospital for Sick Children
St Michael's Hill
Bristol BS2 8BJ

Prof Geoffrey Chamberlain
Dept of Obstetrics and Gynaecology
St George's Hospital Medical School
Cranmer Terrace
London SW17 0RE

Dr J. David Erickson
Chronic Diseases Division
Center for Environmental Health
Centers for Disease Control
Atlanta
Georgia 30333
USA

Miss Ann Foster
EMAS Branch D
Health and Safety Executive
25 Chapel Street
London NW1 5DT

Dr Steven G. Gabbe
Hospital of the University of Pennsylvania
Woman's Hospital Division
3400 Spruce Street
Philadelphia, Pa 19104
USA

Ms Jo Garcia
National Perinatal Epidemiology Unit
Radcliffe Infirmary
Oxford OX2 6HE

Dr F. E. Hytten
Division of Perinatal Medicine
Clinical Research Centre
Medical Research Council
Watford Road
Harrow, Middlesex
HA1 3UJ

Dr E. Marshall Johnson
Director
Daniel Baugh Institute of Anatomy
Jefferson Medical College
Thomas Jefferson University
1020 Locust Street
Philadelphia
Pa 19107
USA

Prof Marvin S. Legator
Dept of Preventive Medicine and
    Community Health
Division of Environmental Toxicology
The University of Texas Medical Branch
25 Keiller Building, F-19
Galveston
Texas 77550
USA

Mr Steven Lorber
North Islington Law Centre
161 Hornsey Road
London N7 6DU

Mr M. E. McDowall
Medical Statistics Division
Office of Population Censuses and Surveys
St Catherine's House
10 Kingsway
London WC2B 6JP

Dr James McEwen
Academic Dept of Community Medicine
King's College Hospital Medical School
Denmark Hill
London SE5 8RX

Ms Sheila McKechnie
Health and Safety Officer
ASTMS
Whitehall Office
Dane O'Coy's Road
Bishops Stortford
Herts

Dr N. Mamelle
INSERM – U170
Université Claude Bernard – Bâtiment 710
La Doua
43 Boulevard du Onze Novembre
69100 Villeurbanne Cedex
France

Dr Donald R. Mattison
Building 10, Room 8C313
Pregnancy Research Branch
National Institute of Child Health and
    Human Development
National Institutes of Health
Bethesda
Maryland 20205
USA

Dr Robert Murray OBE
Consultant in Occupational Health
120 Temple Chambers
Temple Avenue
London EC4Y 0DT

Dr Ann Oakley
National Perinatal Epidemiology Unit
Radcliffe Infirmary
Oxford
OX2 6HE

Mr Jonathan Plaut
Environmental Affairs
Allied Corporation
PO Box 1057R
Morristown
NJ 07960
USA

Sir James Watt
President
Royal Society of Medicine
1 Wimpole St
London W1M 8AE

Foreword

Sir James Watt
President, Royal Society of Medicine

Sir Richard Doll once warned crusaders about the formidable hurdles they can expect to encounter in their attempts to protect patients against health hazards. The value of preventive measures may be extremely difficult to prove: they necessarily enter the cost-benefit equation, but costs and benefits are as much susceptible to subjective assessment as to objective quantification. Ultimately, preventive measures may prove so expensive that authorities might prefer to spend the money on clinical care with its more tangible benefits[1]. Nevertheless, despite such discouragement, Williams has suggested that we are effectively safeguarding the patient's welfare when 'the most valuable thing that we are not doing is less valuable than the least valuable thing that we are doing'[2].

One problem in our modern society is that more women are working in pregnancy in a wide variety of occupations. They are concerned about the effects of their work on the outcome of pregnancy. What information there is about the hazards of working at this time is spread diffusely, and large areas exist where we have no firm answers. Because of the importance of this aspect of preventive health, the Royal Society of Medicine and the Royal Society of Medicine Foundation made it the subject of their 1983 Anglo-American Conference. The idea was inspired by the interest of Professor Geoffrey Chamberlain, who has drawn attention to apparent anomalies and conflicting observations which raise many questions, but provide few answers[3]. Strictly comparable data have been difficult to obtain, owing to the large number of variables, such as age, social class, marriage patterns, family size, social benefits, antenatal screening, the nature of the work and the transportation conditions, management philosophy, staffing facilities, diet, national traditions of employment and the effectiveness or otherwise of safety regulations in different countries.

The participants of the conference obviously realised this during the spirited discussion, the hallmark of a meeting's success; the speakers were subjected to searching probes and suggestions for action from a particularly well-informed and perceptive audience. It became evident that a collaborative and integrated

ix

approach to the problems of pregnant women at work will be necessary, involving practical industrial measures, effective legislation, education and research. The Editor, Professor Geoffrey Chamberlain, is therefore to be congratulated upon arranging the publishing of the proceedings of this symposium with a minimum of delay.

REFERENCES

1. Doll, Sir Richard (1982). *Prospects for Prevention. The Harveian Oration*, Royal College of Physicians, London
2. Williams, A. (1978). Efficiency and welfare. In *Providing for the Health Services*, Black, D. and Thomas, S. P. (Eds.), Croom Helm, London
3. Chamberlain, G. and Garcia, J. (1983). Pregnant women at work. *Lancet*, 1, 228–230

Preface

The catalyst for this book was the Anglo-American Conference held in the summer of 1983 at the Royal Society of Medicine in London. These conferences are held alternately in London and Washington, their purpose being to bring together experts from both sides of the Atlantic to discuss subjects which have repercussions in each country. On this occasion the subject chosen was that of how the work a woman does in pregnancy may affect her health or that of her unborn child. It was decided that we should take the opportunity of bringing so many experts together to produce a volume on the subject in parallel with the meeting. Those speaking came from many disciplines, including obstetrics, epidemiology, pathology, toxicology, occupational health and the law. They each had at their fingertips original and published material from their own discipline, much of which was unknown to those who worked in other aspects of the subject. In consequence, each speaker was asked to contribute a chapter on that aspect of the subject in which he or she was expert, so that one volume could be produced containing material that would be of help to anyone wishing to look into the subject in the future. Particular value is in the large numbers of references given by each contributor, which may lead to further reading.

One of the values of a conference such as 'Pregnant Women at Work' is that it stimulates ideas for doing further research. Each of us realises the deficiencies of our own present knowledge, and the stimulation of meeting other people with slightly different approaches to the same subject produces ideas for new projects. It is hoped that, by disseminating more widely the ideas of the contributors to this conference, others might be able to react to the stimulation. It was decided not to publish the discussion which occurred after each paper, but the editor has grouped together some of the issues considered in a concluding chapter entitled 'Adverse influences of the working environment'.

No volume of this nature could be produced without a lot of co-operation from many workers. The editor is grateful to all the contributors who produced their manuscripts so promptly and allowed publication to proceed at a brisk pace. He is grateful to The Macmillan Press, the publishers, for their expeditious dealing with the matter. Finally, all of us owe a debt to Miss Muriel Mitchell of the Royal Society of Medicine, who so ably organised the conference and whose grasp of the principles and details of running such a meeting has proved invaluable to many at the RSM.

London, 1984   G. C.

Part 1
The Current Situation

1

Women at Work in Pregnancy

GEOFFREY CHAMBERLAIN

In all countries of the Western World two changes in work patterns can be seen: more women are working in pregnancy than 30 years ago and the pregnant workers are staying in employment later into pregnancy than previously. The position in the UK is exemplified in table 1.1. In 1946 Douglas[1] surveyed all the deliveries of one week in England and Wales in the National Birthday Trust study *Maternity in Great Britain*. He reported that 28 per cent of women worked in pregnancy and 10 per cent of these went on to work into the last 10 weeks of pregnancy. Daniels[2], in a randomised study of 2700 pregnant women during 1979, found that the proportion at work had increased to 48 per cent, of whom three-quarters were working into the last trimester. This represents almost a doubling of those working and a much greater proportion of pregnant workers continuing later in gestation.

Table 1.1 Percentage of women in two surveys reported as working in pregnancy and working in the last 10 weeks of gestation. 1946 data from reference 1; 1979 data from reference 2

	1946	1979
Percentage working in pregnancy	28	48
Percentage working after 30 weeks' gestation	10	75

There are probably two main driving forces for this increase of work in pregnancy. First, many couples now enter marriage with increased financial commitments and so need two incomes to satisfy the demand. Mortgages and the buying of furniture would erode a single salary too deeply for most young people and so both pay packets are needed, irrespective of family plans. Second, the years of child-bearing correspond roughly to those of advancement in most

3

professions and occupations. Many women who are going to achieve success in their chosen way of work lay the foundations for this between 20 and 35, yet these are the years when women have children. While one can debate the capacity of males to bring up children, it is a biological fact that only women give birth to them, and so pregnancy and child-bearing would interfere with the progress up the promotion ladder; many women find this inacceptable.

To have a baby is a normal event which should fit into a normal life style, but modern Western life has superimposed a series of social restrictions which can hardly be called natural. Professional advancement and bringing in a share of the family income do not fit with all plans for child-bearing, and it is sometimes difficult for women to fulfil all three sets of functions.

WHAT ARE THE PROBLEMS?

One might wonder whether the combination of pregnancy and work really is a problem with which medical people should involve themselves; there are several aspects to justify our examination of this aspect of life.

(1) There are easily defined toxicological and physical noxious agents which may be teratogenic to a fetus in the first 10 weeks of pregnancy, so that a woman should not be working in early pregnancy in such an environment—for example, the effects of irradiation in early pregnancy, a well-known teratogenic agent. X-rays are used not just in hospitals, but also in security check points and in many industries to inspect products. Similarly, certain defoliants and insecticides may have teratogenic effects[3].

(2) There are other chemicals which may have a less obvious effect in later pregnancy: for example, working with anaesthetic agents may affect fetal growth (Pharaoh et al.[4]).

(3) Similarly, there may be physical agents which affect the unborn fetus. Recently, apparently unnecessary anxiety has been engendered in the popular press about environmental hyperthermia[5], ambient noise[6], optical radiation from video display terminals used in computer analyses[7] and industrial ultrasound[8]. All have produced newspaper headlines but the scientific rebuttal did not make such good copy, and so was often not seen by the newspaper readers or radio and television users.

(4) In addition to those physical and chemical agents that have been investigated, there is much that we do not know about fetal pharmacology and we would do well to remind ourselves of past environmental factors that were thought to be safe but later have been shown to be dangerous. An example might be found in the parallel field of neonatal care: an increased oxygen environment for premature babies was thought to be beneficial in the early 1950s until the problems of retrolental fibroplasia made themselves apparent.

(5) The effects of fatigue following standing for long hours or performing

physically strenuous work is not well understood in the pregnant woman; common-sense would consider this to be detrimental, for blood flow would be relatively diverted from the placental bed circulation, but in practice this shift might be capable of compensation.

In consequence, there are good theoretical grounds for investigating all aspects of a pregnant woman's environment; if work outside the home is becoming an increasing part of that environment, then it, too, needs investigation.

In addition to the above physiologico-pathological justifications, society is demanding better results from pregnancy. With lower birth rates in the Western World, couples are expecting the perfect product at delivery. The dead or abnormal baby which would have been taken as an Act of God by a previous generation is now considered blameworthy, the fault being laid at the door of society or its medical advisers. Consumers are expecting more of their doctors and are pressing the matter increasingly, even to the extent of seeking legal redress if an unhappy result comes from a pregnancy. Usually congenital abnormalities and infants of low birth weight are not the fault of an individual obstetrician, but society needs to know more about environmental factors which might be associated with fetal problems, and these include happenings during the pregnant woman's work. Thirty years ago we considered cigarette smoking in pregnancy to be probably harmless, and it needed the work of Butler and Alberman[9] to convince us that this is a potent and preventable feto-placental toxin.

As with most problems in society, other social pressures come into play. Some women wish to work into pregnancy and resent being told that they should not. They feel that mostly male doctors and male employers are being overprotective and unnecessarily restrictive. It seems sensible, therefore, to know more precisely what the real risks are and to refine our knowledge of them so that a more truthful situation can be presented to the woman worker in pregnancy. It might be that some work in pregnancy does not put most women or their fetuses at any increased risk. If so, it is important to tell women of this and let them continue their chosen life. There is possibly even some educational advantage to children whose mothers continue work during pregnancy. If one puts restrictions on a pregnant woman that are seen to be unnecessary when she regards herself as a healthy individual, there may be resentment when she is given other advice in the antenatal period by the same medical team, even if this later advice is based on sounder principles — for example, the risks if pre-eclampsia supervenes.

WORK PATTERNS IN PREGNANCY

Before considering paid employment, we must remember that whatever else they do, all women work in the home.

Domestic work

Most pregnant women have a home to look after. House maintenance takes up much time and energy — washing clothes, cleaning the house, preparing and tidying up after meals are all conventionally women's work. In addition, in many homes there are other children to look after as well as the intrauterine one. These make demands, and although it is probable that the individual load per child decreases with each new infant, the total load increases with the larger family. Further, in many Western societies the parents and parents-in-law of the woman share the home. In the pregnancy age group, such parents are usually fit and may even be helpers in housework, but older parents (and even some of the younger ones) are an added burden to the load that the woman bears in the home.

Although not considered as work in the psychological sense, physical load may be imposed in pregnancy by sporting activities. Women having babies are young and often still taking an active part in games. Measures of excessive efficiency show them to be as efficient as the non-pregnant with no alteration in their ability to ventilate[10]. In early pregnancy women compete and win at international sports meetings, and probably with the exception of the bumping and compressing sports can continue activity almost to term[11]. All this may add to the work load of a pregnant woman.

As well as these loads on the housewife, if she should stay at home for her day's work, there is less access to such institutional facilities as meals prepared or cleared up by other people and to rest rooms. A woman in her home cannot take time off for being sick; she is there all the time, caring for her family, without the breaks in the grind of housework which the woman who goes out to work manages to enjoy for an hour or two.

Work outside the home

Women who work away from the home differ in educational background, family size and socio-economic grouping from those who stay at home in pregnancy. It might be expected, therefore, that there is a complex relationship between pregnancy outcome and work outside the home which needs sorting out by epidemiological methods.

Of the nine million women working in the United Kingdom, about a third are at office work, two million do service jobs such as catering and cleaning, and over a million work in the health services and in education. Within each of these general categories of posts there is a wide spectrum of physical and mental work actually done, from the lightest of effort to the heaviest. The number of hours worked varies greatly, for many more married women are in part-time employment than single women (table 1.2). The proportion of part-time women workers diminishes as the family grows up (table 1.3).

Table 1.2 Percentage of women aged 16–59 who work, by marital status (source: *General Household Survey*, 1981)

	Full time	Part time
Single	57	5
Married	25	32
Widowed, divorced or separated	31	25
All women	33	25

Table 1.3 Working mothers aged 16–59, by age of youngest child

	Full time	Part time
0–4 years	6	18
5–9 years	13	43
10 years or more	26	43
No dependent child	48	18
All women	33	25

In addition to effects at the place of work itself, there are many other aspects of working out of the home in pregnancy. The pregnant woman has to get to and from work; this may involve little effort in a small village or town, but should she work in a large metropolitan area, it may involve an hour or more of difficult travel on crowded public transport at each end of the day, increasing the stress imposed by a woman's activities in pregnancy[12,14]. It is generally believed that a balanced diet should be eaten by pregnant women, but the food provided at the place of work is usually more renowned for its bulk and filling capacity than for its nutritional value. Since pregnant women often wish and need to rest more in the working day, the availability of rest places at work should be considered also.

It seems logical that if a pregnant woman has an extra physiological load and she has work to do either in the home or outside it, she should get some help with the housework. This is unusual: Douglas in 1946[1] and Daniels in 1979[2] both showed the same picture in the UK — that those with the greatest need had the least help in the home. In the former study the household tasks were done less often by the men whose wives had many children or were in the lower socio-economic classes; in the latter study women married to men in social classes IV and V were less likely to have help during and just after delivery than those in social classes I, II and III. Other countries, such as Holland and Finland, have put great effort into providing domiciliary help to the pregnant and recently delivered, and it may be that some of the excellent results in the perinatal period that these countries report are associated with this help in the home. Perhaps this is a field which could be examined urgently in the UK by those who organise and arrange government health and social programmes. Pregnant women are very badly off for help in the home, and a small infusion of monies into this area might result in a great benefit.

HOW COULD WE MEASURE THE PROBLEM?

We know that pregnancy involves great surges of steroid hormones secreted by the mother in response to hormone signals from the growing trophoblast. This causes sweeping changes to all physiological systems of the mother; those to her cardiovascular system, renal system and endocrine systems are fairly well documented[10], but we know less about the effects on the musculo-skeletal system and are even poorer in the measurement of psychological changes or the response to stress. These are combined physiologico-psychological changes difficult to measure. In consequence, some new assessment needs to be made of the response of a woman's body and mind to pregnancy, and this needs to be set against some measures of outcome.

Outcome measures themselves present difficulties. The firm data measures of *perinatal mortality rates* (PNMR) are becoming less useful as the numbers of perinatal deaths drop; in consequence, softer data are used and in chapter 8 Peters and co-authors review some other measures of outcome in relation to work and events that may happen in pregnancy. It would be possible to consider both *stillbirth* and *neonatal death rates* separately, so extending the time surveyed by 3 weeks. PNMR are stillbirths and first-week neonatal deaths only, while neonatal mortality rates include all deaths in the first 4 weeks of life. Extrapolating from this, some would seek to examine *rates of abortion* (the expulsion of a dead embryo or fetus before the 28th week of gestation) as a measure of outcome, while others would sum abortion rates with stillbirth and neonatal death rates to arrive at a *reproductive wastage rate*. Both the last two measures depend on an accurate knowledge of the numbers of spontaneous abortions — an important but an inexact area. We only know of those who seek medical aid at spontaneous abortion, and even then the diagnosis is often uncertain. An even larger source of error is the unknown number of women who conceive but whose embryo dies and is aborted even before 14 days of gestation (i.e. before the next period is due)[13]. In consequence, abortion rates are imprecise and any index derived from them cannot be very exact.

Another measure of outcome in early pregnancy has been attempted by judging *teratogenesis rates*. The embryo is developing and organogenesis is occurring in the early weeks; external constraints acting now can affect organs permanently, so that congenital abnormalities could result. X-rays, certain chemicals and some infections have been shown to affect fetal development.

Johnson considers this in detail in Chapter 11, describing methods of detecting hazards to the conceptus and interpreting the extrapolation of animal work to the human — an area which must always be taken with care. Teratogenesis rates should be examined with reserve: some malformations may be so severe that the embryo dies and is aborted, with all the statistical problems that causes. Other congenital abnormalities are not detected until many years after the neonatal period, and so would be missed from any assay made within a few weeks of birth.

The birth weight of the infant and the relation of birth weight to gestational age are both measures of outcome depending upon fetal growth and placental bed perfusion in pregnancy. Longer-term measures may be of educational attainments. These are valuable measures of a woman's contribution to her child's health, but such studies are difficult, needing time and producing results long after the event. Peters and co-authors describe some of these long-term measures of outcome in Chapter 8. New measures of outcome and new ways of measuring a woman's reaction to pregnancy are needed.

In addition to all this, the background of the woman needs careful assessment. Her age, parity and socio-economic class are three established criteria used in epidemiology to assess a woman's reproductive capacity. They all have separate effects on the chances of producing a live baby (see figures 1.1, 1.2 and 1.3) and are factors that the mother brings to pregnancy which cannot be altered. These features interact with other medical factors — for example, the perinatal mortality rate in pre-eclampsia (figure 1.4). All these variables might produce an even higher risk to the pregnancy of the working mother but yet might be modified by the work she does. It is important to know of their contribution to any fetal harm which might have been attributed incorrectly to the narrower aetiological features associated only with the work itself.

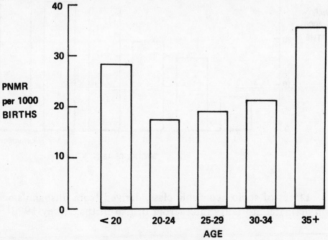

Figure 1.1 Effect of maternal age on perinatal mortality rates (from British Births Survey 1970[15])

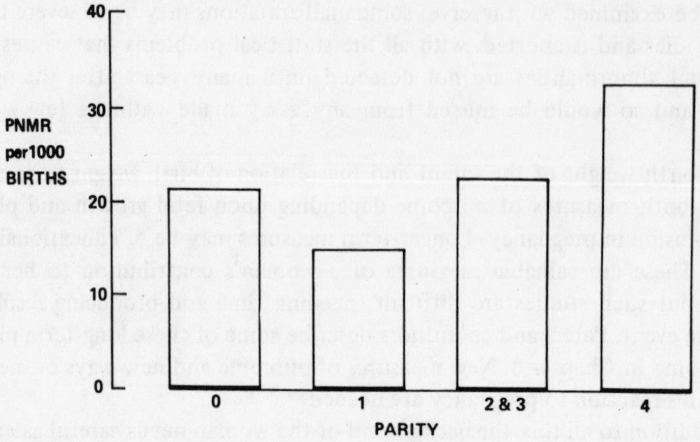

Figure 1.2 Effect of parity on perinatal mortality rates (from British Births Survey 1970[15])

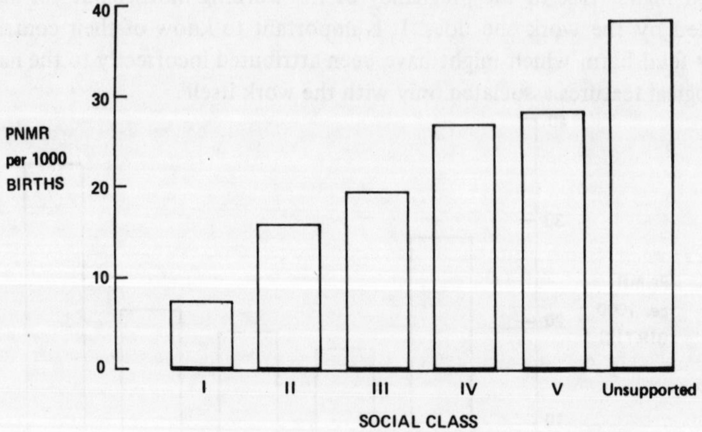

Figure 1.3 Effect of socio-economic class, derived from husband's occupation, on perinatal mortality rates (from British Births Survey 1970[15])

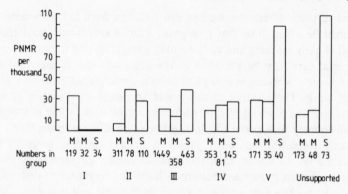

Figure 1.4 Effect of socio-economic class and pre-eclampsia on perinatal mortality rates. Effects of severe pre-eclampsia are seen at their worst in social class V and the unsupported mothers. MMS means mild, moderate and severe, respectively. (From British Births Survey 1970[15])

WHAT HAS BEEN DONE?

Many researchers in the Western World have taken an interest in the subject of work in pregnancy and some are contributing to this volume. Efforts have been made to improve the collection of data about women who are pregnant and work (Chapter 7). The occupational health services (Chapter 19) are involved in this, and the trade unions are taking an active interest in the care of their members while pregnant and working (Chapter 14).

Patterns of antenatal care may need to be re-examined. Formal programmes laid down in the 1920s are still being carried out in most UK antenatal clinics. They presuppose that every pregnant woman is a middle-class lady who has nothing else to do but listen to the advice given by her well-meaning doctors and midwives. There is not the same amount of time in this decade, and pregnancy has to be fitted into the role of the couple's life.

There can be problems in the diagnosis of the pregnancy of the woman at work. She will have her own doubts for some weeks and may be unwilling to pass on information to her employer until she is fairly certain of the diagnosis. In early pregnancy many women have the misery of vomiting, which, although considered normal by those in obstetrics, is still a great interference with the life style of the woman. This comes at a time when she is loth to inform her employer about the possible reasons for sickness.

Throughout pregnancy, it is important that the woman's nutritional needs be considered carefully; many people who work do not have adequate time for meals nor, if the meals are provided in a works canteen, are these prepared for the nutritional needs of a pregnant woman. Rest may be required in pregnancy;

this needs a place where the woman can be away from her workmates. Work hours might be adjusted so that a pregnant woman avoids rush hour travel and the crush of early morning and early evening going from and to home.

Antenatal care may be practised in the place of work if there are enough pregnant women working in one place or in a clinic placed close to a group of places of work. Thus, antenatal care could be nearer to the place of work or living than to the place of birth. This needs organisation; while not impossible in a small country such as the UK, it might be more difficult in the USA.

Recently legislation has been passed in Britain entitling pregnant women to paid time off to obtain antenatal care. In certain circumstances they have the right to maternity pay and maternity leave and to return to their jobs after maternity leave. Pregnant employees have these rights and it is good that they should know all of them[16].

Maternity benefits and allowances are paid on a niggardly scale in the UK and this problem needs re-examination to help those who need it most (see table 1.4). To avoid paying money unnecessarily to those who have less need, it might be possible to involve the much-derided means test, but if this could be seen to bring benefits to those whose needs were greatest, it would be acceptable if introduced in a confidential fashion.

Table 1.4 Maternity grants from selected countries in 1981 and 1982[a] (from *Annual Report*, Maternity Alliance, 1983)

Country	£ per annum
France	525[a]
Luxembourg	500[a]
Austria	482
East Germany	209
Greece	173[a]
Czechoslovakia	89
Poland	32
Portugal	28
UK	25[a]
Ireland	6[a]

CONCLUSIONS

It is probable that women are going to continue working in pregnancy and that this issue will exist until well into the next century. It might be that they will take on heavier work and be employed in industries which may present specific risks to the fetus in pregnancy. As time goes by, we may find more environmental factors currently considered safe which are actually fetotoxic. We need to sort out this problem so that we can advise women before pregnancy seeking answers to their questions at the pre-pregnancy clinics and later in pregnancy. If the hazards of working in pregnancy are overexaggerated, we should say so and thus reassure women, helping them to continue what they naturally want to do. If, however, hazards are there, they should be quantified more precisely, so that pregnant women may be informed accurately, and then they may minimise the risk to themselves and the unborn child.

REFERENCES

1. Douglas, W. B. (1948). *Maternity in Great Britain*, Oxford University Press, Oxford
2. Daniels, W. W. (1980). Maternity rights: the experience of women. London Policy Studies Institute
3. Barlow, S. and Sullivan, F. (1982). *The Reproductive Hazards of Industrial Chemicals*, Academic Press, London, New York
4. Pharoah, P. O. D., Alberman, E., Doyle, P. and Chamberlain, G. (1977). Outcome of pregnancy among women in anaesthetic practice. *Lancet*, 1, 34–36
5. Harvey, M., McRorie, M. and Smith, D. (1981). *Canadian Medical Journal*, 125, 50–53
6. Edmonds, L., Layde, P. and Erickson, J. (1979). Airport noise and teratogenesis. *Archives of Environmental Health*, 34, 243–247
7. Research Reports on Health Issue in V.D.U. Operations (1981). NIOSH Center of Disease Control, U.S. Department of Health, Cincinnati, Ohio
8. Herman, B. and Powell, D. (1981). *Airborne Ultrasound*. DHSS Publication 8108163
9. Butler, N. and Alberman, E. (1969). *Perinatal Problems*, Livingstone, Edinburgh and London, p. 74
10. Seitchik, P. (1967). Body energy expenditure at work in pregnancy. *American Journal of Obstetrics and Gynecology*, 97, 701
11. Bruser, M. (1968). Sporting activities during pregnancy. *Obstetrics and Gynaecology*, 32, 721–725
12. Hytten, F. and Chamberlain, G. (1981) *Clinical Physiology in Obstetrics*, Blackwells Medical, Oxford, London
13. Edmunds, D., Lindsay, K., Muller, J., Wilkaren, E. and Wood, P. (1982). Early embryonic mortality in women. *Fertility and Sterility*, 38, 447–453
14. Rodrigues-Escudero, R., Belanstegreguria, A. and Gutierrez-Martinez, S. (1980). Perinatal complications of work in pregnancy. *Anales Espania Pediatrica*, 13, 465–476
15. Chamberlain, R., Chamberlain, G., Hewlett, B. and Claireaux, A. (1974). *British Births 1970*, Heinemann, London
16. Maternity Allowance (1981). *Pregnant at Work*, A checklist for employers, personnel officers and trade union representatives

2

The Effect of Work on Placental Function and Fetal Growth

FRANK E. HYTTEN

The effects of work in pregnancy on placental function and fetal growth can be approached in two ways: (1) by an examination of what is known about the physiological background – the effect of pregnancy on the response to exercise, and the effect of exercise specifically on the uterus and its contents; (2) by looking at the observed clinical effects of physical work on the well-being of the pregnancy. The quality of the information available is extremely variable, much of it indirect or circumstantial, but it is possible to support an argument that hard physical work by the pregnant woman probably harms the fetus.

THE PHYSIOLOGICAL BACKGROUND

The physiological response to exercise and thermal stress

Few systems of the body escape the effect of physical exertion, and many of the widespread consequences are bound to have some influence on the uterus and its contents. However, in the context of this chapter one effect predominates: it is that 'sympathetic vasomotor activity is increased to non-working tissues in proportion to the severity of exercise'[1].

Cardiac output rises, and the increased flow of blood is directed specifically towards those organs which are primarily involved in exercise, such as the working muscles and the heart, and away from areas which have no immediate priority, such as the skin and splanchnic area (figure 2.1). Sympathetic activity causes dilatation of the blood vessels in muscle and constriction in the viscera and skin.

Compared with four-legged animals, human beings are particularly vulnerable, for while they can often maintain blood pressure during exertion by raising cardiac output, the human upright posture presents a formidable challenge to the maintenance of blood pressure and diversion of blood from non-essential

15

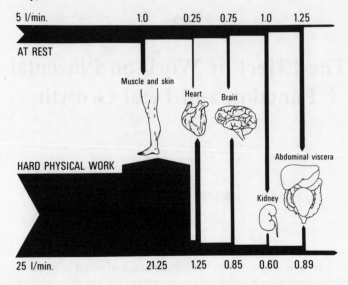

Figure 2.1   Distribution of the resting cardiac output of 5 l/min contrasted with the distribution of cardiac output raised by muscular exercise to 25 l/min (from reference 1)

fields is necessary to preserve an adequate venous return to the heart. Whether the human uterine circulation is included among other abdominal viscera in the sympathetic constriction of blood supply cannot be said with certainty, but it is undoubtedly true in several other species, including the rhesus monkey[2]. The pregnant ewe is the favoured experimental animal and is generally accepted as an appropriate model. In that animal the uterine vessels appear to be almost totally dilated in the resting state[3,4] and are powerfully constricted by both adrenaline[3,5] and noradrenaline[6]. Further evidence, supported by clinical observation in women, is that maternal haemorrhage results, as would be expected, in uterine vasoconstriction[7,8].

The only human data are indirect: the findings of Morris *et al.*[9] that the clearance of radioactive sodium injected into the uterine wall was significantly slower when the supine pregnant woman exercised her legs than when she was at rest. The relation between clearance of an injected tracer from a tissue and the local blood flow is not particularly close, but the conclusion supports the other evidence: exercise reduces blood flow to the uterus.

An additional factor in the equation is the effect of heat. Exercise alone tends to constrict blood vessels in the skin, but as body temperature rises, they dilate, so that prolonged exercise or exercise in a hot environment causes dilatation in both muscle and skin vessels. Thus, there is even greater need to isolate non-essential vascular beds and the splanchnic area is still further constricted[1] (figure 2.2).

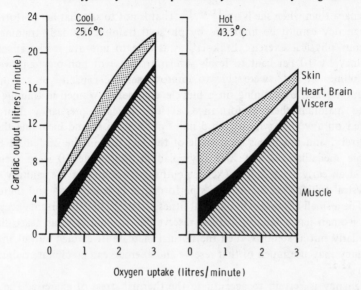

Figure 2.2   Distribution of cardiac output with increasing exercise (measured as oxygen uptake) under cool and hot conditions (from reference 1)

Heat has another effect: water loss by sweating, which may be considerable and is greater and more rapid in persons acclimatised to a hot environment[10]. Prolonged heavy exercise in a high ambient temperature can reduce plasma volume by as much as 10 per cent or more, and that is an additional reinforcement to the mechanisms which must try to preserve circulating volume by sacrificing blood flow to non-essential areas.

The effect of pregnancy on the body's response to exercise

Subjectively the average pregnant woman becomes progressively less able to perform physical exercise. She finds the daily round of housework and shopping more tiring and her badly distributed extra weight makes her cumbersome and awkward, particularly when that extra weight must be lifted, as in climbing stairs. For that reason, and also because of a progesterone-induced lassitude, women tend to be less active in late pregnancy[11,12]; that is true even in rural Africa where, because the demands of agriculture are relatively inescapable, leisure activities are sacrificed[13].

If a pregnant woman chooses to exercise, pregnancy does not seriously impair its efficiency. As would logically be expected, there is no doubt that physical activity costs the average pregnant woman more. For a given amount of physical work cardiac output, heart rate and oxygen uptake increase more when a woman is pregnant than when she is not[11,14,15]. That is not to say that her performance in pregnancy cannot be improved by physical training. By daily training with strenuous physical exercise Erkkola[16] was able to improve work capacity in pregnancy by 10 per cent to levels similar to those of non-pregnant women, and Collings *et al.*[17] were able to improve aerobic capacity in a group of pregnant women by training on a bicycle ergometer. Women in training seem able to maintain their performance, at least in early pregnancy. Korcok[18] reported on a woman who jogged 5 miles per day up to and including the day of delivery, and much has been made of the fact that of the 26 female Soviet Olympic medallists of the XVI Olympiad in Melbourne 10 were pregnant, albeit at an early stage[19]. The exercise enthusiasts point out the salutary effect of physical training on the mother's performance in labour[16,20] and there may indeed be a small advantage in physical fitness. There is one important exception: if the woman has a reduced cardiac reserve due to mild valvular heart disease, particularly mitral stenosis, then the normal increase of cardiac output in early pregnancy may use much of that reserve and exercise can precipitate pulmonary oedema[21,22].

Pregnancy is certain to accentuate the thermal stress of exercise. The body temperature at rest is already somewhat raised above the non-pregnant level and there is a considerable and widespread dilatation in skin vessels[23,24].

THE EFFECT OF EXERCISE ON THE FETUS

Physiological observations

Evidence that maternal exercise has a measurable effect on the fetus is probably unanimous but there is less agreement about its interpretation.

Detailed and elegant data from experimental sheep[25] showed that sustained low-level treadmill exercise, 1–3 mile/h for 1–3 h, had little effect on the fetus until the ewe became clinically exhausted, by which time her body temperature and pulse rate had risen conspicuously. Both uterine blood flow and fetal arterial P_{O_2} fell with exercise, but the difference was only significant for the exhausted group and was without evidence of fetal compromise. With more severe treadmill exercise, 2–2.5 mile/h for 30–60 min, Emmanouilides *et al.*[26] showed a fall in fetal arterial P_{O_2} and a rise in fetal heart rate which was tolerated well. If the fetus was 'chronically distressed' by having had one umbilical artery ligated, then the fall in P_{O_2} was greater.

Human evidence is necessarily less comprehensive but points in a similar direction. In one of the earliest studies Hon and Wohlgemuth[27] examined the fetal heart rate pattern before and after 26 women in late pregnancy had undertaken a 3 min step test. There was little or no effect in 20, moderate changes in 5 and a marked effect – a profound and prolonged bradycardia – in one fetus at 43 weeks, which showed a hypoxic pattern during the subsequent normal short labour. Soiva *et al.*[28] also recorded fetal heart rate patterns after moderately severe exercise on a cycle ergometer. In general, there was a slight increase in rate which settled within 10 min, but in three women with hypertensive complications there was a major disturbance, with changes of -25, -19 and $+42$ beats per minute (bpm), respectively, which took much longer to return to normal. A similar study was reported by Pomerance *et al.*[29], who subjected 54 healthy women at 35–37 weeks of pregnancy to exercise on a bicycle ergometer. Only five fetuses showed a subsequent change in heart rate of plus or minus 20 bpm or more, and four of these five subsequently showed fetal distress in labour. A more recent study[17], in which a group of healthy pregnant women were subjected to exercise training on a bicycle ergometer, examined the effect on fetal heart rate of exercising until maternal heart rate was raised to 150–160 bpm. Fetal heart rate was always raised, albeit not very much, and the authors claim that there was no effect on fetal growth. The rise in fetal heart rate was attributed to three possible causes – arousal of the fetus, transfer of catecholamines and a rise in maternal temperature – but the implication is strongly made that the fetus was not harmed by the mother's exercise.

A similar finding was reported by Hauth *et al.*[30], who studied seven women in late pregnancy, who jogged at least 1.5 miles per day three times per week before and during pregnancy. Immediately after the jogging, fetal heart rate was always raised, to as much as 180–204 bpm in 9 of 15 tests, and it took 12–30 min for fetal heart rate to return to pre-jogging levels. All tests showed a reactive fetal heart rate pattern.

Other possible effects of exercise have not been examined. For example, Schaeffer[31] pointed out that with marathon running body temperature would be considerably raised and that could be teratogenic if it occurred in very early pregnancy. Indeed, increased body temperature itself, apart from exercise, is likely to be hazardous for the same reason as exercise: the diversion of blood from the splanchnic area. Pystynen[32] looked at the effect on fetal heart rate of the mother taking a Finnish sauna bath at a mean dry bulb temperature of 64 °C for 10–25 min. In a considerable proportion the fetal heart rate was seriously disturbed, especially so in two women with mild anaemia, and one woman who was 2 weeks past term delivered a stillborn infant the following day.

Another possibility appears never to have been considered. It is that maternal plasma lactate levels rise even with relatively mild exercise[30]. If the fetal levels also happened to be raised because of intrauterine hypoxia, then the fetus would have more difficulty in unloading lactate to the mother because of the diminished gradient, and lactate could accumulate in the fetus. If it is lactate accumulation rather than hypoxia itself which damages the fetal brain[33], then maternal exercise could increase the possibility.

To summarise the evidence so far: it is apparent that the uterine circulation is subject to sympathetic vasoconstrictive control and will be reduced in circumstances which divert blood from the splanchnic area. Therefore, physical activity, particularly in the upright position and in a hot environment, can be expected to reduce blood flow to the uterus. Because the placenta and its blood supply almost certainly enjoy a large margin of safety in normal circumstances, everyday physical activity, even including the less vigorous sporting pursuits, will not seriously diminish the supply. But if exercise is severe, or if the margin of safety is for any reason reduced, then the fetus may be in peril. Other possible but lesser hazards are an increase in maternal, and therefore fetal, body temperature and the accumulation of lactate.

The clinical consequences

If, as has been suggested, the margin of safety in blood supply to the pregnant uterus is reduced by physical work, then data from population groups should reveal trends in fetal growth and viability. Trends are indeed apparent and credit must be given to André Briend[34] for drawing attention to them. It is salutary to recall that when birth weight and perinatal mortality were first related to differences in social class of the mother more than a century ago, hard physical work among the lower-class women, particularly in the factories, was the environmental element held responsible. That led, at the turn of the century, to a great deal of important legislation to protect pregnant women from the demands of industrialised society. It was much later that the social class gradient in reproductive performance was attributed to nutritional differences — an exaggerated concept which is with us still.

Women have always carried more than their share of physical work in the home and in the fields. No doubt, it is because the origins of that tradition were firmly established in the mists of evolutionary time that no folk-lore appears to have developed which would suggest that pregnant women might benefit from rest. A component of male chauvinism is probably involved, and those assiduous anthropologists H. H. Ploss and M. and P. Bartels[35] noted that in Greenland and in some Amazon tribes, when a woman is pregnant, the husband is forbidden to undertake strenuous work.

The importance of rest in late pregnancy was pointed out in 1895 by the French obstetrician Pinard[36]. He observed that infants born to 500 mothers who had rested for at least 10 days in a Parisian Council refuge for the indigent were, on average, 280 g heavier than infants born to a further 500 women who came directly to the maternity hospital for delivery.

That observation was followed up by another Frenchman, Letourneur, who made a detailed study of 627 deliveries in Paris in 1896[37]. His material was published *in extenso* in a thesis and the data have been reworked by Briend[34]. The results of multiple regression analysis are shown in table 2.1. The effect on birth weight of fetal sex and maternal parity, not examined by Letourneur himself, was as one would expect, but the biggest difference was an advantage

Table 2.1 Factors influencing birth weight in 627 deliveries in Paris reported by Letourneur in 1896 and calculated by Briend[34]

Factors influencing birth weight	Mean value of effect	SEM
Rest before delivery	+ 202 g if > 8 days	37 g
Parity	+ 193 g if mother multiparous	37 g
Sex of infant	+ 100 g if male	37 g

of about 200 g if the mother had rested for 8 days or more before delivery. Among women who had physically demanding work, such as domestic servants, the effect of rest was to increase birth weight by 238 g, compared with an increase of 161 g for those women with a less tiring occupation such as needlewoman; that difference was not statistically significant.

Some years later Peller[38] reported similar effects of rest in a maternity home in Vienna. He showed not only an effect on birth weight, but also a dramatic effect on mortality (table 2.2).

Table 2.2 Effect of duration of stay in a maternity home on stillbirth and neonatal death rates[38]

Duration of stay (day)	n	Stillbirths (%)	Neonatal deaths (%)
< 2	1925	4.7	4.8
2–7	223	5.8	4.0
8–28	417	1.9	1.9
> 28	203	2.3	0.5

Conclusions about the benefit of rest in late pregnancy drawn from those early French and Austrian data must be tentative, but Briend has given cogent reasons why they are likely to be sound. For example, women who were admitted to rest homes before delivery were certainly from the most deprived strata of society, with a high proportion of primigravidae and the unmarried, so that, if anything, their results might have been expected to be much worse than the others.

More recent data all point in the same direction. For example, Balfour and Talpade[39] collected data from India which showed that women working in textile mills, although they had a higher average energy intake from food than the general population, had babies of lower birth weight. Their work was not physically arduous but they worked all day standing beside a machine. The mean birth weight of infants born to mill workers was only 2441 g, almost 200 g below the weight of babies delivered to the wives of mill workers who lived in the same social conditions but did not work; mill workers who had been laid off as the result of a strike had infants almost as big as did the non-workers (table 2.3).

Table 2.3   Effect of maternal work on birth weight in India[39]

	n	Mean birth weight (g)	SD
Mill workers	134	2441	407
Mill workers during and after strike	89	2594	414
Wives of mill workers	236	2639	390

Balfour[40] was subsequently able to confirm the effect of standing work in an English textile factory where women of similar social background and doing similar jobs could be divided into those who stood to work and those who sat. Sitting workers not only had larger babies, but also had a very much lower stillbirth rate (table 2.4). Hirsch[41], reporting from Berlin in 1927, also found a much lower stillbirth rate in textile workers who sat at work, compared with those who stood.

Table 2.4   Effect of posture of textile mill workers on birth weight and stillbirth rate[40]

	n	Mean birth weight (g)	SD	Stillbirth rate (%)
Sitting workers	236	3468	537	6.4
Standing workers	1074	3386	476	20.3

In the only recent study, Tafari and his colleagues[42] collected detailed information on a group of relatively poor Ethiopian women. Those whose daily work outside the home was strenuous gained less weight in pregnancy and had considerably smaller infants than those whose work was considered to be light.

CONCLUSIONS

Direct human evidence that strenuous activity impairs blood flow to the uterus and has a deleterious effect on the fetus is not available but a great many straws are blowing in that direction.

Physical activity, particularly while standing and in a hot environment, undoubtedly causes the diversion of blood away from the abdominal viscera, and the uterus is not spared from that general physiological response. In the ordinary course of events the large margin of safety enjoyed by the placental blood supply ensures that no harm comes to the fetus, but with severe exercise, or if the fetus is already compromised, harm seems likely to occur. The evidence for that is that some infants show cardiographic signs of distress when the mother exercises and in conditions where the mother habitually works hard in a standing position there is convincing statistical evidence of reduced fetal growth.

It is probable that the small babies characteristic of many peoples in the developing countries are not because of shortage of food but because the women exist under the worst possible circumstances for ensuring a free blood flow to the pregnant uterus: a hard daily grind, mostly standing and in hot conditions.

REFERENCES

1. Rowell, L. B. (1974). Human cardiovascular adjustments to exercise and thermal stress. *Physiological Reviews*, **54**, 75–159
2. Misenhimer, H. R., Margulies, S. I., Panigel, M., Ramsey, E. M. and Donner, M. W. (1972). Effects of vasoconstrictive drugs on the placental circulation of the rhesus monkey. *Investigative Radiology*, **7**, 496–499
3. Greiss, F. C. (1953). The uterine vascular bed: effect of adrenergic stimulation. *Obstetrics and Gynecology*, **21**, 295–301
4. Greiss, F. C. (1972). Differential reactivity of the myoendometrial and placental vasculatures: adrenergic responses. *American Journal of Obstetrics and Gynecology*, **112**, 20–30
5. Rosenfeld, C. R., Barton, M. D. and Meschia, G. (1976). Effects of epinephrine on distribution of blood flow in the pregnant ewe. *American Journal of Obstetrics and Gynecology*, **124**, 156–163
6. Rosenfeld, C. R. and West, J. (1977). Circulatory response to systemic infusion of norepinephrine in the pregnant ewe. *American Journal of Obstetrics and Gynecology*, **127**, 376–383
7. Greiss, F. C. (1966). Uterine vascular response to haemorrhage during pregnancy. *Obstetrics and Gynecology*, **27**, 549–554
8. Assali, N. S. and Brinkman, C. R. (1973). The role of circulating buffers in fetal tolerance to stress. *American Journal of Obstetrics and Gynecology*, **117**, 643–652
9. Morris, N., Osborn, S. B., Wright, H. P. and Hart, A. (1956). Effective uterine blood flow during exercise in normal and pre-eclamptic pregnancies. *Lancet*, **2**, 481–484
10. Fox, R. H. (1965). Heat. In Edholm, O. G. and Bacharach, A. L. (Eds.), *The Physiology of Human Survival*, Academic Press, London, pp. 53–79
11. Blackburn, M. W. and Calloway, D. H. (1976). Basal metabolic rate and work energy expenditure of mature, pregnant women. *Journal of the American Dietetic Association*, **69**, 24–36
12. Hytten, F. E. (1980). Nutrition. In Hytten, F. E. and Chamberlain, G. V. P. (Eds.), *Clinical Physiology in Obstetrics*, Blackwell Scientific, Oxford, p. 176

13. Roberts, S. B., Paul, A. A., Cole, T. J. and Whitehead, R. G. (1982). Seasonal changes in activity, birth weight and lactational performance in rural Gambian women. *Transactions of the Royal Society of Tropical Medicine and Hygiene*, **76**, 668–678

14. Guzman, C. A. and Caplan, R. (1970). Cardiorespiratory response to exercise during pregnancy. *American Journal of Obstetrics and Gynecology*, **108**, 600–605

15. Pernoll, M. L., Metcalfe, J., Schlenker, T. L., Welch, J. E. and Matsumoto, J. A. (1975). Oxygen consumption at rest and during exercise in pregnancy. *Respiration Physiology*, **25**, 285–293

16. Erkkola, R. (1976). The influence of physical training during pregnancy on physical work capacity and circulatory parameters. *Scandinavian Journal of Clinical and Laboratory Investigation*, **36**, 747–754

17. Collings, C. A., Curet, L. B. and Mullin, J. P. (1983). Maternal and fetal responses to a maternal aerobic exercise program. *American Journal of Obstetrics and Gynecology*, **145**, 702–707

18. Korcok, M. (1981). Pregnant jogger: what a record! *Journal of the American Medical Association*, **246**, 201

19. Bruser, M. (1968). Sporting activities during pregnancy. *Obstetrics and Gynecology*, **32**, 721–725

20. Zaharieva, E. (1972). Olympic participation by women. *Journal of the American Medical Association*, **221**, 992–995

21. Ueland, K., Novy, M. J. and Metcalfe, S. (1972). Hemodynamic responses of patients with heart disease to pregnancy and exercise. *American Journal of Obstetrics and Gynecology*, **113**, 47–52

22. Szekely, P. and Snaith, L. (1974). *Heart Disease and Pregnancy*, Churchill Livingstone, Edinburgh, p. 60

23. Hytten, F. E. and Leitch, I. (1971). *Physiology of Human Pregnancy*, 2nd edn, Blackwell Scientific, Oxford, p. 191

24. deSwiet, M. (1980). The cardiovascular system. In Hytten, F. E. and Chamberlain, G. V. P. (Eds.), *Clinical Physiology in Obstetrics*, Blackwell Scientific, Oxford, pp. 23–26

25. Clapp, J. (1980). Acute exercise stress in the pregnant ewe. *American Journal of Obstetrics and Gynecology*, **136**, 489–494

26. Emmanouilides, G. C., Hobel, C. J., Yashiro, K. and Klyman, G. (1972). Fetal responses to maternal exercise in the sheep. *American Journal of Obstetrics and Gynecology*, **112**, 130–137

27. Hon, E. and Wohlgemuth, R. (1961). The electronic evaluation of fetal heart rate. IV. The effect of maternal exercise. *American Journal of Obstetrics and Gynecology*, **81**, 361–371

28. Soiva, K. Salmi, A., Grönroos, M. and Peltonen, T. (1964). Physical working capacity during pregnancy and effect of physical work tests on foetal heart rate. *Annales Chirurgiae et Gynaecologiae Fenniae*, **53**, 187–196

29. Pomerance, J. J., Gluck, L. and Lynch, V. A. (1974). Maternal exercise as a screening test for uteroplacental insufficiency. *Obstetrics and Gynaecology*, **44**, 383–387

30. Hauth, J. C., Gilstrap, L. C. and Widmer, K. (1982). Fetal heart rate reactivity before and after maternal jogging during the third trimester. *American Journal of Obstetrics and Gynecology*, **142**, 545–547

31. Schaeffer, C. F. (1979). Possible teratogenic hyperthermia and marathon running. *Journal of the American Medical Association*, **241**, 1892

32. Pystynen, P. (1961). Effect of the Finnish sauna bath on the maternal blood circulation and fluid and electrolyte balance in toxaemia of late pregnancy. *Acta Obstetrica et Gynecologia Scandinavica*, **40**, supplement 3

33. Myers, R. E. (1978). Lactic acid accumulation as cause of brain edema and cerebral necrosis resulting from oxygen deprivation. In Korobkin, R. and Guilleminault, C. (Eds.), *Advances in Perinatal Neurology 1*, SP Medical and Scientific, New York, 85–114

34. Briend, A. (1980). Maternal physical activity, birth weight and perinatal mortality. *Medical Hypotheses*, **6**, 1157–1170

35. Ploss, H. H., Bartels, M. and Bartels, P. (1935). *Woman*, Vol. II, Heinemann, London, p. 446

36. Pinard, A. (1895). Note pour servir à l'histoire de la puériculture intrautérine. *Annales de Gynécologie et d'Obstétrique*, **44**, 417–422

37. Letourneur, L. (1897). De l'influence de la profession de la mère sur le poids de l'enfant. Thèse, Paris

38. Peller, S. (1931). Erfordert die Bekamfung der prä-, intra- and post-natalen Sterblichkeit medizinische der sozialmedizinische Reformen? *Zentralblatt für Gynäkologie*, **55**, 268–275

39. Balfour, M. I. and Talpade, S. K. (1930). The maternity conditions of women mill-workers in India. *Indian Medical Gazette*, **65**, 241–249

40. Balfour, M. (1938). The effect of occupation on pregnancy and neonatal mortality. *Public Health Journal of the Society of Medical Officers of Health*, **51**, 106–111

41. Hirsch, M. (1927). Weiterer Beitrag zur gewerblichen Pathologie von Schwangerschaft und Geburt. *Zentralblatt für Gynäkologie*, **51**, 136–141

42. Tafari, N. Naeye, R. L. and Gobezie, A. (1980). Effects of maternal undernutrition and heavy physical work during pregnancy on birth weight. *British Journal of Obstetrics and Gynaecology*, **87**, 222–226

3

The Hazards of Work in Pregnancy

ROBERT MURRAY

The title of this chapter, which seemed deceptively simple originally, has given a lot of trouble. The main problem has been the word 'work'. 'Hazard' is straightforward as meaning a potential risk to health in particular circumstances of exposure; 'pregnancy' means the period between implantation and involution; but 'work' has overtones and harmonics which make it necessary to examine it more closely. For example, the difference between work and leisure is that work is generally regarded as the time one is paid for and leisure as the time one is not paid for. It bears no relation to the amount of physical or mental effort.

Women have always been an essential part of the labour force. In the past the average woman had far more pregnancies than she has now, except in the most primitive societies; pregnancy is nowadays more of an interruption of a career rather than a career in itself.

An American paperback a few years ago was entitled *Work is Dangerous to Your Health*. Similarly, it could be said that 'Pregnancy is dangerous to your health'. The state of pregnancy has always had its inherent dangers, modified by the life style of the pregnant woman, and in too many cases, through ignorance or neglect, has led to death or damage to the mother or baby. To what extent such damage or death has been attributable to the work which women inevitably had to do is impossible to say, as there are no data, but it is certainly true that at the present time, for whatever reason, fewer mothers and babies are dying than at any time in our history, even though more mothers go out of their home to work and work longer throughout their pregnancy.

This very fact of survival accentuates the cases that do arise. When women in the pottery industry experienced abortion and stillbirth, there was little social outcry: what were a few additional deaths due to lead when the normal perinatal mortality was 200 per thousand total births? As it came down to the present level of 12 per thousand and people regarded a normal pregnancy as their birthright, a dramatic event such as the thalidomide story captured the conscience of the world and intensified research into the hazards of the repro-

27

ductive process arising out of environmental exposure. Paid employment, as distinct from the work which women have always done, can involve different kinds of environmental exposures, so that the question to be addressed is: 'Are there any factors in the employment of women which present special dangers during pregnancy?'

The special dangers which we are anxious to avoid are abortion, stillbirth, teratogenesis and mutagenesis, together with any other metabolic or biochemical defects. The environmental factors which may affect these dangers can be divided into physical, chemical, biological and psychosocial. The difficulty is that the dangers and the environmental factors have existed since the world began and it is very difficult to prove any cause and effect relationship. The normal environment involves all of these factors, but the ingenuity of man has intensified them, particularly in the working environment, to such an extent as to represent potential dangers to the health of people exposed.

PHYSICAL HAZARDS

Noise and vibration

There is no evidence that noise causes any more problems in pregnancy than at any other time, apart from intensifying mental stress. Local vibration from hand-held vibrating tools has been reported as causing autonomic nervous system effects[1], but the evidence is unsupported by any epidemiological studies, and in any case it is doubtful whether this would be more important during pregnancy than at any other time. Whole-body vibration has been said to be associated with menstrual disorders but there are no reports of its effects on pregnancy[2]. Low-frequency (18–30 kHz) high-power ultrasound is extensively used in industry for cleaning of watches and machine parts. Workers exposed to this type of ultrasound have complained of headache, earache, vertigo and general discomfort[3], but there are no reports of effects on pregnancy. The effect of high-frequency ultrasound (100–10 000 kHz) on pregnancy has been extensively investigated, particularly as the technique is used specifically in obstetrics. No effect on chromosomes has been detected[4].

Thermal stress

Many industrial jobs involve exposure to heat or cold, and there has been a great deal of investigation on the differences in reaction to thermal stress among men and women[5]. There is more interindividual variation than intersex variation, and no reports have been made of any effects in pregnancy.

Electromagnetic spectrum

Microwaves

Possible effects on the fetus from the thermal effect of microwave radiation have been reported, but there is an absence of data on depth–dose distribution in tissues. Reports of miscarriages and impaired embryo development are difficult to evaluate. A WHO Report[6] decided that the evidence was inadequate to reach any conclusions. The authors were equally unable to reach any conclusions about the effect of high-frequency electromagnetic fields.

Ionising radiation

With ionising radiation the situation seems clear. Stewart and her colleagues[7] have pointed to a clear dose–response relationship between irradiation of the fetus and leukaemia in the first 10 years of the child's life. Apart from radiologists, many women are exposed to ionising radiations, from isotopes for thickness gauges in cigarette factories to X-rays for non-destructive testing of Christmas puddings. X-radiography in shoe shops has been abandoned because of the risk to shop assistants. Security X-radiography at airports is done with high-voltage sets and image intensifiers, so that there is no risk. Because of the potential hazard, it is necessary to limit radiation exposure of any woman known to be pregnant. The main problem is that the fetus is at its most sensitive during the early stages of pregnancy, when the woman may be unaware of the situation.

Gravity

As pregnancy advances, while the woman's mind and fingers still remain nimble, her body becomes progressively less so. This is particularly important if her job involves lifting and carrying, but problems also arise even when sitting at a typewriter. It is important where there is any occupational health doctor or nurse in the factory that they collaborate with the physician in charge of the case so that suitable arrangements can be made for appropriate ergonomic adaptations of the job where this is possible. The American College of Obstetricians and Gynecologists[8] have produced guidelines on pregnancy and work which accent this need for collaboration with the occupational health services. Their scheme is summarised in figure 3.1.

CHEMICAL HAZARDS

In this important group of potentially hazardous environmental factors lead, in particular, has a long history as an abortifacient, and during the last century

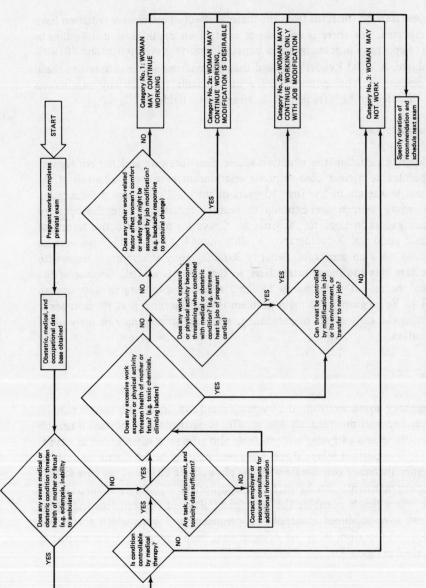

Figure 3.1 Summary of American College of Obstetricians and Gynecologists' guidelines on pregnancy and work

women employed in white lead works and the pottery industry suffered severely (and so did their unborn children) from the effects of lead[9]. The result has been that women are now prohibited from working in many lead processes. The EEC Directive on Lead suggests a standard for men of 70 μg/100 ml of blood[10]. These figures are based, not on epidemiological studies of the effect of different concentrations of lead, but on the feasibility of achieving such concentrations in various lead processes.

The reproductive effects of exposure to mercury were highlighted by the epidemic of mercury poisoning in Minamata, Japan[11]. The epidemic was caused by a factory voiding a mercury effluent into Minamata Bay. The mercury was ingested by fish and shellfish, where it was converted into methyl mercury. There were several deaths among people who ate the contaminated fish but 23 children were born with severe signs of brain damage, even though the mothers had little or no symptoms. In Iraq similar cases arose from the consumption of bread made from wheat treated with a mercury fungicide[12]. While these circumstances were environmental rather than occupational, they provide a danger signal concerning the handling of mercury preparations by pregnant women.

Apart from lead and mercury, there are reports of an increased frequency of spontaneous abortions and malformations among women employed in a copper smelter, where, in addition to exposure to copper, there was also exposure to lead, arsenic, cadmium and sulphur dioxide. According to Hemminki *et al.*[13], the reliability of the data on spontaneous abortions was in question. Exposure to solder fumes was suggested as the reason for an increased incidence of spontaneous abortions among workers in the production of radio and television sets.

One of the most important industries so far as potential reproductive effects are concerned is the health industry. The first suggestion of possible reproductive hazards in operating theatres came from a Russian questionnaire study in 1967[14], but since then there have been a number of studies which agree that there is an increased risk of spontaneous abortions in theatre staff. The possible causes are suggested to be nitrous oxide and halothane. It has also been suggested that there is a higher risk of malformations in children born to women exposed to anaesthetic gases during pregnancy. According to Hemminki[15], the existing evidence of an increased risk of malformation caused by operating theatre exposure rests on a weaker basis than does the evidence on spontaneous abortions. A number of sterilising agents, including ethylene oxide, formaldehyde, propylene oxide, glutaraldehyde, methyl bromide, β-propiolactone, hexachlorophene and sodium azide, have been shown to produce mutagenicity and carcinogenicity in experimental animals[16]. Of these, hexachlorophene and ethylene oxide have come under suspicion in two human studies — one connecting the hospital use of hexachlorophene with the occurrence of malformations and the other suggesting an association between ethylene oxide and a risk of spontaneous abortion. Formaldehyde exposure has been linked to an increased frequency of spontaneous abortions in a Russian study.

The preparation and administration of cytotoxic drugs, most of which are mutagenic *in vitro*, represents a potential hazard for hospital personnel.

Several other substances have come under suspicion.

Phthalates (dioctyl and dibutyl) as plasticisers in the manufacture of plastics.

Styrene as a solvent in the manufacture of glass-reinforced plastics.

Carbon disulphide in the manufacture of viscose rayon.

Chloroprene in the manufacture of synthetic rubber.

Perchloroethylene as a dry cleaning agent, which has largely replaced trichloroethylene.

Vinyl chloride: the monomer is used to make polyvinyl chloride (PVC). There is little free monomer left in the product used for making plastics articles and it is not released on heating PVC.

Carbon monoxide is frequently evolved when any carbon-containing material (from coal to natural gas to cigarettes) is burned in an oxygen-deficient atmosphere.

In addition to these substances, a recent EEC publication[17] mentions the following as producing mutagenic or teratogenic effects such that the employment of pregnant women in contact with them requires careful supervision: acridine; antimony; benzene; dimethyl formamide; formaldehyde; vanadium; methyl chloroform (1,1,1-trichloroethane). In most of these cases the evidence for an effect on pregnancy is based on animal experiments.

BIOLOGICAL HAZARDS

Several infections, particularly rubella, are known to produce effects on the fetus, although few infections are associated with occupation. Two cases of chlamydial infection were reported by Beer *et al.*[18] in farmers' wives who had helped their husbands with lambing. In view of possible infections, special care must be taken with pregnant hospital workers with regard to exposure to cytomegalovirus, herpes simplex, *Toxoplasma*, varicella and syphilis. Isolation procedures should be developed which specifically prohibit pregnant hospital workers from entering isolation areas, although this presents considerable difficulties, especially in the early weeks of pregnancy, when, as with radiation exposure, the effect is likely to be greatest while the woman may be still unaware of her pregnancy.

PSYCHOSOCIAL HAZARDS

Pregnancy is a mystical state surrounded by a whole series of taboos, many of which are likely to affect the mental health of the pregnant worker. The subject is a complex one because of its multifactorial and subjective nature and because of the great individual differences that exist. There is no good epidemiological evidence of any effect on mental health, although one study in the USA suggested that nurses, waiters, secretaries, personnel service workers and inspectors in manufacturing industries had significantly elevated rates of mental illness[19]. The WHO Report (World Health Organization, 1983) advises caution in drawing any inferences from these findings.

CONCLUSIONS

Pregnancy of itself is a potentially hazardous condition, in that, within any group of pregnant women, there may be complications, some well and some badly understood, that will affect the health of mother and child. The question we have to answer is whether under modern conditions, when women are working in commerce and industry, there exist particular hazards – physical, chemical, biological or psychosocial – that might act as a bar to employment in certain circumstances or require special care to be taken during the pregnancy. Moreover, are there factors at work which present such a potential danger to the fetus that steps should be taken to eliminate them?

This chapter introduces the topic and indicates some possible areas of interest. Other chapters in this volume will discuss more deeply some of these aspects. The main problem is that occupational epidemiology on spontaneous abortions and malformations is still in its early stages, although, with an increasing female work force in industry and a recognition of the reproductive hazards, there is an urgent need to uncover any occupational attribution so that appropriate advice can be given to employers and workers.

REFERENCES

1. Futatsuka, M., *et al*. (1980). Vibration hazards in forestry workers. *J. Sci. Lab.*, **56** (Pt II), 27–48
2. World Health Organization (1983). *Women and Occupational Health Risks*, EURO Reports and Studies 76, WHO, Copenhagen, p. 32
3. Hu, H. (1983). In Levy, B. S. and Wegman, D. H. (Eds.), *Occupational Health*, Little, Brown, Boston, p. 225
4. World Health Organization (1983). *Op. cit.*, p. 34. Several references
5. World Health Organization (1983). *Op. cit.*, p.31
6. World Health Organization (1983). *Op. cit.*, p.33
7. Bethell, J. F. and Stewart, A. M. (1975). Prenatal irradiation and childhood malignancy. *Br. J. Cancer*, **31**, 271
8. American College of Obstetricians and Gynecologists (1977). *Guidelines on Pregnancy and Work*, NIOSH, Rockville, Md.
9. Oliver, T. (1908). *The Diseases of Occupation*, Methuen, London, pp. 198–199
10. Official Journal of the European Community. Directive 80/1107 EEC

11. Harada, Y. (Ed.) (1968). *Congenital Minamata Disease*, Kuonamoto University
12. Kavoussi, N. (1977). The effects of industrialisation on spontaneous abortion in Iran. *J. Occup. Med.*, **19**, 419–423
13. Hemminki, K., *et al.* (1983). Assessment of methods and results of reproductive occupational epidemiology: spontaneous abortion and malformations in the offspring of working women. *Am. J. Ind. Med.*, **4**, 300–301
14. Vaisman, A. I. (1967). Working conditions in surgery and their effect on the health of anaesthesiologists. *Eksp. Khir. Anesteziol.*, **3**, 44–49
15. Hemminki, K., *et al.* (1983). *Op. cit.*, 303
16. Hemminki, K., *et al.* (1983). *Op. cit.*, 303
17. Commission of the European Communities (1983). *Activities of the ECDIN Project in Relation to Preventive Medicine: Occupational Health Guidelines for Chemical Risk*, CEC, Luxembourg
18. Beer, R. J. S., *et al.* (1982). Pregnancy complicated by psittacosis acquired from sheep. *Br. Med. J.*, **284**, 1156–1157
19. World Health Organization (1983). *Op. cit.*, p. 26

4

Women Workers at Higher Risk of Reproductive Hazards

RAJA W. ABDUL-KARIM

The interest and approach to possible work-related health hazards must be an international endeavour transcending geographical, social and ideological boundaries. The waters, the air and the food chains do not follow any prescribed geographical boundaries, but mingle and interwind to act as one body on which the survival of living beings ultimately depends. Even were this not so, and if geographical limits defined and contained the hazard limits, a society can not and must not be impervious to the health hazards in another society, for, as has been so aptly stated, 'No man is an island . . .'.

The issue of the working woman cannot be isolated from the overall concern of toxicology and other health hazards. A substance demonstrating toxicity to health cuts across the spectrum of human development and gender. Only the temporal relationships and the nature and severity of the effect may differ. This will be the overriding theme of this chapter on the woman worker. This is an expression of concern about an issue that must be forthrightly addressed and resolved. In the search for the solution one cannot rely on science alone, for the code of human behaviour and interaction is outside the realm of the scientific method.

The concern about occupational disease is not new. Hippocrates taught his pupils to heed the environment of their patients. In the fifteenth century illnesses among metallurgists and miners were recognised, and in the seventeenth century Ramazzini added an enquiry as to a person's occupation among the questions patients should be asked. He may thus be regarded as the founder of occupational medicine. In the USA it is particularly significant that the first American physician devoted to industrial medicine was a woman: Alice Hamilton.

In a rather limited context, until relatively recently occupational diseases were primarily a man's domain. This is no more the case. With the shift of employment outside the home, millions of women, seeking equal opportunities with men, have now joined the work force. Even the home, a traditional bastion of safety and shelter, has become a place of potential health hazard

35

with the introduction of sprays, paints, oven cleaners and microwave ovens. Data from *Employment and Earnings* (**30**, No. 1, United States Department of Labor) show the dramatic increase in women in the labour force during the past 35 years. In the USA during 1947 the total non-institutional population of women 16 years and over was close to 52 million, with only a little over 16 million (32 per cent) in the labour force. By 1965 only 40 per cent of the female population 16 years and over were in the labour force. By 1979 the corresponding figure was 51 per cent and in 1982 it rose to 52.7 per cent or 47 944 000 women. These women are employed in diverse occupations, including mechanics, metal craft workers, printers, locomotive engineers, furnace tenders, textile industries, garbage collectors, farm workers, photography, pharmaceutical industries and research laboratories, in addition to the teachers, clerics, physicians, stockbrokers — to name only a few. Assuming that the rate of pregnancy is the same in the employed and in the unemployed, a reasonable estimate is that 8–12 per cent of the women in the reproductive years would be pregnant. It is expected, therefore, that a significant number of employed women would be pregnant.

The topic of possible adverse consequences to health related to a person's occupation involves complex issues which are multifaceted and often represents a conflict of rights. Time and space will only permit of a brief mention of some of these.

There is the right of women for equal opportunities and access to employment and their right to be protected from exposure to work-related health hazards. There is also the right of the employer to hire the most suitable and productive person for a particular job. There is the right for industry to pursue progress. Progress not only affects the particular industry, but also has an impact on nations and on the work force. Progress as viewed nowadays is virtually synonymous with new products which may result in or be accompanied by the release of pollutants into our environment. Growth is an essential feature of the industrial process and so to constrain this growth process will place any particular industry at an unfair disadvantage. There is the right of the worker to be fully informed, the right to know what is injurious and what is not, the right to know what to expect, and the right to have fears and anxieties allayed. The all too frequent qualifications that something could be, may be or is possibly hazardous without the necessary supporting data can truly represent the state of the art, but are neither illuminating nor comforting. The counsellor may feel relieved after giving such advice, but the subject is none the wiser. Finally, there is the right of the conceptus to a toxin-free gestation and to grow in an optimal environment.

The preceding issues notwithstanding, there is the problem of identification of the reproductive hazards in the work place. Reproductive wastage is a major health hazard issue that people as a whole, and the health professionals in particular, have to deal with. In the USA 7 per cent and perhaps up to 10 per cent of newborns have defects. It is estimated that 10 per cent of congenital malformations are caused by environmental factors and after other known causes (e.g. genetic or chromosomal) are included, the preponderance of birth defects (65–70 per cent) remains unexplained. One must add to these statistics reproductive wastage due to sexual dysfunction, infertility, premature and early menopause, spontaneous abortions, prematurity, intrauterine growth retardation, and the long-term sequelae of prenatal exposure to toxic agents[1]. While at present it is not how much of this reproductive wastage is due to environmental exposure, the latter will remain a suspect until the issue is resolved.

The list of toxic or potentially toxic substances to which working women may be exposed is rapidly increasing and, within the confines of this chapter, it is counter-productive to list them. Suffice it to say that the potential for exposure is widespread: the list of occupations would include those of painters; printers; woodworkers; and workers in hospitals, agriculture, textile and cloth industries, laundry and dry cleaning. Exposure is to a variety of biological and chemical agents, such as carbon tetrachloride, aniline, chloroprene, trichloroethylene, perchloroethylene, chloroform, lead, arsenic, mercury and the polychlorinated biphenyls. For example, in the USA 81 per cent of arsenic is used in agriculture, 8 per cent in ceramics and glass, 5 per cent in chemicals and 6 per cent for other purposes[2]. Arsenic is used in fungicides, insecticides, metallurgy, pigment production, glass manufacturing, rodent poisons and semiconductors.

The exposure of women workers is not limited to biological and chemical hazards but also includes the physical hazards. There is convincing experimental evidence of the detrimental effect of noise and heat on reproduction. Many workers are exposed to these conditions in carrying out their duties. Radiation, microwaves and ultrasound are other examples.

The problems of identifying environmental factors hazardous to reproduction and intrauterine development are well known to all researchers in the field. Exposure to a multitude of potential harmful agents makes it sometimes difficult to single out the causative agent or agents. This, coupled with the fact that direct human experimentation is unethical, presents an almost insurmountable difficulty in assessing potential reproductive human toxins. Where and how, then, are we to get the necessary information? Reliance on animal data is not always dependable; experimentation on humans is unethical; there is often a long interval between exposure and an observed effect; and, finally, should these obstacles be somehow surmountable, there is always the plethora of new chemicals and other variables occurring at a rate that all but defies appropriate biological testing in a reasonable length of time. In the USA several hundred new chemicals are introduced annually. As reviewed by Fishbein[3], there are nearly 3 500 000 known chemicals. In the USA alone 25 000–30 000 chemicals are produced in significant amounts. The plastics industry alone reportedly uses nearly 2500 chemicals or mixtures. The yearly number of new industrial chemicals is staggering — estimated to be between 700 and 3000. The effects of most of these chemicals on human health in general (as well as plant and animal life on which we are dependent) is unknown, and, more specifically, their effect on reproduction.

The majority of these chemicals do not have safety limits of exposure set forth by the Occupational Safety and Health Administration (OSHA)[4]. Thus, we find that the deep and appropriate concern among the public in general has far outstripped the science. As health providers we are called upon increasingly frequently to supply answers to questions where only conjecture exists. Exposure is not limited to employment but includes other everyday products such as drugs, food additives, exhaust emissions and pesticide sprays.

SPECIFIC SITUATIONS OF WOMEN AT INCREASED RISK FOR REPRODUCTIVE HAZARDS

The preceding overview has attempted to outline the complex issues faced by the woman worker. Occupation may adversely affect her reproductive potential in one or more of the following areas:

Decreased libido.
Menstrual irregularity: oligo/anovulation.
Luteal phase deficiency.
Premature ovarian failure.
Increased incidence of abortion.
Increased incidence of congenital malformations.
Increased incidence of fetal growth retardation.
Increased fetal and postnatal carcinogenesis.
Poor survival after birth.
Embryo-fetal lethal effects.
Marital discordance.

The husband's occupation and health

Any woman married to a man himself exposed to reproductive hazards is by default a woman at higher risk to reproductive failures. There is mounting evidence of occupational reproductive toxicity in the male, varying all the way from loss of libido to loss of potency, disturbance in ejaculation and varying degress of abnormalities in the semen. A woman worker (and a housewife or homemaker is a woman worker) married to such a man is at increased risk for decreased conception rates and a decreased likelihood for a pregnancy to reach a normal and successful outcome. Among the compounds that are known to affect adversely male reproduction are vinyl chloride, organic lead, inorganic mercury, chlordecone, chloroprene and dibromochloropropane.

The possible reproductive hazard as a result of male exposure to anaesthetic gases has raised much controversy. Spence and co-workers reported data from the USA and the UK[5] pertaining to operating room physicians. Their analysis strongly suggested that the live-born of male anaesthetists had an increased incidence of congenital malformations. This association was evident in both the US and the UK data. With respect to the rate of spontaneous abortions, the combined data showed a non-statistically significant increase among the wives of anaesthetists. A significant increase was noted in the UK data when adjusted for age and smoking habits.

Tomlin[6] reported on the health problems of anaesthetists and their families. His report also found an increased incidence of spontaneous abortions (more pronounced if the wife was the anaesthetist); a higher incidence of malformations, particularly in the central nervous and musculo-skeletal systems; and a lowering of the birth weight. Significantly, the reduction in birth weight was confined to the female offspring, who also showed a disproportionately higher incidence of malformations compared with the males. It should be emphasised that, strictly speaking, a cause–effect relationship between anaesthetic gases and the reproductive outcome is not proved by any of these studies. Whatever the aetiology, however, there is an apparent relationship between paternal occupation and adverse effects on reproduction.

Finally, medications and illness in the male may constitute a reproductive hazard. There is evidence suggesting that the offspring of male epileptics ingesting hydantoin are at an increased risk for malformations. The drug has been found in the semen of these men and is judged to be at least a contributing cause[7].

Women workers exposed to anaesthetic gases

Medical and paramedical women exposed to anaesthetic gases seem at a greater risk for adverse reproductive outcomes, although there is still controversy about the nature and extent of the hazards. Two principal adverse effects have been described: (1) an increase in the rate of spontaneous abortions; (2) an increased risk for congenital malformations. The available evidence strongly supports the former and the link to congenital malformations is weak.

It is realised that the population studied in these epidemiological surveys represents operating room personnel that may or may not be directly involved in the administration of anaesthetic agents. The direct link, therefore, between anaesthetic gases and the increased abortion rate is, strictly speaking, implied but not proved. We are unaware of controlled studies where the reproductive outcome of exposure to specific anaesthetic gases, including the effect of duration, dosage, maternal blood levels, and so forth, has been examined. Nonetheless, on the basis of personal observation and the available literature, we advise women exposed to anaesthetic gases to modify their jobs when desiring a pregnancy.

Synthetic hair dyes

We are unaware of specific studies addressing the issue of reproductive hazards among synthetic hair dye users. Sufficient related information is available, however, to make this aspect worthy of consideration. This may represent an occupational hazard not only among those whose job is to colour hair, but also among the recipients. The dyes are absorbed through the skin. It is estimated that in the USA more than 30 million persons dye their hair, the majority being women. Among the adverse effects noted that could impair reproduction are the possibilites of increased chromosomal damage and cancer of the breast[8,9].

Despite the paucity of information on the relationship, if any, between the use of synthetic hair dyes and reproduction, there is a reasonable body of evidence showing that some of the constituents of hair dyes can be hazardous to health. The benzenes and toluenes may be taken as examples.

Benzene

Benzene is a commonly used agent in the manufacturing of dyes, varnishes, solvents, medicinal chemicals and other compounds. Its reproductive toxicity in humans and various animal species is still not well delineated. In animals, benzene at maternally toxic doses does not seem to increase the incidence of congenital malformations. However, reductions in fetal body weight, delayed ossification and a possible increase in fetal haemorrhages are observed. These effects appear more pronounced in the female than in the male fetus.

The observations in humans pertaining to benzene exposure are coloured by the concomitant exposure to other chemicals. Women seem more susceptible than men to the toxic effects of benzene, probably owing to its slower elimination by virtue of the higher body fat content in women[10]. Maternal-to-fetal transfer of benzene does occur[11]. Workers in industries where exposure to benzene, petroleum, chlorinated hydrocarbons exists (e.g. leather, rubber products and glue) have an increased rate of menstrual disturbances and possibly abortions. Chromosomal damage can occur, apparently after exposure to toxic levels or prolonged high levels.

Toluene

There are no clear-cut studies on the toxicity of toluene in humans. Women workers exposed to toluene, as in the manufacture of electrical insulating material, or in the production of mica insulating materials or varnished cloth, may show a higher rate of menstrual dysfunction but are also concomitantly exposed to other chemicals.

It thus appears that while at present the specific reproductive toxicity of benzene and toluene cannot be ascertained, broadly speaking, exposure to these and other agents can constitute a reproductive hazard that should be part of the evaluation in women whose employment exposes them to these agents.

Ethylene oxide

There is an increase in spontaneous abortions among women involved in sterilising instruments in hospitals and in those working in textile plants. The main offending agent in the former seems to be ethylene oxide[12,13].

Passively carried agents

The reproductive hazards from parental exposure to a noxious environment should also include the harmful effects on normal children, for, in the last analysis, they are the fruit of reproduction. Here one may cite the adverse effect on other family members of asbestos, lead and other agents carried by the parents on their clothing. Nor is the nursing infant immune from potentially hazardous chemicals, for many of these are known to be secreted and even concentrated in breast milk[14].

Strenuous physical activity

Women whose occupations require constant and excessive physical activity are at increased risk for disturbance in their reproductive system. Women predisposed to these disturbances include long-distance runners, competitive swimmers, ballet dancers and military cadets. The observed effects include: delayed menarche, amenorrhoea, menstrual irregularities and luteal phase defects[15-17]. Although it appears that these disturbances are reversible, the long-term effects are not understood. Nor is the aetiology well delineated, but, as Rebar and Cumming[18] have postulated, the observed effects may be the result of several factors – psychological, nutritional, hormonal and environmental.

The effect of activity on reproduction is not limited to the non-pregnant worker. As reviewed elsewhere[19], exercise can alter uterine blood flow. The decrease in flow can be particularly hazardous to the fetus with growth retardation or to one where the potential for growth retardation is present (e.g. in pregnancy with chronic hypertension). In these and other situations we are firmly convinced of the beneficial effects to the fetus of prolonged periods of maternal rest. This in many instances will be disruptive to the working woman's ability to carry out her responsibilities effectively and, hence, will raise the issue of her rights versus the rights of the fetus versus those of her employer.

CONCLUSIONS

The preceding discussion has attempted to outline the complexities involved in addressing the issue of women workers and reproductive hazards. The problem is real, the solution elusive. While the primary concern may centre around exposure to various chemicals, we have attempted to show that exposure to possible reproductive hazards is limited to neither chemicals nor a woman's occupation.

A list of known or potential toxins in this chapter is not helpful, and many are referred to in other chapters of this book. The issue, however, is how to reconcile the fact of health hazards with the right to employment.

It is a well-recognised fact that the necessary information fully to appreciate and place in proper perspective the possible health hazards of workers and non-workers is either unknown or incompletely known; nor is it possible with our current systems of subjecting all existing and newly created agents to comprehensive testing. The numbers are staggering; animal testing is not necessarily applicable to humans; and human testing is slow and, except with truly informed consent, unethical. The long latent period which is sometimes present before an effect is noted makes providing the appropriate answers hard. Agents with a weak expression require large numbers of observations before an effect can be verified. Furthermore, our current practice allows products to be marketed without an appreciation of their reproductive toxicity. In the USA the Toxic Substances Control Act describes four levels of investigation[20]. The information pertaining to reproduction is required at Level IV, at which time the product is already on the market. Furthermore, as mentioned by Koeter[21], safety limits of exposure based on the subchronic studies do not necessarily indicate safety from adverse reproductive effects. In many instances the threshold for reproductive toxicity may be lower than the limits set by subchronic studies.

In recommending guidelines to resolve the multifaceted aspects of the woman worker, one must realise that the question of reproduction cannot be isolated from the overall issue of health hazards to humans and of health hazards to animals and plants on which human survival depends. Secondly, a distinction must be made between inacceptable occupational exposure under normal operational conditions and exposure due to unforeseen accidents. The latter is an occupational risk, true of all professions, which should be accepted by all those seeking employment. The risk should be minimal, but nevertheless present-day reality dictates its possibility.

Exposure under normal operational conditions is a different matter. The appropriate containment of known and potential hazardous compounds is a major public health issue taxing the ingenuity of man. There must be appropriate safeguards, including attire and ventilation, with the appropriate back-up system to contain and appropriately dispose of what has been washed or ventilated.

It is time to pause, to assess where we are and where we would like to be, and to reflect on the problems at hand before we face new ones. A major effort should now be made to take stock of what hazards exist and to know how to deal with them. We cannot maintain the current pace of exposure to the new, for it is far outstripping our ability to comprehend and assess its impact. Scientists and health officials should address existing hazards and their impact on human health, including reproduction, with the same zeal and fervour as is seen in creating new and better things. Employment will not be curtailed — just channelled in new directions. Such an approach cannot be regional but must be global — but then, so is the problem.

REFERENCES

1. Manson, J. (1978). Human laboratory animal test systems available for detection of reproductive failure. *Prevent. Med.*, **7**, 322–331
2. Dickerson, O. B. (1981/1982). Arsenic poisoning from occupational and environmental exposure. *Occup. Med.*, **4**, Winter
3. Fishbein, L. (1979). *Potential Industrial Carcinogens and Mutagens*, Elsevier, Amsterdam, p. 1
4. Greenberg, J. (1980). Implications for primary care providers of occupational health hazards on pregnant women and their infants. *J. Nurse Midwif.*, **25**, 21–29
5. Spence, A. A., Cohen, E. N., Brown, B. W., Knill-Jones, R. P. and Himmelberger, D. U. (1977). Occupational hazards for operating room-based physicians. *J. Am. Med. Assoc.*, **238**, 955–959
6. Tomlin, P. J. (1979). Health problems of anaesthetists and their families in the West Midlands. *Br. Med. J.*, i, 779–783
7. Abdul-Karim, R. W. (1981). *Drugs During Pregnancy: Clinical Perspectives*, Stickley, Philadelphia, pp. 45–51
8. Kirkland, D. J. and Lawler, S. D. (1978). Venitts chromosomal damage and hair dyes. *Lancet*, ii, 124–128
9. Nasaca, P. C., Lawrence, C. E., Greenwald, P., Chorost, S., Arbuckle, J. T. and Paulson, A. (1980). Relationship of hair dye use, benign breast disease, and breast cancer. *J. Natl Cancer Inst.*, **64**, 23–28
10. Sato, A., Nakajima, T., Fujiwara, Y. and Murayama, N. (1975). Kinetic studies on sex differences in susceptibility to chronic benzene intoxication with special reference to body fat content. *Br. J. Ind. Med.*, **32**, 321–328
11. Dowty, B. J., Laseter, J. L. and Storer, J. L. (1976). The transplacental migration and accumulation in blood of volatile organic constituents. *Ped. Res.*, **10**, 696–701
12. Hemminki, K., Mutanen, P., Saloniemi, I., Niemi, M. L. and Vainio, H. (1982). Spontaneous abortions in hospital staff engaged in sterilizing instruments with chemical agents. *Br. Med. J.*, **285**, 1461–1463
13. Hemminki, K., Kyyronen, P., Niemi, M., Koskinen, K., Sallmen, M. and Vainio, H. (1983). Spontaneous abortions in an industrialized community in Finland. *Am. J. Pub. Hlth*, **73**, 1, 32–36
14. Rogan, W. J., Bagniewska, A. and Damstra, T. (1980). Pollutants in breast milk. *New Engl. J. Med.*, **302**, 1450–1453
15. Anderson, J. L. (1979). Women's sports and fitness program at the U.S. Military Academy. *Phys. Sports Med.*, **7**, 72–78
16. Frisch, R. E., Wyshak, G. and Vincent, L. E. (1980). Delayed menarche and amenorrhea in ballet dancers. *New Engl. J. Med.*, **303**, 17–19
17. Shangold, M., Freeman, R., Thysen, B. and Gatz, M. (1979). The relationship between long distance running, plasma progesterone and luteal phase length. *Fertil. Steril.*, **31**, 130–133

18. Rebar, R. W. and Cumming, D. C. (1981). Reproductive function in women athletes. *J. Am. Med. Assoc.*, **246**, 1590
19. Bruce, N. W. and Abdul-Karim, R. W. (1974). Mechanisms controlling maternal placental circulation. *Clin. Obstet. Gynec.*, **17**, 135–151
20. Ellison, T. (1983). Toxicological effects testing. In Domingues, G. S. (Ed.), *Guidebook: Toxic Substances Control Act*, CRC Press, Cleveland (cited by Koeter, (1983)
21. Koeter, H. B. W. M. (1983). Relevance of parameters related to fertility and reproduction in toxicity testing. In Mattison, D. R. (Ed.), *Reproductive Toxicity*, Alan R. Liss, New York, pp. 81–85

5

Reproductive Hazards of the American Life Style

STEVEN G. GABBE

Perinatal morbidity and mortality due to many treatable disorders, such as rhesus isoimmunisation and diabetes mellitus, have decreased. It is only logical, therefore, to turn attention to those environmental factors encountered in day-to-day lives which represent reproductive hazards. This chapter will focus on elements of the American life style which have been linked to poor reproductive outcome. It should be remembered that, although life in the USA has many aspects unique to that society, other countries in today's world share these problems. Furthermore, while some studies have demonstrated risks to female reproductive performance, similar factors may pose equal if not greater threats to men.

STRESS

Life in the USA, particularly in large urban centres, is most often characterised as frenetic and anxiety-provoking – a life style in the fast lane. When rhesus monkey mothers are stressed, fetal bradycardia and hypoxia result. Such stress undoubtedly leads to catecholamine release, with impairment of the utero-placental circulation and increased uterine activity[1]. Poor reproductive performance is also well known in animals that are crowded. Human gestation complicated by interpersonal tension and stress may also be associated with childhood morbidity in the form of behaviour disorders, including hyperactivity, neuroses and mental retardation[2]. Such pressure can often be attributed to the increasingly common problem of divorce and of wife-battering. Economic hardships associated with pregnancy due to rising health care costs or loss of the woman's income may fuel such conflicts. Obviously separating the contribution of stress itself from other significant aetiological variables such as low socioeconomic status and poor nutrition is extremely difficult[3].

45

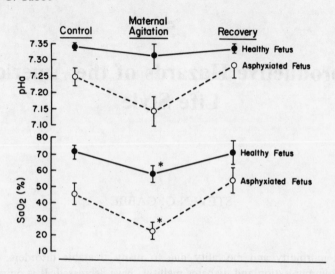

Figure 5.1 Excitement of the pregnant rhesus monkey mother is associated with fetal hypoxia, probably resulting from catecholamine release with impairment of the utero-placental circulation and increased uterine activity (data from reference 1)

ACCESS TO HEALTH CARE

In the USA funds available for health care programmes for the poor have been cut as a result of the economic recession. In the Hospital of the University of Philadelphia during the past year, the number of women who have not had prenatal care prior to delivery doubled to 13 per cent of all those delivered. At Parkland Memorial Hospital in Dallas 16 per cent of all women delivering in 1980 had received no prenatal care. The incidence of infants of low birth weight, stillbirths and neonatal deaths was three times higher in this group than in those women attending the prenatal clinic[4]. Kessner's analysis of perinatal outcome in New York City also emphasised that the quality of prenatal care could be correlated with perinatal outcome[5]. Unfortunately, those patients who by virtue of their low socio-economic status required prenatal care the most often received the least. Of 22 000 black and Puerto Rican mothers at risk, less than 2 per cent secured adequate prenatal care.

MATERNAL AGE

In the USA one in five births is to a woman 18 years or younger[6]. Although births to older teenagers have decreased, an increase of 22 per cent has occurred

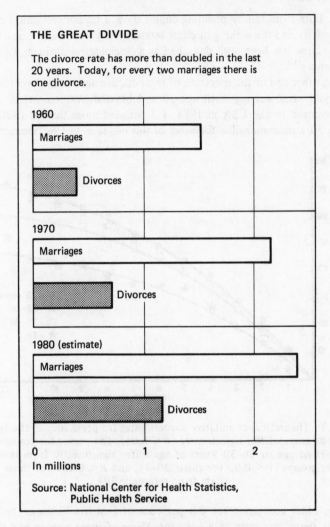

Figure 5.2 In the past three decades the frequency of divorce has risen dramatically (data from reference 58)

in women age 15–17 in the past 10 years. These pregnancies are associated with an increased risk of pregnancy-induced hypertension and pelvic-inlet contraction, as well as inadequate nutrition and poor health before gestation[7]. Approximately 50 per cent of urban teenage women engage in premarital sex, and few are using the most effective contraceptive techniques, the oral contraceptive or intrauterine device[8]. Of all pregnancies among unmarried teenagers, half occur in the first 6 months after they become sexually active and over one-fifth in the first month[9]. Data from family planning clinics show a lag between onset of teenage sexual activity and the seeking of clinic services – a year in some cases. The teenage pregnancy has been well described as a 'sociological problem with medical consequences'[10].

At the other end of the spectrum of reproductive age, many American women are delaying child-bearing until age 30 and beyond. Approximately 3 646 000 births occurred in the USA in 1981, 1.3 per cent more than in 1980. Women over age 30 were responsible for most of this increase. In 1960 women 30 years

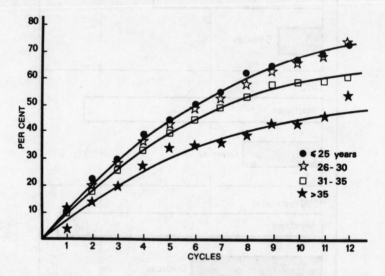

Figure 5.3   Theoretical cumulative success rates for pregnancy in the age groups shown. The curves differ significantly ($P < 0.01$). The curves for younger women ≤ 25 years of age or 26–30 years of age differ significantly from those of the two older groups ($P < 0.03$ for those 30–35, and $P < 0.001$ for those over 35) (data from reference 59)

of age or older accounted for 6.8 per cent of first live births in the USA; by 1979 this figure had risen to 8 per cent. Many of these women had elected to pursue their careers before beginning a family. However, this choice may lead to a decrease in fecundity or reproductive potential[11]. Furthermore, pregnancies in older women are associated with an increased risk of Down's syndrome and other genetic abnormalities, as well as hypertension and gestational diabetes mellitus.

PERINATAL INFECTIONS

During the past two decades sexual promiscuity has increased in virtually all socio-economic classes of the American society. Not surprisingly, venereal diseases now occur in epidemic proportions. Gonorrhoea ranks first among the reported communicable diseases in the USA. From 1971 to 1976 the reported cases of gonorrhoea increased from more than 600 000 to over 1 000 000, and it has been estimated that only one-third of all cases were actually reported[12]. Gonorrhoeal infection not only can limit reproductive potential by damaging the fallopian tubes, but also during pregnancy causes chorio-amnionitis, with premature rupture of the membranes and premature delivery, neonatal ophthalmitis and sepsis, and maternal endometritis[13]. Cases of syphilis have nearly quadrupled since 1957, while herpes simplex and cytomegalovirus may be isolated from 0.65 and

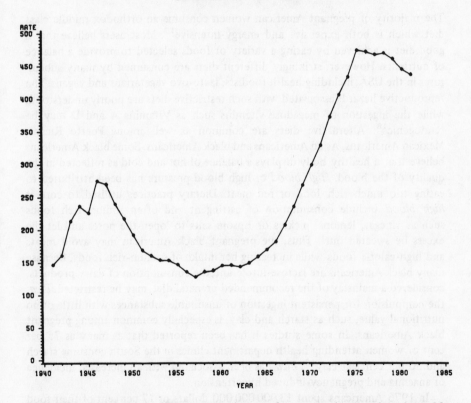

GONORRHEA – Reported civilian cases per 100,000 population, by year, United States, 1941-1981

Figure 5.4 Beginning in 1966, reported gonorrhoea cases increased at about 12 per cent per year until 1973, when over 800 000 cases were reported. A sharp increase of reported cases in the late 1960s and early 1970s is felt to represent an actual increase in the occurrence of the disease as well as improved case detection procedures. Since 1973 the number of reported cases has levelled off at about 1 000 000 cases per year. Levelling off of reported cases since 1975 is felt to be due to disease-intervention activities initiated in 1973 (data from reference 14)

3 per cent of obstetrical patients, respectively. The percentage of congenital syphilis cases reported in children less than 1 year old increased from 38.6 per cent of all cases of congenital syphilis in 1980 to 55.7 per cent in 1981[14]. This increase in reported cases was probably caused by a greater frequency of early syphilis in American women and by lack of medical care and serological testing in the prenatal period. Of newborns infected with cytomegalovirus, 5-10 per cent may later be found to be deaf and mentally retarded[15]. Most recently, a new syndrome of acquired immunodeficiency has been identified in children whose mothers were sexually promiscuous or drug addicts[16].

DIET AND EXERCISE

The majority of pregnant American women consume an orthodox middle class diet which is both expensive and energy-intensive[17]. Most users believe that a good diet is achieved by eating a variety of foods selected to provide a balance of nutrients. However, strikingly different diets are consumed by many subcultures in the USA, including health foodists, lacto-ovo vegetarians and vegans. The reproductive hazards associated with such restrictive diets are poorly understood, while the ingestion of megadose vitamins such as Vitamins A and D may be teratogenic[18]. Alternative diets are common as well among Puerto Ricans, Mexican Americans, Asian Americans and black Americans. Some black Americans believe that a healthy body displays a balance of hot and cold as reflected in the quality of the blood. *High blood* or high blood pressure has been attributed to eating too much rich food or red meat. Dietary practices utilised to correct *high blood* include consumption of astringent and often sodium-rich foods such as vinegar, lemons, pickles or Epsom salts to 'open the pores and let the excess be sweated out'. Thus, the pregnant black American may avoid meats and high-calorie foods while increasing her intake of sodium-rich foods. Because many black Americans are lactose-intolerant, the consumption of dairy products, considered a mainstay of the recommended prenatal diet, may be restricted. *Pica*, the compulsion for persistent ingestion of unsuitable substances with little or no nutritional value, such as starch and clay, is especially common among pregnant black Americans. In some studies it has been reported that as many as 75 per cent of women attending health department clinics in the South consume starch and 50 per cent eat clay[17]. *Pica* has been associated with an increased incidence of anaemia and pregnancy-induced hypertension.

In 1976 Americans spent 13 900 000 000 dollars or 17 per cent of their food dollar on fast foods. By 1985, it is estimated that Americans will spend approximately 50 per cent of their food dollar outside the home. While fast food meals may provide adequate protein, their caloric content may be excessive and they are high in sodium, cholesterol and saturated fats[19].

Exercise and competitive sports have become an increasingly important part of day-to-day life for the American woman. In 1970 one woman started the

New York City marathon but failed to finish. Ten years later, 2578 women entered this 26.2 mile race and over 60 per cent completed the event. In 1975 the Women's Sports Federation estimated that over 50 million American women actively engaged in athletic recreation. Although older studies found little effect of exercise on reproductive performance in women, recent investigations have

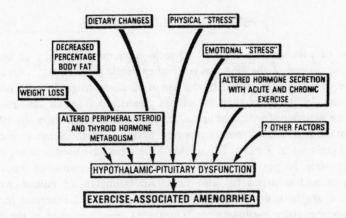

Figure 5.5 Factors which may contribute to exercise-associated amenorrhoea (data from reference 60)

confirmed significant alterations in menstrual function. Intensive training in the premenarcheal years can result in delayed menarche[20]. Serious runners, cyclists, swimmers and ballet dancers may also experience amenorrhoea as well as a shortened luteal phase. Such menstrual dysfunction is most common in runners and has been documented in 12–43 per cent of these women. The precise aetiology of such abnormalities has not been determined but may be due to physical and emotional stress, dietary changes, altered hormonal secretion during acute and chronic exercise, weight loss and a decreased percentage of body fat[21]. The effect of exercise-related amenorrhoea on subsequent fertility is not known.

Pregnant women are also participating in athletics in increasing numbers. Concern has arisen that exercise during pregnancy can reduce uterine blood flow and lead to fetal growth retardation. Clapp has observed that in the near-term pregnant ewe sustained, low-level exercise to exhaustion produced significant falls in both uterine and umbilical blood flow. However, uterine and umbilical oxygen uptakes were unchanged[22]. Both Collings and co-workers[23] and Metcalfe[24] have observed that fetuses of normal pregnant women participating in an aerobic exercise programme demonstrated no evidence of impaired growth. Yet Clapp and Dickstein have recently reported that frequent, vigorous endurance exercise during pregnancy will limit maternal weight gain, reduce gestational length and increase the incidence of fetal growth retardation significantly[25].

Little information is available on the effects of sudden repetitive peak exercise such as experienced during a tennis match, the effects of exercise in early pregnancy, or the effects of exercise on pregnancies with a compromised utero-placental circulation.

PSYCHOACTIVE DRUG ABUSE

The use of psychoactive drugs by all socio-economic classes, by all age groups and in all regions of the USA has reached epidemic proportions[26]. An explosive increase of about twentyfold in the use of all illicit drugs occurred during the 1960s and 1970s. More than 50 million Americans from all age groups have had some experience with marijuana, and 20 million use it daily. In 1981 59.5 per cent of high school seniors reported having used the drug, an increase of over 40 per cent in 3 years. Ten million Americans have used cocaine, including approximately 30 per cent of 18–25-year-olds. Consumption of tranquillisers, stimulants and sedatives has also risen. An estimated 13 million Americans have used amphetamines without medical supervision. The increase in sedative ingestion, especially methaqualone (Quaalude), may be linked to the dramatic rise in cocaine use, as the drug is taken to bring the cocaine user down. At the present time almost half a million Americans are addicted to heroin. It has been suggested that increased psychoactive drug abuse may be attributed to changes in child-rearing practices and family stability in the USA.

Both clinical and animal research studies have linked drug abuse to alterations in sexual behaviour, infertility due to inhibition of ovulation or prevention of implantation, embryotoxicity, impaired parturition, lactation failure, and maternal neglect of offspring[27]. Marijuana use has been documented in 13 per cent of obstetrical patients in a Southern California clinic[28]. It was thought to increase both uterine activity and the fetal passage of meconium. In men marijuana may inhibit spermatogenesis and testosterone secretion. Little information is available on the consequences of cocaine consumption in pregnancy, although anorexia among cocaine users is common and could certainly limit prenatal nutrition. Maternal cocaine abuse has been associated with abruptio placentae[29]. In evaluating the effects of drug abuse, one must consider the pharmacological alterations produced by the drug itself as well as the ecologic effects[30]. For example, women addicted to heroin may contract hepatitis or skin infections from contaminated needles or pelvic inflammatory disease as a result of prostitution taken up to finance their drug habit. Menstrual dysfunction has been documented in 60–90 per cent of heroin addicts. Their pregnancies are marked by poor nutrition and inadequate prenatal care, contributing to premature delivery and intrauterine growth retardation[31]. Infants born to heroin-addicted mothers also suffer a high incidence of neonatal abstinence reactions.

ALCOHOL

The incidence of alcoholism among American women has steadily increased in the past 20 years. There are at present 2.25 million alcoholic women in the USA and most are of child-bearing age[32]. It has now been clearly recognised that heavy alcohol use during pregnancy is associated with poor reproductive outcome[33]. Fetal risks associated with moderate or minimal alcohol consumption have not been as well established. Fetal alcohol syndrome (FAS), a triad of facial dysmorphology, antenatal and postnatal growth deficiency and central nervous system involvement including mental retardation, has been observed in from 1 in 300 to 1 in 2000 live births. It has been described in 30-40 per cent of infants of alcoholic mothers. The State of New York has estimated a yearly cost of 155 million dollars directly related to the birth of children damaged by alcohol[34]. Maternal alcohol use also significantly increases the risk of spontaneous abortion[35,36].

The mechanism by which alcohol alters fetal development remains controversial. Exposure in the first trimester appears critical for dysmorphology, in the second trimester for fetal loss, and in the third trimester for impaired intrauterine growth. Both acute and chronic fetal poisoning may cause spontaneous abortion. Fetal growth retardation may result from impaired umbilical circulation, effects of placental amino acid transport, decreased absorption of nutrients across the maternal intestinal mucosa and altered hepatic metabolism in the mother[37,38].

Many studies have attempted to define the dose–response curve for maternal alcohol ingestion and teratogenicity. Heavy drinkers, those women who consume at least five drinks on some occasions and no fewer than 45 drinks per month, are at greatest risk. (One drink has usually been defined as 15 ml of absolute ethanol.) Studies performed throughout the USA and in varied socioeconomic classes have documented heavy drinking in from 1.5 per cent (Loma Linda, California) to 14.1 per cent (Seattle, Washington) of the pregnant population[39]. Heavy drinkers tend to be older, live alone, receive limited prenatal care, smoke heavily, use psychoactive drugs and associate with men who drink heavily. The paternal contribution to FAS remains controversial. Moderate alcohol consumption has been associated with spontaneous abortions, behavioural dysfunction, adverse mental and motor development, and impaired conditioning in newborns[33]. Studies in animals suggest that binge drinking, the giving of short-term doses of alcohol of critical size, may also have deleterious effects[40]. Thus, there may be a continuum of fetal damage dependent not only upon the dose of alcohol, but also on when in gestation it is consumed and its metabolism by the mother[41]. As stressed by Kalter and Warkany, '... the whole story of the possible impact on prenatal life of maternal alcohol consumption, combined with smoking, coffee, drugs of abuse, unfavourable demographic characteristics, low social status, poor nutrition, and other factors still remains to be told'[42].

Recent data indicate that drinking patterns may be changing in some American women. Streissguth *et al.* have compared alcohol consumption of pregnant women in Seattle, Washington, between 1974/75 and 1980/81[43]. The number of women who reported any alcohol use around the time of the first prenatal visit dropped from 81 per cent to 42 per cent. Fifty-eight per cent of the women interviewed in 1980/81 reported that they were already abstaining by the first prenatal visit, a threefold decrease over 6 years. These behavioural changes were attributed to public education programmes with heightened awareness of the dangers of alcohol. On the other hand, no significant change was observed in heavy drinking or binge drinking around the time of conception.

CIGARETTE SMOKING

It has been stated that 'Cigarette smoking, one of the first manifestations of women's social emancipation, is emerging as a possible threat to her procreative role'[44]. Smoking became widespread among women after World War II. Between 1965 and 1976 approximately one-third of all American women smoked[45]. Since 1976 the proportion of women smokers has declined to 28 per cent. The annual per capita cigarette consumption in the USA has also decreased, from 4528 in 1965 to 3900 in 1979. Nevertheless, cigarette smoking has increased among adolescent girls, so that in the 17–19-year age group there are now five female smokers for every four male smokers.

Cigarette smoking has emerged as a threat to both general health and reproductive function in women. It is associated with one-fifth of newly diagnosed cancer cases and one-fourth of cancer deaths in women. Women who smoke manifest an increased frequency of menstrual dysfunction and a lower age at menopause[46]. Smoking may alter the motility of the female reproductive tract, increasing uterine tone, and may impair implantation. In men smoking has been associated with a reduction in sperm count and a greater frequency of abnormal sperm morphology[47].

The pregnant smoker is at increased risk for the spontaneous abortion of an otherwise normal fetus, fetal death associated with placental abruption or placenta previa, premature delivery and premature rupture of the membranes, symmetrical fetal growth retardation, and the delivery of infants who subsequently have behaviour and cognitive development problems and are at greater risk for Sudden Infant Death Syndrome[48]. There is a clear dose-response relationship, with heavier smokers experiencing these problems with greater frequency. Delivery of infants of low birth weight increases by 30 per cent in women smoking less than one pack of cigarettes daily and by more than 100 per cent in those smoking at least one pack per day[49].

Cigarette smoke contains over 1000 separate chemical constituents, including nicotine, carbon monoxide, polycyclic aromatic hydrocarbons and hydrogen cyanide. The adverse effects on fetal growth and development have been attri-

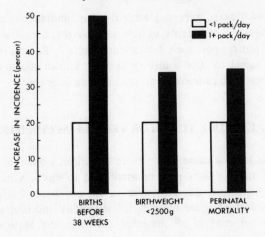

Figure 5.6 Incidence of several complications for the fetus and newborn infant increases as a function of the amount the mother smokes (data from reference 61)

buted primarily to fetal hypoxia resulting from exposure to carbon monoxide and nicotine. Carbon monoxide combines with haemoglobin in the smoking mother and her fetus, forming carboxyhaemoglobin and reducing oxygen-carrying capacity[50]. Fetal carboxyhaemoglobin levels are usually 15–20 per cent higher than maternal levels. Therefore, in heavy smokers fetal oxygen-carrying capacity may be reduced by as much as 25 per cent. Nicotine exerts its deleterious fetal effects through a catecholamine-mediated reduction in utero-placental perfusion and decreased fetal oxygenation[51].

Attention has recently been directed to the pregnant passive smoker, the nonsmoker exposed to air contaminated with tobacco smoke. Bottoms has demonstrated that thiocyanate levels, which correlate well with the number of cigarettes smoked per day, are significantly higher in the fetus whose mother does not smoke but who lives in a household with smokers[52]. The possible clinical effects of passive smoking during pregnancy have not been established.

CAFFEINE

It has been estimated that in a typical year Americans consume nearly 1 000 000 000 kg of coffee[53]. Depending on the method of brewing, each cup of coffee may contain from 75 to 300 mg of caffeine. Caffeine is also ingested in tea, Cola and cocoa beverages, and in many over-the-counter drug preparations. A study of primarily white, married, college-educated pregnant women revealed that only 5 per cent consumed four or more cups of coffee daily and less than 1 per cent drank seven or more cups each day[54]. Although it had been suggested that heavy coffee drinkers were at greater risk for spontaneous abortion, fetal death and the delivery of infants of low birthweight, a carefully performed investigation did not support such deleterious effects[54]. Rather, heavy caffeine use should be a signal to elicit a history of other known contributors to poor pregnancy outcome, such as smoking or psychoactive drug abuse.

TRAUMA DUE TO MOTOR VEHICLE ACCIDENTS

Accidents are the leading cause of death in American women of reproductive age, and half of these deaths may be attributed to motor vehicle crashes[55]. Overall, 50 000 Americans die each year in car accidents. Such trauma has emerged as an important cause of maternal morbidity and mortality. In 1977 approximately 1 per cent of all maternal deaths in the State of Oklahoma

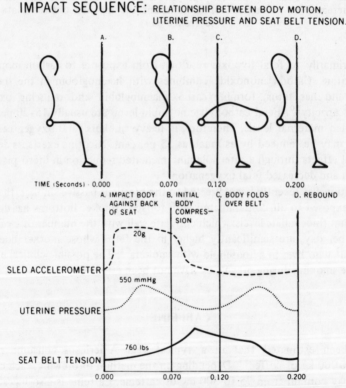

Figure 5.7 After an automobile collision the lower part of the body remains more or less stationary. The pelvis absorbs the restraining force of the lap belt and forces the body to decelerate with the car seat in the car. The upper body, however, is free to rotate on the lower spine. Marked increases in uterine pressure can occur, as well as rupture of other viscera, including bladder, bowel, liver and spleen (data from reference 62)

resulted from automobile accidents[55]. Although ejection from the vehicle is the leading cause of death in such cases, two-thirds of drivers and passengers fail to use seat belts. During pregnancy the use of such restraints is reduced, as mothers may fear the belt will injure their fetus. Lap belts alone allow the body of a passenger to flex forward on impact and may focus the decelerative forces on the maternal abdomen[56]. However, combination lap and shoulder belts, when properly worn, can significantly reduce fetal loss.

CONCLUSIONS

Having reviewed current trends in the American life style, one can only become increasingly concerned about the hazards presented to the population of the USA and their reproductive potential. Life has become more stressful, and economic pressures have limited the financial resources for all health care. One million teenage girls become pregnant each year; 650 000 are unmarried; 20 000 are 14 or younger; 400 000 have abortions. Sexual freedom has brought rising rates of gonorrhoeal infection, syphilis and herpes. If the cocaine trade were included by *Fortune* in its list of the 500 largest industrial corporations, cocaine would rank seventh in volume of domestic sales at between 27 000 000 000 and 32 000 000 000 dollars. In 1978 880 million dollars of promotion and advertising encouraged Americans to smoke. The fetal alcohol syndrome is now the third most common cause of mental handicap after Down's syndrome and neural tube defects. While it is true that women who are poor and receive inadequate prenatal care are often the same women who smoke, drink and use drugs, it is also clear that these social plagues have infected all socio-economic groups within American society. And they are problems which have emerged in the past 20–30 years. It is unrealistic to expect that alcoholism, drug abuse and smoking can be eliminated, but it is reasonable that their use prior to and during pregnancy can be halted. It is encouraging that, during gestation, women appear voluntarily to decrease cigarette, alcohol and psychoactive drug use. Research must continue to not only elucidate the maternal and fetal effects of these practices, but also develop techniques to control their abuse. In a recent survey almost half of the American women polled had no knowledge that smoking significantly increased perinatal risks. Only one in four pregnant smokers reported receiving any advice from a physician to stop smoking. Obviously, therefore, education of health care providers, the general population and legislators must be expanded[57].

REFERENCES

1. Morishima, H. O., Pedersen, H. and Finster, M. (1978). The influence of maternal psychological stress on the fetus. *Am. J. Obstet. Gynecol.*, **131**, 286–290

2. Stott, D. H. (1973). Follow-up study from birth of the effects of prenatal stresses. *Develop. Med. Child Neurol.*, **15**, 770–787

3. Seiden, A. M. (1979). Psychologic trauma and stress. In Buchsbaum, H. J. (Ed.), *Trauma in Pregnancy*, Saunders, Philadelphia, pp. 204–235

4. Leveno, K., Roark, M. and Nelson, S. (1983). The human and economic consequences of no prenatal care and low birthweight. Presented at *Society of Perinatal Obstetricians Third Annual Meeting, January, 1983, San Antonio, Texas*, Abstract 31B

5. Kessner, D. M., Singer, J., Kalk, C. E. and Schlesinger, E. R. (1973). *Infant Death: An Analysis by Maternal Risk and Health Care*, Institute of Medicine, National Academy of Sciences, Washington, D. C., p.3

6. Hollingsworth, D. R. and Kreutner, A. K. K. (1980). Teenage pregnancy solutions are evolving. *New Engl. J. Med.*, **303**, 516–518

7. Duenhoelter, J., Jimenez, J. and Baumann, G. (1975). Pregnancy performance of patients under 15 years of age. *Obstet. Gynaecol.*, **46**, 49–52

8. Zelnik, M. and Kantner, J. F. (1980). Sexual activity, contraception use and pregnancy among metropolitan-area teenagers: 1971–1979. *Fam. Plann. Perspect.*, **12**, 230–237

9. Zabin, L. S., Kantner, J. F. and Zelnik, M. (1979). The risk of adolescent pregnancy in the first months of intercourse. *Fam. Plann. Perspect.*, **11**, 215–222

10. Hollingsworth, D. R. (1982). The pregnant adolescent: A sociologic problem with medical consequences. In Burrow, G. N. and Ferris, T. F. (Eds.), *Medical Complications during Pregnancy*, Saunders, Philadelphia, pp. 546–564

11. DeCherney, A. H. and Berkowitz, G. S. (1982). Female fecundity and age. *New Engl. J. Med.*, **306**, 424–426

12. Monif, G. R. G. (1978). Gonorrhea and pregnancy. *Perin. Care*, **2**, 12–16

13. Edwards, L. E., Barrada, M. I., Hamann, A. A. and Hakanson, E. Y. (1978). Gonorrhea in pregnancy. *Am. J. Obstet. Gynecol.*, **132**, 637–641

14. Anon. (1982). Annual Summary 1981. *Morbidity and Mortality Weekly Report*, **30**, 86

15. Sever, J. L., Larsen, J. W. Jr. and Grossman, J. H. III (Eds.), *Handbook of Perinatal Infections*, Little Brown, Boston, p. 23

16. Rubinstein, A., Sicklick, M., Gupta, A., Bernstein, L., Klein, N., Rubinstein, E., Spigland, I., Fruchter, L., Litman, N., Lee, H. and Hollander, M. (1983). Acquired immunodeficiency with reversed T_4/T_8 ratios in infants born to promiscuous and drug-addicted mothers. *J. Am. Med. Assoc.*, **249**, 2350–2356

17. Cassidy, C. M. (1982). Subcultural prenatal diets of Americans. In *Alternative Dietary Practices and Nutritional Abuses in Pregnancy*, National Academy Press, Washington, D.C., pp. 25–60

18. Pitkin, R. M. (1982). Megadose nutrients during pregnancy. In *Alternative Dietary Practices and Nutritional Abuses in Pregnancy*, National Academy Press, Washington, D.C., pp. 203–211

19. Young, E., Brennan, E. and Irving, G. (1978). Perspective on fast foods. *Dietet. Curr.*, **5**, 24–30

20. Frisch, R. E., Gotz-Welbergen, A. V., McArthur, J. W., Albright, T., Witschi, J., Bullen, B., Birnholz, J., Reed, R. B. and Hermann, H. (1981). Delayed menarche and amenorrhea of college athletes in relation to age of onset of training. *J. Am. Med. Assoc.*, **246**, 1559–1563

21. Rebar, R. W. and Cumming, D. C. (1981). Reproductive function in women athletes. *J. Am. Med. Assoc.*, **246**, 1590

22. Clapp, J. F. III (1980). Acute exercise stress in the pregnant ewe. *Am. J.*

Obstet. Gynecol., **136**, 489–494
23. Collings, C. A., Curet, L. B. and Mullin, J. P. (1983). Maternal and fetal responses to a maternal aerobic exercise program. *Am. J. Obstet. Gynecol.*, **145**, 702–707
24. Metcalfe, J. M. Personal communication
25. Clapp, J. F. and Dickstein, S. (1983). Maternal exercise performance and pregnancy outcome. Presented at the *Society for Gynecologic Investigation Thirtieth Annual Meeting, March 1983*, Abstract 195
26. Nicholi, A. M. Jr. (1983). The nontherapeutic use of psychoactive drugs. A modern epidemic. *New Engl. J. Med.*, **308**, 925–933
27. Schardein, J. L. (1976). *Drugs as Teratogens*, CRC Press, Cleveland
28. Greenland, S., Staisch, K. J. and Brown Gross, S. J. (1982). The effects of marijuana use during pregnancy. I. A preliminary epidemiologic study. *Am. J. Obstet. Gynecol.*, **143**, 408–413
29. Acker, D., Sachs, B., Tracey, K. and Wise, W. (1983). Abruptio placentae associated with cocaine use. *Am. J. Obstet. Gynecol.*, **146**, 220–221
30. Lee, R. V. (1982). Drug abuse. In Burrow, G. N. and Ferris, T. F. (Eds.), *Medical Complications during Pregnancy*, Saunders, Philadelphia, 538–545
31. Connaughton, J. F., Reeser, D., Schut, J. and Finnegan, L. P. (1977). Perinatal addiction: Outcome and management. *Am. J. Obstet. Gynecol.*, **129**, 679–686
32. Noble, E. P. (Ed.) (1978). *Alcohol and Health: Third Special Report to Congress 1978* U.S. Department of Health, Education, and Welfare, Washington, D.C.
33. Council on Scientific Affairs (1983). Fetal effects of maternal alcohol use. *J. Am. Med. Assoc.*, **249**, 2517–2521
34. Russel, M. (1980). The impact of alcohol-related birth defects (ARBD) on New York State. *Neurobehav. Toxicol.*, **2**, 277–283
35. Harlap, S. and Shiono, P. H. (1980). Alcohol, smoking, and incidence of spontaneous abortions in the first and second trimester. *Lancet*, ii, 173–176
36. Kline, J., Stein, Z., Warburton, D., Shrout, P. and Susser, M. (1980). Drinking during pregnancy and spontaneous abortion. *Lancet*, ii, 176–180
37. Mukherjee, A. B. and Hodgen, G. D. (1982). Maternal ethanol exposure induces transient impairment of umbilical circulation and fetal hypoxia in monkeys. *Science, N. Y.*, **218**, 700–702
38. Rosett, H. L., Weiner, L., Lee, A., Zuckerman, B., Dooling, E. and Oppenheimer, E. (1983). Patterns of alcohol consumption and fetal development. *Obstet. Gynaecol.*, **61**, 539–546
39. Weiner, L., Rosett, H. L., Edelin, K. C., Alpert, J. J. and Zuckerman, B. (1983). Alcohol consumption by pregnant women. *Obstet. Gynaecol.*, **61**, 6–12
40. Sulik, K. K., Johnson, M. C. and Webb, M. (1981). Fetal alcohol syndrome: embryogenesis in a mouse model. *Science, N. Y.*, **214**, 936–938
41. Anon. (1983). Alcohol and the fetus – is zero the only option? *Lancet*, i, 682–683
42. Kalter, H. and Warkany, J. (1983). Congenital malformations. Major environmental causes. *New Engl. J. Med.*, **308**, 491–496
43. Streissguth, A. P., Darby, B. L., Barr, H. M., Smith, J. R. and Martin, D. C. (1983). Comparison of drinking and smoking patterns during pregnancy over a six-year interval. *Am. J. Obstet. Gynecol.*, **145**, 716–724
44. Anon. (1978). Cigarette smoking and spontaneous abortion. *Br. Med. J.*, i, 259–260
45. Harris, J. E. (1980). Patterns of cigarette smoking. In *The Health Conse-*

quences of Smoking for Women, U.S. Department of Health and Human Services, Washington, D.C., pp. 17–42

46. Mattison, D. R. (1982). The effects of smoking on fertility from gametogenesis to implantation. *Environ. Res.*, **28**, 410–433

47. Campbell, J. M. and Harrison, K. L. (1979). Smoking and infertility. *Med. J. Aust.*, **1**, 342–343

48. Hasselmeyer, E. G., Meyer, M. B., Longo, L. D. and Mattison, D. R. (1980). Pregnancy and infant health. In *The Health Consequences of Smoking for Women*, U.S. Department of Health and Human Services, Washington, D.C., pp. 191–249

49. Meyer, M., Jonas, B. and Tonascia, J. (1976). Perinatal events associated with maternal smoking during pregnancy. *Am. J. Epidemiol.*, **103**, 464–476

50. Longo, L. D. (1977). The biological effects of carbon monoxide on the pregnant woman, fetus, and newborn infant. *Am. J. Obstet. Gynecol.*, **129**, 69–103

51. Resnick, R., Brink, G. W. and Wilkes, M. (1979). Catecholamine-mediated reduction in uterine blood flow after nicotine infusion in the pregnant ewe. *J. Clin. Invest.*, **63**, 1133–1136

52. Bottoms, S. F., Kuhnert, B. R., Kuhnert, P. M. and Reese, A. L. (1982). Maternal passive smoking and fetal serum thiocyanate levels. *Am. J. Obstet. Gynecol.*, **144**, 787–791

53. Punke, H. H. (1974). Caffeine in America's food and drug habits. *J. Sch. Hlth*, **44**, 551–562

54. Linn, S., Schoenbaum, S. C., Monson, R. R., Rosner, B., Stubblefield, P. G. and Ryan, K. J. (1982). No association between coffee consumption and adverse outcomes of pregnancy. *New Engl. J. Med.*, **306**, 141–145

55. Crosby, W. M. (1979). Automobile injuries and blunt abdominal trauma. In Buchsbaum, H. J. (Ed.) *Trauma in Pregnancy*, Saunders, Philadelphia, pp. 101–12

56. Crosby, W. M., Snyder, R. G., Snow, C. C. and Hanson, P. G. (1968). Impact injuries in pregnancy. I. Experimental studies. *Am. J. Obstet. Gynecol.*, **101**, 100–110

57. Roper Report (1980). Federal trade commission staff report on the cigarette advertising investigation (1981), Washington, D.C.

58. Rachlin, C. Z. (1983). Divorce statistics. *Newsweek*, Jan 10

59. Federation CEDOS, Schwartz, D. and Mayaux, M. J. (1982). Female fecundity as a function of age. Result of artificial insemination in 2193 nulliparous women with azoospermic husbands. *New Engl. J. Med.*, **306**, 404

60. Cumming, D. C. and Rebar, R. W. (1983). Exercise and reproductive function in women. *Am. J. Ind. Med.*, **4**, 113–125

61. Longo, L. M. (1982). The health consequences of maternal smoking. Experimental studies and public policy recommendations. In *Alternative Dietary Practices and Nutritional Abuse in Pregnancy. Proceedings of a Workshop Committee on Nutrition of the Mother and Preschool Child*, National Academy Press, Washington, D.C., 139

62. Crosby, W. M. *et al.* (1968). *Am. J. Obstet. Gynecol.*, **101**, 108

6

Birth Defects and Parental Occupation

J. DAVID ERICKSON

The purpose of this chapter is to describe some of the epidemiological activities at the Centers for Disease Control (CDC) in the field of birth defects and parental occupation. A decade ago little evidence about hazard or safety was available and concerns about possible associations between occupational exposures and birth defects seemed relatively new. Perhaps the dearth of evidence stemmed from the recent trend of women moving into fields of employment that had been traditionally the exclusive preserves of men, fields which were perceived as being potentially inimical to a female's reproductive function. Further, we are still more or less at the same point, although many investigations have been started in the past few years in the USA; perhaps much evidence will be available in the relatively near future. At CDC a major study will soon be completed which has as its primary purpose the assessment of the birth defects risks of a very special type of occupational setting: the Vietnam war. It is ironic that the trend to female employment in traditionally male occupations has also generated an interest in the possibility of male-mediated reproductive problems deriving from those occupational exposures.

This chapter is concerned with three main topics: first, the previous studies on parental occupation and birth defects; second, the ongoing study aimed at Vietnam veterans, mostly because the design of this study will permit of the examination of a much broader range of occupational exposures than just those connected with military service and the focus will be on some exciting methodological progress in data collection techniques; third will be described a major obstacle to progress in the US in this field, an impediment which keeps us from learning as much as we could about the role of occupational exposures as causes of birth defects.

61

EPIDEMIOLOGICAL STUDIES

Studies of occupational hazards to reproduction, including the occurrence of birth defects, usually begin in one of two ways.

(1) *The case control study*: one begins with cases having the reproductive outcome of interest and controls without such an outcome and looks back in time to compare the relative frequency of a particular occupational exposure in each group.

(2) *The cohort study*: one starts with persons exposed in a particular occupational setting and uses controls who are not exposed, so comparing the frequency of reproductive outcome of interest in the two groups.

In each case the question of interest is the same: Is the exposure associated with an increase (or decrease) in the frequency of the outcome being studied? Each of these two types of study have advantages and disadvantages. The case control study can, in some circumstances, be done quicker and more cheaply than can a cohort study. It can also give a more sensitive or powerful study for a fixed expenditure – it can give us 'more bang for the buck'. In addition, since the study begins with those with and without the condition of interest, a wide variety of exposures can be assessed. Also, there is usually little potential for bias in the determination of the disease status. However, there are possibilities for bias in the determination of the exposure of interest, and this becomes a major concern if the exposure information is derived from the memory of those who have had the misfortune to have a poor reproductive outcome, such as a child with a birth defect.

The cohort study can be expensive. It can take a long time to collect the information of interest, although the shortness of the human gestational period helps to mitigate this problem, and there are strategies which epidemiologists frequently use to overcome this disadvantage. Because the cohort study starts out with groups separated by exposure, there is usually little concern about bias in exposure determination, and there is no limit to the number of different health outcomes which may be assessed relative to the exposure. However, particularly for some reproductive outcomes, such as spontaneous abortion, there is a possibility for biases to affect the ascertainment of the reproductive outcomes.

It must be stressed that case control studies are cheaper than cohort studies, but it is generally considered that the cohort study is preferable to the case control study. In part, this is because the cohort study proceeds logically from cause – exposure – to disease, whereas the case control study approaches the problem backwards, proceeding from effect – the poor reproductive outcome – to the putative cause – the exposure.

It seems impossible for an epidemiologist to discuss work with a general group without starting out with all the caveats, as this makes it seem that we do not believe in the methods of our discipline. However, it is patently obvious that if one is to make inferences about human illness, it is only reasonable that one ought to study human illness. For all its real and imagined faults, the epidemiological study does deal with humans and their diseases. The exhortations of those who advocate the use of animal and other laboratory techniques of doubtful prognostic value for humans in place of good epidemiology are not, in our opinion, to be embraced uncritically. The epidemiologist loves randomisation of treatments, strict control of extraneous variation and all the other trappings of 'hard' science, but he also likes quick answers. Good non-epidemiological techniques are needed and have a valued place in our armamentarium of tools which can be used to help ensure a safe work place, but questions of human prognostic relevance, such as species specificity, will be forever with us. Thus the enthusiasm for the use of techniques which have not been shown to be valid predictors of human ill-health is to be greeted with scepticism.

PREVIOUS CDC STUDIES OF BIRTH DEFECTS AND OCCUPATION

Our studies began with CDC's Metropolitan Atlanta Congenital Defects Program, which is primarily a hospital-based record review system in which an attempt is made to ascertain all babies with structural congenital malformations born to mothers residing in a five-county area including and surrounding the city of Atlanta[1]. The data included in our occupational analyses were a subset of the total roster – they were derived from interviews with mothers of babies with selected defects, including central nervous system defects, oro-facial clefts, intestinal atresias, chromosomal anomalies and abdominal wall defects. Most interviews were done in the homes of the babies' parents within 6 months of the birth of the affected child. Information gathered during the interviews included an employment history for the mother beginning 2 years prior to conception and ending at the time of birth, and for the father at the time of conception.

The information collected about occupation was coded according to the system of the US Census Bureau[2]. This system is quite comprehensive and provides an industry code as well as an occupational code. The occupational classification includes 417 categories and the industrial code has 215 categories. The Census Bureau has compiled a very lengthy list of job and industry titles (23 000 and 19 000, respectively) which are cross-referenced with the codes.

Since only the parents of affected babies were interviewed and not the control parents of unaffected babies, the occupational distribution of parents of babies with one particular type of defect was compared with the distribution of parents of babies with all other types of defects. This approach is illustrated in table 6.1. The computer program was set to display only those 2×2 tables where the odds ratio was at least 2 and the chi-square was not less than 3.84 (i.e. $P \leqslant 0.05$). The parental exposure comparisons were made for each malformation type, and for each occupation, each industry and each occupation-industry cross-classification.

Table 6.1 Analytical layout for association between occupation and birth defects in previous CDC studies

| | Exposure status | |
| | Specific | All other |
Disease status	occupation/industry	occupations/industries
Specific defect	a	b
All other defects	c	d

Analytical criteria: Odds ratio = ad/bc; chi-square $\geqslant 3.84$.

Because the interviewed women had all been pregnant, it was not surprising that the overall percentage who were employed (38 per cent) was lower than the corresponding figure for all Atlanta women 16 years of age and over (47 per cent). Undoubtedly, both these percentages have since risen. Among those study mothers who were employed during the first trimester, the occupational distribution was similar to that of all Atlanta women, except that there were more study women who were health workers (10 per cent compared with 5 per cent). This could be due to a selection bias whereby malformed babies born to health workers were more likely to be ascertained by the surveillance programme, and/or these women were more likely to grant an interview (about 85 per cent of targeted women completed an interview). These women could also have been inclined to work during pregnancy more than women in other occupations. Finally, it could be that this apparent excess is due to an increased risk of having babies with birth defects. The occupational distribution for study fathers was very similar to that of all Atlanta men. Unfortunately, there were no sex-specific industry of employment figures available from the Census Bureau for Atlanta with which to compare the study parents.

Tables 6.2 and 6.3 show two of the more striking findings of our study. Table 6.2 shows an association between maternal employment in nursing with cleft lip with or without cleft palate; none of these nurses worked in an operating theatre. Table 6.3 shows exomphalos and gastroschisis as specific defects of

Table 6.2 Association between maternal first trimester employment in nursing and cleft lip with or without cleft palate

	Nursing	All other occupations
Clefts	6	154
All other defects	10	819

Odds ratio = 3.2; chi-square = 4.0.

Table 6.3 Association between maternal first trimester employment in the printing trade and abdominal wall defects

	Printing trade	All other occupations
Abdominal wall defects	3	71
All other defects	1	914

Odds ratio = 38.6; chi-square = 17.6.

concern in association with maternal employment in the printing trade; two of the three mothers of babies with the abdominal wall defects operated printing presses, while the other was a binder and a press operator. The fourth member working in this trade was also a press operator, and had a baby with microcephaly, cleft lip and limb defects. There were no really striking paternal associatons apparent in this study.

In these analyses there were a number of employment categories which were seemingly over-represented among the parents of babies with particular malformations, in addition to the examples noted above, but there are a number of difficulties in interpreting those results. First, there is heterogeneity within the occupational and industrial categories which we used to classify the study parents. We took the approach of looking first at the associations between specific malformation groupings and the occupational or industrial codes, and delving further if there appeared to be an association on the crude classification. This approach may have helped to mitigate another problem, namely that we made many defect–occupation and industry comparisons and one would expect quite a number to appear to be statistically significant owing to chance alone. It is difficult to know how to balance such problems, but these data ought to be used primarily to generate hypotheses to be tested in new studies.

To return briefly to the issue of the relative desirability of case control and cohort studies, it has been noted before that cohort studies are generally more expensive than case control studies. This derives in part from the length of time it usually takes for many diseases to becomes manifest once the cohort has been formed. In our context, a more important problem with cohort studies is that most reproductive outcomes are rare and therefore it is necessary to include large numbers of exposed and unexposed to gather a reasonable number of the outcome. In the case control approach the latter problem is of little concern, and for many types of non-occupational studies of reproductive problems the case control study is clearly the method of choice. However, in the occupational study setting the choice is not so clear. In many instances the prevalence of an occupation of interest may be as rare as the reproductive outcome. For example, there has been considerable interest in the possibility that exposure to anaesthetic gases may cause reproductive problems, yet we found not one anaesthetist in our study. In instances such as this the choice of a study design may evolve from consideration of other factors, as, for example, the existence of a useful registry with which to begin a study.

Another specific problem with the design of our study was that we had no interview data from parents who had normal index births. The major reason for gathering our data was to detect associations between maternal drug use and the occurrence of birth defects. We had considerable concern that mothers of babies with birth defects might embellish their memories relative to mothers of normal babies, and therefore it was decided to make comparisons of one type of malformation versus all others. We feel that this is justified, since we know of no human or animal data which would suggest that some exposure causes a uniform increase in the rates of all types of defects. However, the possibilities for memory embellishment for items such as an occupational history do not seem great, and therefore the lack of normal controls was somewhat unsatisfying.

Before leaving description of these old analyses we should recall[1]: 'Use of these data from Atlanta should be regarded as nothing more than casting a net with a very coarse mesh. If we are lucky we may catch some real associations, but most are likely to get away. Further, because of the small numbers involved, this sort of exploration can do virtually nothing to help us in pronouncing an occupation or industry "safe" for reproducing humans . . . . Our approach is less than ideal but does represent a start in a rather barren field.' This is the caveat of the epidemiologist, and an expression of an opinion that, in a field as devoid of data as this, information collected for other purposes should be used to generate hypotheses. We believe that the epidemiological approach requires more, not less, emphasis in the field of occupation and reproduction. Is it a damnation that we will miss finding some associations? It would be wonderful if we could obtain a perfect understanding of the true state of Nature, but we never will, and that should not prevent us from doing what we can with the best tools we have at our disposal, imperfect as they may be.

STUDY OF BIRTH DEFECTS AND MILITARY SERVICE IN VIETNAM

As noted before, the primary purpose of this study is to determine whether veterans of the Vietnam conflict are at increased risk of having babies with birth defects[3]. Many of these veterans have been concerned that they are at such a risk. The major focus of their concern has been on the herbicides (primarily *Agent Orange*) which were used extensively by US forces in Vietnam to deprive the enemy of cover and to destroy crops; herbicides may have been applied to as much as 10 per cent of the land area of South Vietnam over the period 1962–1970. The *Agent Orange* used was a 50–50 mixture of 2,4-dichlorophenoxy and 2,4,5-trichlorophenoxy acetic acids, and was contaminated by the highly toxic 2,3,7,8-tetrachlorodibenzo-p-dioxin.

The extent and duration of US troops' exposure to *Agent Orange* is generally unknown. Moreover, we do not know whether such exposure as did occur would place humans at increased risk of ill-health, including the problem of fathering babies with birth defects. If, over the past decade, the roughly 3 000 000 US men who served in Vietnam were not at increased risk and they had an average of one baby each, then there will have been about 60 000 babies with major structural defects born to them — or 120 000 if these men had an average of two babies each. The point is that even in the absence of an increased risk associated with Vietnam service, a large number of malformed babies will have been born to Vietnam veterans.

This study is similar in design to the studies which we have done before. It is a case control study deriving cases from the Metro Atlanta surveillance programme. In this new study, however, parents of normal index babies are being included as controls. We will be able to make comparisons of parents of normal index births with parents of babies with defects, as well as the malformation–malformation type of contrasts such as were done in our earlier studies. The study is much larger than our previous study and will attempt to include the parents of about 5400 index babies born with major congenital defects and 3000 families of normal index babies; the index babies were born between 1968 and 1980. The imbalance in the number of cases and controls is unusual, since the typical case control study has equal numbers of cases and controls, or more controls than cases. However, the typical case control study is smaller than this study. Our statistical power calculations made during the study design phase indicated that, given the number of cases, we would gain very little power by increasing the number of controls above 3000; we chose to study a large number of cases, since it will be desirable to divide the 5400 into subgroups of specific types of malformations.

Once we locate the selected study families, the mothers and fathers who are willing to co-operate are interviewed by telephone. The mother's two-part interview takes about 45 minutes and the father's about 35. The major components of the mother's interview are listed in table 6.4, the father's two-part interviews are similar. The four parts which comprise a family interview are each done by different interviewers. The purpose of using two interviewers for each parent is to attempt to reduce interviewer bias by blinding the second interviewer (who gathers various kinds of exposure data) to the case control status of the family. Since the first interviewer gathers a complete pregnancy history, blinding is not possible, because every case family will have at least one malformed child, whereas control families will have such a child infrequently. As can be seen in table 6.4, the interviews cover a wide range of topics other than those which specifically deal with military service in Vietnam. Of particular interest here is the occupational history which is being collected from both the mother and the father. The fact that we ask mothers and fathers some identical questions will also be useful in evaluating our methods. Table 6.5 contains some preliminary data on the opinion of mothers and fathers about whether the index pregnancy was planned — these are fascinating and somewhat humorous results.

Table 6.4 Major question areas for mothers, birth defects–Vietnam service case control study

Part 1:	Interviewer 1
	pregnancy history
	outcome
	gestational period
	birth weight
	birth defects
	cancer
Part 2:	Interviewer 2
	about mother
	occupational history
	chronic diseases
	health during index pregnancy
	birth control before index pregnancy
	alcohol
	tobacco
	birth defects in family
	about father
	birth defects in family
	occupational history
	military service, Vietnam
	chronic diseases
	alcohol
	tobacco
	family socio-demographic information

Table 6.5 Mothers' and fathers' answers to question: Was index pregnancy planned? Preliminary data from birth defects–Vietnam service study

		Mothers' answers	
		Yes	No
Fathers' answers	Yes	1716	430
	No	271	1107

The telephone interviewers are aided by a computer-assisted telephone interviewing (CATI) system. Each interviewer has a computer terminal which displays each question in sequence and through which the interviewer records the parent's answers. Some major advantages and disadvantages of using a CATI system are listed in table 6.6. A significant advantage is that the data are checked while the interview is being done, which improves data quality and reduces the

Table 6.6 Computer-assisted telephone interviewing advantages and disadvantages

Advantages

real-time logic, consistency and range checks, better data quality and fewer
  call-backs
real-time modification of questionnaire
automatic skip-pattern implementation
integration with tracing information
edited back-up
improved interviewer monitoring
quick access to data
reduced paper
marginally reduced operating costs

Disadvantages

set-up time and cost
reasonable typing speed required
computer intimidates some interviewers
hardware failures
questionnaires difficult to view in entirety

number of call-backs required. The computer system automatically leads the
interviewer through the appropriate skip patterns of questionnaire branching
in response to the parent's answers, and parts of the questionnaire are modified specifically for each respondent (e.g. certain dates regarding the index
pregnancy are calculated by the computer and inserted into the questions).
The monitoring of interviewers by authorised supervisors is also substantially
enhanced. In a normal telephone interview only the interviewer's and respondent's voices can be monitored; with CATI it is possible, by use of a cathode
ray tube, to see how the interviewer records the parent's answers at the time
at which they are given. The main disadvantage with a CATI system is that
if the computer malfunctions, all interviews in progress have to be stopped
and the parents recontacted. Fortunately, such incidents have been rare in our
study.

NO RECORD LINKAGE POSSIBLE – AN IMPEDIMENT TO PROGRESS IN THE USA

Significant progess in the field of reproductive care and of assessing the effects
of the environment on health in the USA awaits the means for linking individual
data records in various data sets. The means lacking are simple – universal and
unique personal identifiers. Such identifiers are available and regularly used as
a part of reproductive outcome data collection in some parts of the world,
but this is not the case in the U.S.

The American Social Security Number (SSN) is a unique personal identifier but it is not considered a national identification number. SSNs have been used to help locate individuals for various occupational studies. CDC is making use of this capability for the large birth defects study considered. Since 1974 State of Georgia birth certificates have provided for the collection of maternal numbers. With the help of the National Institute of Occupational Safety and Health, we transmit the numbers to the Internal Revenue Service (IRS; the federal tax department). The IRS searches its files of taxpayer records and returns to us the latest address of desired individuals. The system has been a great help to us, but the situation could be better. First, it only helps us to locate people and does not provide us with occupational information. Second, the person for whom we are searching must have filed a tax return recently in order for us to obtain a relatively current address. Third, the SSN was not conceived with computer data processing in mind. As explained earlier, our large ongoing case control study is being supported primarily to assess whether Vietnam veterans are at increased risk of having babies with birth defects. In order to answer this simple question, we must find the families of the case and control babies and question them. How much simpler it would have been if we could have linked CDC's birth defects registry records with military records. We could have done that if fathers' SSNs were regularly found on such documents as birth certificates. However, if this had been possible, then our study would have been much circumscribed and the other data we are collecting, including the non-military occupational information, could not have been gathered, and that would have been a pity.

The situation in the Scandinavian nations, where benefits can accrue from simple record linkages, is enviable. The Norwegian government assigns an unique personal identification number to each of its citizens shortly after birth. This number is subsequently used as an identifier on a variety of official and private records. There are at least three important differences between the Norwegian number and the US SSN.

(1) The Norwegian number is a national identification number and it becomes a part of many record systems.

(2) The Norwegian number is assigned shortly after birth, whereas the SSN is usually assigned at the time a person obtains his or her first job. Early assignment of the numbers makes it possible to evaluate health outcomes which could be the result of problems occurring during, or prior to, pregnancy. For example, early assignment makes the linkage of birth and infant death records very simple. In the USA no national linkage of birth and infant death records is available – an appalling state of affairs. The early assignment of identification numbers also makes other important studies possible. For example, a study is currently under way in Oslo which will evaluate the effects of certain pre-natal and perinatal events on school performance.

(3) The Scandinavians designed their numbers with automated data processing

in mind. The Norwegian number is an eleven-digit number; the first six digits indicate the date of birth and the next three are sequential numbers assigned to those born on any given date, but it is the last two digits which deserve our attention. These are check digits and are the result of a series of arithmetic operations on the first nine digits. These two digits make computer checking for recording and transcription errors possible.

In addition to the ability to link individuals' records together in various data fields, it is also possible to link parental records with children's records. The identification numbers of the mother and of the father appear on the birth certificates of their children. Thus, it is very simple to construct fertility histories for women, men or couples. Since various occupationally oriented registers also contain national numbers, investigations of occupational risks can be quite simple. Some results of a study done by Bjerkedal[4], which involved the linkage of birth records with occupational information gathered during the Norwegian census, are found in table 6.7; as can be seen in the table, women

Table 6.7 First-born 1970–1973 with one or more congenital malformations according to economic activity of mother, November 1, 1970, Norway

	Number of births	Malformations per 1000 births	Relative risk
Not active	29 075	28.6	—
Active	74 719	31.9	1.12[a]

[a]95 per cent confidence interval: 1.03–1.21.

who were economically active prior to, and perhaps during, their first pregnancies had a 12 per cent higher risk of having a baby with a birth defect than those who were not economically active. It should be noted that this excess risk could be due to occupational factors or it could be the result of factors which are merely concomitants of economic activity. There is no way to distinguish between these two hypotheses from the data at hand.

The utilisation of record linkage capabilities requires stringent standards to safeguard the privacy of individuals. My understanding of procedures in Norway suggests that permission to link various data sets requires extensive scientific and lay review to ensure that the linkages proposed are for projects which are worthy of the support of society and that security is such that unnecessary invasions of privacy are not incurred. It may be that in the USA we have not warmly embraced the idea of a national identification number because of fears of loss of privacy. While that is a real concern, without better data sets and without the means for linking them our nation will remain a part of the underdeveloped world in respect of our understanding of how our environment influences our health.

REFERENCES

1. Erickson, J. D., Cochran, W. M. and Anderson, C. E. (1979). Parental occupation and birth defects. A preliminary report. *Contr. Epid. Biostat.*, **1**, 107–117
2. U.S. Bureau of the Census: 1970 Census of Population. *Alphabetical Index of Industries and Occupations*, U.S. Government Printing Office, Washington, D.C., 1971
3. Erickson, J. D., Mulinare, J., James, L. M. and Fitch, T. G. (1983). Design and execution of a very large birth defects case-control study. In *Proceedings of World Conference on Prevention of Physical and Mental Congenital Defects, Strasbourg, 1982* (in press)
4. Bjerkedal, T. (1983). Occupation and outcome of pregnancy. A population-based study in Norway. In *Proceedings of World Conference on Prevention of Physical and Mental Congenital Defects, Strasbourg, 1982* (in press)

7

The Epidemiological Identification of Reproductive Hazards

MICHAEL E. McDOWALL

Epidemiology has so far had limited success in the identification of occupational hazards, be they carcinogenic or teratogenic. Epidemiological methods have of course been vital in the follow-up of clues, but the greater majority of the clues have been provided by the perception of clinicians or pathologists, aided frequently by coincidence[1,2]. The range of potentially dangerous substances encountered in the occupational environment[3,4] is so great that it is difficult to see how reliance on this haphazard approach to health and safety at work will show up more than a few of the dangers. Mortality data have been routinely analysed by occupation since the 1850s[5], but recent years have seen repeated calls for a systematic approach to the search for occupational carcinogens in particular[2,6]. The study of reproductive hazards of occupation has a less extensive history than that of occupational mortality but the same argument can apply. An unsystematic approach to the search for such hazards is likely to be too dependent on luck for revealing all but the grossest effects. We need, therefore, to consider the possibilities for detecting hitherto unsuspected risks due to occupational exposures in a routine and systematic manner.

REPRODUCTIVE HAZARDS

A wide range of reproductive hazards have been associated with parental exposure to environmental (including occupational) substances[7]. It is possible to classify these effects according to the reproductive outcome (e.g. congenital defects or spontaneous abortions) or according to the mechanism involved (mutagenic or teratogenic). Different mechanisms can cause similar effects, and it is clear that some substances may be teratogenic, carcinogenic and mutagenic[8]. Reproductive outcome, while not necessarily the most efficient marker for reproductive hazards, is thus a more manageable measure for surveillance[9] and it is likely to

73

be easier to routinely collect data on, for example, infant mortality than on chromosomal damage. Table 7.1 illustrates adverse reproductive outcomes which have been associated with the occupational exposure of one or other parent[7,9]. This table omits developmental disabilities and behavioural disorders which would clearly be very difficult to monitor routinely and consistently.

Table 7.1 List of adverse possible reproductive outcomes associated with occupational exposure of parents

Childhood cancer	Lowered fertility
Infant mortality	Congenital defect
Stillbirth	Spontaneous abortion
Changed sex ratio	

AVAILABLE DATA

Many of the reproductive outcomes recorded in table 7.1 are routinely measured by national vital statistics; the only outcome not recorded for England and Wales is spontaneous abortion not requiring hospitalisation. The disadvantages of using these data for identifying reproductive hazards are clearly the availability and quality of occupational data (e.g. in England and Wales the father's, but not the mother's, occupation is currently recorded at birth registration) and the lack of any exposure data other than job title. The advantages are its national coverage important when examining such relatively rare events as congenital defects, and its ready availability. The remainder of this chapter examines how the repro- ductive outcomes listed in table 7.1 (excluding spontaneous abortion) can be monitored in relation to parental occupation, assessing how far already-available routine statistics can be used. The emphasis is on England and Wales data but the approaches, and difficulties, would be similar in many other countries. Some general problems, applicable to analysis of most of the data sets, are discussed after the outcomes have been considered in turn.

CHILDHOOD CANCER

The most commonly reported association between childhood cancer and parental occupation relates to fathers in hydrocarbon-related occupations, but there have been several conflicting findings which may be related to the various methods employed[10]. Studies have looked at either incidence or mortality from cancer related generally to parent's occupation at birth. Sanders *et al.*[11] used routine England and Wales mortality data which had been occupation-coded for the

Registrar General's *Decennial Supplements on Occupational Mortality* for the years 1959–63[12] and 1970–72[13], and an association was observed between kidney tumours and hydrocarbon-related fathers' occupations.

The study suffered through its use of paternal occupation at the time of the child's death and through its inability to examine the mother's occupation, which was not recorded on child death certificates. It would be possible in future studies of this sort to link the child death certificate with the birth certificate, thus obtaining the father's occupation at birth (the mother's occupation will not be requested at birth registration until 1985 at the earliest) and from 1983 onwards the mother's occupation has been recorded at child death registration. Although Sanders *et al.*[11] used only the years covered by the decennial occupational mortality analyses, childhood deaths, unlike adult deaths, have been fully occupation coded by OPCS since 1972, so it would be feasible to use the data for routine monitoring, although the linkage of birth to death certificates would make it a fairly expensive exercise.

It has been suggested[14] that the conflicting results obtained in this area may be due partly to the use of cancer mortality or cancer incidence in the various studies. The cancer registration programme in England and Wales records the father's but not the mother's occupation at time of registration, and, while it would be possible to link these records with birth certification, it would be a more difficult task than linking death certificates on both technical and confidentiality grounds.

SEX RATIO

There is a hypothesis that chromosomal damage can affect the sex ratio by a higher *in utero* death rate for males[9]. In principle the measure is easy to monitor from routine vital statistics, but accounting for even large-scale significant deviations from expected ratios has proved difficult or impossible[14]. Currently 10 per cent of live-birth (and 100 per cent of stillbirth) certificates in England and Wales are coded for parent's occupation (i.e. for the father's occupation for legitimate and joint-registered illegitimate, and the mother's occupation for sole-registered illegitimate births). The use of a sample, coupled with the inherent variability of the sex ratio, suggests that monitoring should look for consistency over time or between related occupations. This measure has not been monitored in the past, however: the last published analysis for England and Wales relates to 1931[15]. A new analysis of fathers' occupations on legitimate and joint-registered illegitimate total live births and stillbirths for 1978 has revealed some areas for possible review with further years' data, including the low ratios for the children of agricultural workers shown in table 7.2.

Table 7.2 Sex ratios of total births (legitimate and illegitimate joint registered) for selected fathers' occupations (England and Wales, 1978 10% sample)

Father's occupation[16]	Male births	Female births	Sex ratio (males per 1000 females)
Occupation order I (occupation units 1–6) — farmers, foresters and fishermen	785	821	956
Occupation unit:			
002. Farmers, etc.	329	348	945
003. Agricultural workers	222	235	945
005. Gardeners and groundsmen	129	142	908
All births 1978 (live and still — 100%)	309 722	291 804	1061

CONGENITAL DEFECTS

Congenital defects identified in the first week of life are routinely notified to OPCS as part of the England and Wales monitoring system. The system[17] is designed to identify quickly any significant increase in the incidence of a wide range of conditions. The inclusion of congenital defects identified in the first week of life is intended to ensure a speedy analysis but it does mean that there are serious deficiencies in the data for a number of conditions frequently not identified until later in life.

Parent's occupation is requested on the notification form and these data have recently been analysed for the first time[18]. By relating the congenital defect data to births by the father's occupation, malformation incidence rates were calculated for the father's occupation — malformations by the mother's occupation were analysed proportionately. Because of the reporting deficiencies in the occupation data, both sets of results were expressed as ratios with 100 representing observed malformations equal to the expected. The many deficiencies in the data[18] indicate that they should be treated with reserve at present but further years' analyses will be studied for consistency.

Tables 7.3 and 7.4 show malformations ratio(s) (MR) and proportional malformations ratio(s) (PMR) for a selection of father's and mother's occupations, respectively, for a number of conditions. The data have been analysed over two time periods (1974–1976 and 1977–1979) in order to show up consistency or the lack of it in the results. A brief discussion of some of the results usefully illustrates some of the many influences which have to be considered in interpreting these data and probably others related to reproductive outcome.

Table 7.3 Malformation ratios by father's occupation[16] for selected conditions and occupations (England and Wales 1974-1976, 1977-1979)

Occupation	Malformation					
	Anencephalus and/or spina bifida		Cleft lip and/or palate		Down's Syndrome	
	1974-1976	1977-1979	1974-1976	1977-1979	1974-1976	1977-1979
Miners and quarrymen	131	149ᵃ	110	102	75	82
Engineering and allied workers	122	113	103	100	101	98
Moulders and coremakers	172ᵃ	207ᵃ	–	–	–	–
Clerical workers	104	107	123ᵃ	124ᵃ	130ᵃ	110
Postmen	125	135	63	105	–	221ᵃ
Police	92	108	137	134	–	124
Professional and technical workers	61ᵃ	68ᵃ	82ᵃ	87ᵃ	96	104

ᵃStatistically significant (95 per cent confidence level) difference from 100. A dash indicates fewer than 10 cases.

Table 7.4 Proportional malformation ratios by mother's occupation[16] for selected conditions and occupations (England and Wales; 1974–1976, 1977–1979)

Occupation	Malformation					
	Anencephalus and/or spina bifida		Cleft lip and/or palate		Down's Syndrome	
	1974–1976	1977–1979	1974–1976	1977–1979	1974–1976	1977–1979
Clothing workers	129[a]	128[a]	99	87	56	102
Labourers and unskilled workers, NEC	142[a]	138[a]	104	113	81	116
Clerical workers	94	108	96	94	82	86
Professional and technical workers	69[a]	65[a]	113	105	137[a]	140[a]

[a]Statistically significant (95 per cent confidence level) difference from 100.

Male clerical workers show high rates for their children over a wide range of malformations (with MR for all malformations together of 123 and 127, respectively, for the two time periods), although this is least in evidence in the central nervous system (CNS) conditions. There is no obvious occupational hazard in clerical work to account for these figures and the explanation may be self-selection into clerical work of men with a predisposition to father children with congenital defects. The PMR for mothers in clerical work indicates nothing about their overall rate of malformations. However, if the pattern for clerical mothers was the same as for clerical fathers, some disproportion between the CNS defects and the other conditions should be apparent in table 7.4: this is not so. Clearly, selection effects may vary for men and women.

Selection of a slightly different sort may account for the high proportions of CNS defects in children of mothers who are clothing workers. CNS defects have a high incidence in Ireland[18] and it is possible that clothing workers include proportionately more Irish women than other occupations.

High maternal age in professional women almost certainly accounts for their high PMR for Down's Syndrome – while their low ratios for the CNS defects perhaps reflect a better diet or a higher take-up of screening facilities.

Possibly a more directly occupation-related condition is the very high ratios for moulders and coremakers for CNS defects. Men in this occupation experience near-normal ratios for other conditions and men in related occupations in the same industrial group show no such excess.

Less easy to comment on are the consistently raised (although not statistically significant) ratios for CNS defects for postmen and clefts for policemen.

LOWERED FERTILITY

The examination of fertility rates by occupation is not new in the UK. The then General Register Office (GRO) produced *Decennial Supplements* based on 1921[19] and 1931[15] which looked at fertility by occupation, employing largely the same method as used in the equivalent studies on occupational mortality. The number of children born to men in specific occupations in the study year was compared with the number of men in the respective occupations enumerated at the Census. The major interest of these early studies was to examine the family building habits of different occupations as part of national studies of fertility. The exercise has been repeated using the 1971 Census to assess its usefulness in identifying occupational influences on fertility.

In the present study the analysis was based on legitimate births from the sample (3.3 per cent per year) which had been coded for the father's occupation for the three years 1970-1972). These were compared within age groups with the number of married men in each occupation enumerated in the 1971 Census. Standardised fertility ratio(s) (SFR) were derived by indirect standardisation within the age range 15-24.

There are a number of problems arising from this method which deserve mention. Two sources of data (census and birth registration) are used (unlinked) and the quality from each source may vary. This, however, is unlikely to produce as much bias as the corresponding problem does for the occupational mortality studies, since here it is more likely that the occupation at census and birth registration will be reported by the same person. The major problems in this analysis arise from the range of factors, aside from any occupational influences, which can affect fertility. An approach to the problem would be to compare an occupation's fertility with that of similar occupations, maybe within the same social class, to try to allow for non-occupational influences. However, it has been demonstrated[20] that differences in age at marriage and duration of marriage can seriously affect the results of this type of study and should therefore be allowed for independently, if possible. In the present exercise, the percentage of men in the 15–24 age group who were married in the 1971 Census was used as a guide to age at marriage between the different occupations. A higher percentage married at younger ages would tend to produce a lower SFR for that occupation.

A discussion of two occupation groups showing low fertility illustrates the type of approach to interpretation which can be made and its problems.

The two underground occupations *coal miners, underground* and *other underground workers* showed low SFR – 91 and 74, respectively, compared with 115 and 119 for surface workers in mines and in quarries. However, *other underground workers* show a high percentage (60 per cent) of men aged 15–24 as married, and this might contribute to their lower SFR.

Bleachers and finishers and *dyers* in the textile industry are related occupations in their exposure to chemicals and substances for treating textiles and exhibit low SFR (74 and 73), where the SFR for all *textile workers* as a group is 118. In addition, these two occupations have similar percentages married at 15–24 as the remaining textile workers. Under these circumstances it is possible to hypothesise an association between these occupations and reduced fertility. Such a hypothesis may be reinforced by a recent Danish study[21] associating reduced fertility in women (and possibly men) with exposure to textile dyes.

The many problems of this approach have prompted a search for alternative methods. One possibility being investigated is the use of the 1971 Census fertility questions – this would allow fertility measurement by both mother's and father's occupation and would provide detailed duration of marriage data.

STILLBIRTHS AND INFANT MORTALITY

Both stillbirths and infant deaths are subject to routine vital registration and the father's occupation is recorded as part of the registration (currently 100 per cent of stillbirths and infant deaths are occupation coded). Since 1975 infant deaths in England and Wales have been routinely linked with the child's birth certificate, which enables the analysis to take place on the father's occupation at the infant's birth rather than death (although only 10 per cent of birth certificates are currently routinely coded for occupation).

Table 7.5 shows stillbirths and infant mortality rates by social class for 1978. It can be seen that the rate for both these series varies by a factor of nearly 2 between social classes I and V. It is clearly essential, therefore, to compare an

Table 7.5 Stillbirth and infant mortality rates by social class: legitimate births only (England and Wales, 1978)

Social class		Stillbirths (per 1000 live births and stillbirths)	Infant mortality (per 1000 live births)
I	(Professional, etc.)	6.3	9.8
II	(Managerial, etc.)	6.8	10.1
IIIN	(Skilled, non-manual)	7.5	11.1
IIIM	(Skilled, manual)	8.5	12.4
IV	(Semi-skilled)	9.2	13.6
V	(Unskilled)	12.0	17.2
All		8.2	12.4

Source: OPCS (1982). *Mortality Statistics Perinatal and Infant: Social and Biological Factors 1978, 1979*, Series DH3 No. 7, HMSO, London.

occupation's rates with those expected on the basis of its social class in order to try and separate any purely occupational influences from social factors. The Social Class Classification[22] is formed on the basis of the father's occupation. Once the mother's occupation is collected at birth registration, it will be important to recalculate these rates by the mother's social class before any serious analysis is undertaken. Table 7.6 shows stillbirth and infant mortality rates for fathers in glass and ceramic occupations and furnacemen, showing markedly high rates in both indicators.

SOME GENERAL CONSIDERATIONS

A number of general considerations apply to all, or most, of the data sets considered above when used for identifying reproductive hazards.

(1) The aim of monitoring occupations normally requires the ability to look at all, or some large segment of, the work force. To keep this exercise at a manageable level, it is necessary to group occupations into some form of classification. Classification implies some loss of information and exposures are unlikely

Table 7.6 Stillbirth and infant mortality rates for selected fathers' occupations — glass and ceramic workers (England and Wales, 1975–1978)

Occupation	Stillbirths (per 1000 live births and stillbirths)	Infant mortality (per 1000 live births)
Ceramic formers	10.89 (24)	14.22 (31)
Glass formers, finishers, etc.	11.63 (48)	12.50 (51)
Furnacemen, kilnmen — glass and ceramic	20.98 (18)	23.81 (20)
Ceramic decorators and finishers	13.16　(4)	10.00　(3)
Glass and ceramic workers, NEC	19.61 (12)	16.67 (10)

to cover the fairly wide categories of occupations used. Recent experience[23] has shown that an ill-suited classification can lose up to two-thirds of the cases of interest. No one classification is likely to be ideal for every purpose and the ability to return to the original data record for the full occupation report is valuable. This is possible for the data sets described here but difficult for anything more than a small number of cases.

(2) A major problem in routine data monitoring by a large number of variables (in this case, occupation) is the question of multiple comparisons. If many significance tests are performed, there is a high probability of producing some statistically significant results, even if there are no real associations between occupations and the conditions (in this case, reproductive outcomes) studied[24]. In such circumstances statistics provides no clues as to which significant results (if any) may actually reflect an association. There are some technical approaches to this problem but most of them seriously increase the risk of rejecting real associations, and the only satisfactory answer is to look for a consistency of results between different studies, over time or in related occupations and areas[25]. This approach was particularly adopted in the congenital malformations study reported above.

(3) The discussion on infant mortality and stillbirth measurement mentioned the importance of allowing for social class when looking for occupational associations. Other non-occupational exposures, notably smoking and alcohol consumption, can influence reproductive outcome[7]. If possible, such confounding factors should be taken into account. This will be extremely difficult in the analysis of routinely collected data, and, although social class may allow for some of the variation in these factors, it will generally have to be left to detailed special studies to follow up clues raised by the form of monitoring discussed.

(4) Possible occupational self-selection on health grounds and its effect on congenital malformation rates has been discussed. This is likely to be a general phenomenon in occupational reproductive epidemiology. Recent studies have

reported apparent selection effects in spontaneous abortion incidence[26] and have confirmed the existence of a *healthy worker effect* in women's employment[27] (i.e. that women who are working are on average healthier than those who are not).

CONCLUSIONS

This chapter has considered the relevance of routine data on reproductive outcomes in England and Wales as measures suitable for monitoring and identifying occupational hazards to reproduction. One immediate constraint is clearly the lack of mother's occupation at birth registration – plans are in hand to collect this information but it is unlikely to happen before 1985. The examples given in this chapter show the type of analyses which will then be possible by the mother's occupation – but the study of the potential hazards arising from the father's occupational exposures is, of course, relevant in its own right.

Given the ability, in due course, to carry out these analyses for both parents' occupations, how far does this meet the need for a systematic approach to identifying reproductive hazards? Routine data do not readily allow assessment of the various selection effects that link health and employment, and, partly owing to the healthy worker effect, cannot easily provide an answer even as to whether working in pregnancy carries greater risks to the pregnancy outcome than staying at home[28,29]. The inability to allow for many confounding factors (except perhaps social class) and the loss of occupation precision arising from classification have already been discussed.

Nevertheless, the data are readily available, are fairly cheaply analysed and cover a wide range of outcomes with (in most cases) continuous national coverage. The study of occupational mortality by the *Decennial Supplement* methodology[12,13] suffers general data problems similar to those of the approach considered here – i.e. the inability to account for selection effects and confounding factors and the loss of occupation detail through the use of a classification. The *Decennial Supplements*, however, are felt to have value[6] for the systematic review of occupational hazards to health and for the provision of baseline rates of disease incidence of value to other researchers. This chapter has shown equally that routine data on reproductive outcomes can provide clues or queries for possible follow-up by more specific studies. As in the case of occupational mortality[30], national data sets may be able to contribute to such specific studies.

Acheson[1] has proposed a register of women employed in industry directly linking their occupational exposures to the occurrence of various reproductive outcomes. Such an approach could clearly provide more satisfactory identification of possible problem areas – it would, however, require a fairly large number of women in the register to measure accurately relatively rare adverse reproductive outcomes by occupation, and could raise problems in terms of both confidentiality of data and expense. The approaches outlined in this chapter may suffer many faults but are clearly more practical propositions.

REFERENCES

1. Acheson, E. D. (1979). Record linkage and the identifications of long term environmental hazards. *Proc. R. Soc. Lond.*, **205**, 165–178
2. Siemiatycki, V., Day, N. E., Fabry, J. and Cooper, V. A. (1981). Discovering carcinogens in the occupational environment: A novel epidemiologic approach. *J. Nat. Can. Inst.*, **66**, 217–225
3. Calkins, D. R., Dixon, R. L., Gerber, C. R., Zain, D. and Omen, G. S. (1980). Identification, characterisations and control of potential human carcinogens: A framework for Federal decision making. *J. Nat. Can. Inst.*, **64**, 169–176
4. Barlow, S. and Sullivan, F. (1982). *The Reproductive Hazards of Industrial Chemicals*, Academic Press, London
5. McDowall, M. (1983). William Farr and the study of occupational mortality. *Pop. Trends*, **31**, 12–14
6. Jones, D. R. (1983). The analysis of available statistical sources for the detection of occupational cancer hazards. Summary report of an IARC/City University meeting held at City University, December 1982. City University, London
7. Seven, L. E. (1981). Reproductive hazards of the workplace. *J. Occup. Med.*, **23**, 685–689
8. Hemminki, K., Sovsa, M. and Vainio, H. (1979). Genetic risks caused by occupational chemicals. *Scand. J. Work. Envir. Hlth*, **5**, 307–327
9. Buffler, P. A. and Aase, J. M. (1982). Genetic risks and environmental surveillance: epidemiological aspects of monitoring industrial populations for environmental mutagens. *J. Occup. Med.*, **24**, 305–314
10. Gold, E. B., Diener, M. D. and Szklo, M. (1982). Parental occupations and cancer in children. *J. Occup. Med.*, **24**, 578–584
11. Sanders, B. M., White, G. V. and Draper, G. V. (1981). Occupations of fathers of children dying of neoplasms. *J. Epidemiol. Comm. Hlth*, **35**, 245–250
12. OPCS Registrar General (1971). *Decennial Supplement on Occupational Mortality 1959–63*, HMSO, London
13. OPCS Registrar General (1978). *Decennial Supplement on Occupational Mortality 1970–72*, HMSO, London
14. Walby, A. L., Merrett, J. D., Dean, G. and Kirke, P. (1981). Sex ratio of births in Ireland in 1978. *Ulster Med. J.*, **50**, 83–87
15. GRO Registrar General (1953). *Decennial Supplement – Occupational Fertility 1931 and 1939*, HMSO, London
16. OPCS (1970). *Classification of Occupations*, HMSO, London
17. Weatherall, J. A. C. and Haskey, J. C. (1976). Surveillance of malformations. *Br. Med. Bull.*, **32**, 39–44
18. OPCS (1982). Congenital malformations and parents' occupations. *OPCS Monitor* MB3 82/1
19. GRO Registrar General (1927). *Decennial Supplement – Occupational Fertility 1921*, HMSO, London

20. Hopkin, W. A. B. and Hajnal, J. (1947). Analysis of births in England and Wales by father's occupation. *Pop. Studies*, 1, 187-203, 275-300
21. Rachootin, P. and Olsen, J. (1983). The risk of infertility and delayed conception associated with exposure in the Danish workplace. *J. Occup. Med.*, 25, 394-402
22. Leete, R. and Fox, J. (1977). Registrar General's social classes: origins and uses. *Pop. Trends*, 8, 1-7
23. McDowall, M. (1983). Leukaemia mortality in electrical workers in England and Wales. *Lancet*, i, 246
24. Gardner, M. J. (1973). Using the environment to explain and predict mortality. *J. Roy. Statist. Soc. Series A*, 136, 421-440
25. Jones, D. R. and Rushton, L. (1982). Simultaneous inference in epidemiological studies. *Int. J. Epidemiol.*, 11, 276-282
26. Hemminki, K., Niemi, M. L., Kyyronen, P., Kilpikavi, I. and Vainio, H. (1983). Spontaneous abortions and reproductive selection mechanisms in the rubber and leather industry in Finland. *Br. J. Ind. Med.*, 40, 81-86
27. Waldron, I., Herold, J., Dunn, D. and Staum, R. (1982). Reciprocal effects of health and labour force participation among women: evidence from two longitudinal studies. *J. Occup. Med.*, 24, 126-132
28. McDowall, M., Goldblatt, P. and Fox, J. (1981). Employment during pregnancy and infant mortality. *Pop. Trends*, 26, 12-15
29. Chamberlain, G. and Garcia, J. (1983). Pregnant women at work. *Lancet*, i, 228-230
30. Fox, A. J. (1979). The role of OPCS in occupational epidemiology: some examples. *Am. Occup. Hyg.*, 21, 393-403

8

The Effects of Work in Pregnancy: Short- and Long-term Associations

TIMOTHY J. PETERS, PHILIPPA ADELSTEIN, JEAN GOLDING
AND NEVILLE R. BUTLER

Ruskin[1] has suggested: 'In order that people may be happy in their work, these three things are needed: They must be fit for it. They must not do too much of it. And they must have a sense of success in it.' Unfortunately, perhaps, few epidemiological studies have collected data on such aspects of employment. In this chapter we present previously unpublished information from the 1958 British Cohort Study on the hours worked per week, the gestation at which the job was given up and the actual job involved.

Although occupational health monitoring has been largely concerned with long-term effects such as the morbidity and mortality of workers employed in certain industries, few studies have been concerned with the effect of the occupation of the mother on her unborn fetus. In a study of the outcomes of 3179 pregnancies, McDonald[2] noted an increased rate of congenital defects among laundry workers. More recently, an increased risk of abortions and of malformations has been suggested for anaesthetists[3,4], and other studies have suggested that infants with congenital defects are more likely to be born if the mother has been a laboratory worker[5].

In this chapter we examine whether there are demonstrable associations with outcomes such as the development of toxaemia, or the birth of an infant who is growth-retarded, of pre-term gestation or with a major malformation. We shall examine associations with perinatal death as well as with the growth and educational achievement of the survivors.

THE DATA

The *1958 British Perinatal Mortality Survey*[6,7] was concerned with two populations. First, it studied in depth the pregnancies terminating in a live birth or a stillbirth in the first week of March 1958, in the whole of England, Scotland and Wales. In all, it is estimated that about 98 per cent of the total births entered the study. The population of births identified in this way is known as the *control week population*. The second part of the study was concerned with the stillbirths and neonatal deaths (i.e. deaths within 28 days of birth) occurring in the same area over the whole of the 3 month period March, April and May, 1958. It has been estimated that the ascertainment in this part of the study was approximately 95 per cent[7]. This population is known as the *three-month deaths*. In order to estimate death rates for the cases occurring in the 3 months, the population at higher risk has been taken to be 12 times that of the control week.

For both samples, detailed questionnaires completed by the midwife at birth included a question concerning the mother's paid job (if any) during pregnancy, the hours worked and the date on which the work was given up. Information on blood pressure was also recorded. This consisted of the dates and readings of the first, the last and the maximum diastolic measurements during pregnancy. The presence of albuminuria in the absence of urinary infection was also recorded, as was the occurrence of eclamptic fits.

Definitions of the toxaemia groups are as in reference 6. *Normotensive* refers only to patients with all recorded diastolic blood pressures below 90 mm and no proteinuria. *Pure essential hypertension* refers to mothers with a diastolic pressure of 90 mm or more before the 20th week of pregnancy with no rise of more than 10 mm thereafter, and no proteinuria. *Mild toxaemia* is defined as a maximum diastolic pressure of 90–99 mm and no proteinuria; in *moderate toxaemia* the maximum is 100–109 mm without proteinuria; for *severe toxaemia* either the maximum blood pressure was over 109 mm, or proteinuria was found in a woman with a diastolic pressure of 99 mm or more, or eclampsia developed. Cases with some form of albuminuria but normotensive throughout or with insufficient blood pressure recordings are in the group *unclassified proteinuria*.

Parity is defined as the number of previous pregnancies with a gestation of 28 weeks or more. A *primipara* (parity 0) is a woman with no such previous pregnancies, although she might have had one or more preceding abortions.

Throughout this chapter only singleton pregnancies have been included. We have omitted all cases where the mother's employment history was not recorded.

At the age of 7 years 85 per cent of the children in the control week population who survived were contacted. They were examined by a clinical medical officer, their heights and head circumferences were measured and educational tests of various types were carried out[8]. In the present study we shall be considering the results of the reading test, the problem arithmetic score, and the child's height and head circumference.

WORKING MOTHERS

Almost 40 per cent of the 16 994 mothers delivering in the control week had worked during pregnancy. Of these, one-half continued to work until they were at least 6 months pregnant (figure 8.1). Of those who were employed, half were in non-manual and half in manual occupations. Most were working for more than 30 hours per week, and one-sixth were working for over 45 hours per week (figure 8.2).

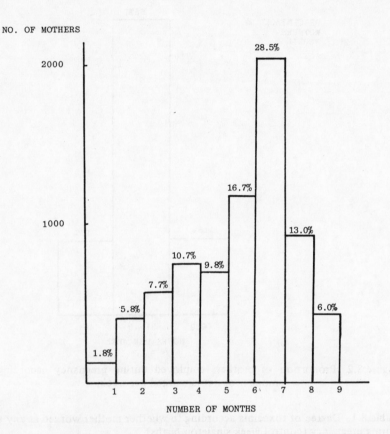

Figure 8.1 Distribution of the number of months worked during pregnancy: control week population

TOXAEMIA

While for many years the obstetrician has advised the pregnant woman with a rising blood pressure to rest as much as possible and, if working, to give up her job, the scientific evidence that work *per se* has an effect on the development of severe toxaemia has been lacking.

Table 8.1 shows the prevalence of all classes of toxaemia for the working mothers compared with the rest of the control week population. For mild, moderate and severe toxaemia there is an increased rate among the mothers who worked. This increase is, however, misleading. Parity is one of the main

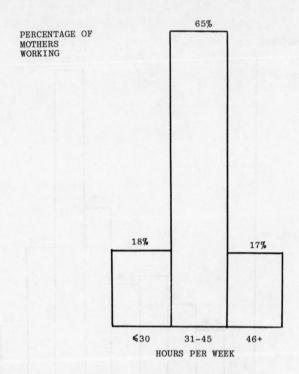

Figure 8.2 Proportion of mothers employed during pregnancy according to number of hours worked per week

Table 8.1 Degree of toxaemia according to whether mother worked at any time during pregnancy (control week singleton births)

Degree of toxaemia	Mother worked	Mother did not work
Normotensive	3996 (60.8%)	6944 (67.2%)
Pure essential hypertension	100 (1.5%)	184 (1.8%)
Mild	1119 (17.0%)	1536 (14.9%)
Moderate	294 (4.5%)	382 (3.7%)
Severe	520 (7.9%)	511 (4.9%)
Unclassified proteinuria	170 (2.6%)	227 (2.2%)
Unknown	373 (5.7%)	547 (5.3%)
Total	6572 (100.0%)	10 331 (100.0%)

$P < 0.0001$.

factors known to influence the incidence of toxaemia in Britain[9] and, as might be expected, the primiparae are far more likely to be working at the start of pregnancy than are women of other parities (figure 8.3).

In table 8.2 we compare the incidence of toxaemia within parity groups. It can be seen that there is now no hint of any significant difference in risk of toxaemia between women who worked and those who did not.

In considering the number of hours worked each week in early pregnancy, parity has again been taken into account (table 8.3). Numbers became relatively small, but it can be seen that there is certainly no evidence of an increase in toxaemia with increased hours of work. In fact, if anything, the reverse is true, the woman being more likely to be normotensive if she worked more than 35 hours per week. Only hours worked in early pregnancy have been considered here; therefore, this result is unlikely to be a reflection of the obstetric advice given to hypertensive pregnant women working such hours.

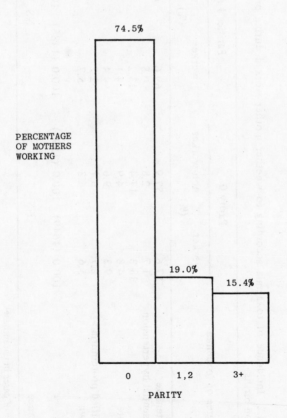

Figure 8.3 Proportion of mothers of each parity group known to be working at start of pregnancy

Table 8.2 Incidence of toxaemia according to whether mother worked during pregnancy, within parity groups (control week singleton births)

Degree of toxaemia	Parity 0		Parities 1 and 2		Parities 3+	
	worker (%)	non-worker (%)	worker (%)	non-worker (%)	worker (%)	non-worker (%)
Normotensive	57.6	57.9	69.6	69.3	65.3	67.9
Pure essential hypertension	1.7	2.8	0.8	1.5	1.8	1.8
Mild	18.3	17.4	13.2	14.3	16.6	14.6
Moderate	4.8	4.9	4.1	3.5	2.3	3.4
Severe	9.3	9.6	4.4	4.1	4.8	4.1
Unclassified proteinuria	2.7	3.1	2.2	2.0	2.8	2.1
Unknown	5.6	4.3	5.7	5.3	6.4	6.1
Total[a]	100.0 (4649)	100.0 (1593)	100.0 (1488)	100.0 (6351)	100.0 (435)	100.0 (2386)
Significance	NS		NS		NS	

[a] Number of cases in parentheses.

Table 8.3 Incidence of toxaemia among working mothers according to hours worked per week, by parity

Degree of toxaemia	Parity 0		Parities 1 and 2		Parities 3+	
	Under 35 h (%)	35 h+	Under 35 h (%)	35 h+	Under 35 h (%)	35 h+
Normotensive	55.3	57.9	67.8	70.0	61.0	68.3
Pure essential hypertension	2.4	1.6	1.3	0.6	1.9	2.0
Mild	20.3	18.1	13.9	13.0	21.1	13.2
Moderate	5.9	4.6	5.4	3.3	2.4	2.4
Severe	9.4	9.3	4.3	4.6	5.6	3.4
Unclassified proteinuria	2.3	2.8	2.8	2.0	2.8	2.9
Unknown	4.4	5.7	4.5	6.5	5.2	7.8
Total[a]	100.0 (575)	100.0 (4025)	100.0 (534)	100.0 (895)	100.0 (213)	100.0 (205)
Significance	NS		NS		NS	

[a]Number of cases in parentheses.

In table 8.4 the data are presented for primiparae according to the date when the mother stopped work. We have taken only the deliveries at term (38–41 completed weeks) for this analysis, so that the first period of time (June–November) roughly corresponds to the first two trimesters and the second time period can be taken as the third trimester. It can be seen that there is no difference in the incidence of toxaemia among the group of mothers who continued to work until the third trimester relative to those stopping in the first two trimesters.

Table 8.4 Incidence of toxaemia according to date primiparae stopped work (deliveries 38–41 weeks only, control week births)

Degree of toxaemia	Parity 0	
	June–Nov. (%)	Dec.–delivery (March 3–9) (%)
Normotensive	59.4	57.3
Pure essential hypertension	2.3	1.4
Mild	18.5	20.0
Moderate	5.3	4.7
Severe	7.5	9.3
Unclassified	2.6	2.7
Unknown	4.4	4.6
Total[a]	100.0 (1744)	100.0 (1950)

[a] Number of cases in parentheses.

Thus, the present study indicates that the woman who has worked during her pregnancy is at no greater risk of developing toxaemia than a woman of the same parity who has not worked.

This finding supports an earlier observation by Stewart[10] on a sample of 1318 singleton first pregnancies in Northamptonshire. She found that the incidence of toxaemia of pregnancy was evenly distributed between housewives not gainfully employed, women gainfully employed at some period up to the 28th week and women gainfully employed beyond the 28th week. She, too, concluded that it was difficult to believe that employment influenced the development of this particular hazard of pregnancy.

It must be emphasised, however, that this does not necessarily mean that once toxaemia has developed, the policy of advising the women to stop work is wrong. The present data cannot give a meaningful answer on this point.

PRE-TERM DELIVERY

In spite of intensive investigation, little is known of the mechanisms which result in some women going spontaneously into labour before term. In the

1958 control week population, 283 infants (1.7 per cent) were delivered after spontaneous onset of labour prior to 37 completed weeks gestation and were of low birth weight (< 2500 g). Although there were strong association with factors such as maternal youth, low maternal pre-pregnant weight, low social class and illegitimacy[11] there were no statistically significant differences according to history of maternal employment (table 8.5).

Table 8.5 Proportion of women spontaneously going into labour pre-term and delivering an infant < 2500 g

Parity	Employment in pregnancy	
	Yes	No
0	1.6% (75)	2.3% (36)
1	1.9% (37)	1.6% (138)

Number of term low-birth-weight births in parentheses.

GROWTH RETARDATION AT TERM

In a similar way we examined information concerning births of all infants of low birth weight (< 2500 g) delivered at term (37 completed weeks or more) and showed that the major associations were with primiparity, short maternal height and low pre-pregnant weight, low social class and maternal smoking[12]. Table 8.6 shows that the infants of the employed mothers appeared to be slightly more likely to be growth-retarded, but the differences were not statistically significant.

Table 8.6 Rate of low-birth-weight term delivery according to whether mother was employed at start of pregnancy

Parity	Employed in pregnancy	
	Yes	No
0	3.5% (163)	2.8% (45)
	NS	
1	2.8% (54)	2.3% (203)
	NS	

Number of term low-birth-weight births in parentheses.

PERINATAL DEATH

The 7117 stillbirths and neonatal deaths for which data were obtained were compared with the infants delivered in the control week. It can be seen from table 8.7 that among primiparae the death rate did not differ according to whether the mother worked or not, but there was a statistically significant difference for multiparae – the death rate was increased by 25 per cent if the mother worked.

Table 8.7 Numbers of stillbirths and neonatal deaths compared with numbers of births in control week according to history of employment at some time during pregnancy (rates per thousand total and live births, respectively)

Parity		Employment in pregnancy	
		Yes	No
0	No. control week births	4660	1596
	No. deaths	2059	715
	Death rate	**36.8**	**37.3**
	Significance	NS	
1+	No. control week births	1921	8744
	No. deaths	936	3393
	Death rate	**40.6**	**32.3**
	Significance	$P < 0.0001$	

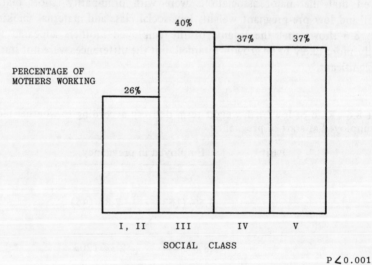

Figure 8.4 Proportion of mothers working during pregnancy by social class (based on husband's occupation)

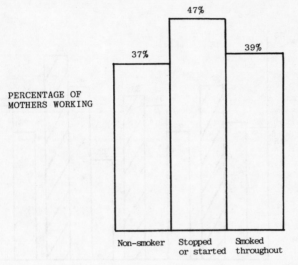

47%

39%

37%

PERCENTAGE OF
MOTHERS WORKING

Non-smoker   Stopped   Smoked
or started   throughout

P∠0.001

Figure 8.5 Proportion of mothers working during pregnancy by smoking habit
during pregnancy

The mothers who worked differed from those who did not work in a number of respects. Working mothers were less likely to be in social classes I and II (figure 8.4) and more likely to have stopped or to have started smoking during pregnancy (figure 8.5). The latter finding did not account for the excess of deaths in the working group. We therefore examined the importance of both the father's occupation and the type of job in which the mother was employed.

In table 8.8 we show the rates of stillbirth and neonatal death according to whether the mother worked or not, within social class groups based on the father's occupation. It can be seen that within each of the husband's social classes the infants of the mothers who worked were at greater risk than those who did not. In addition, figure 8.6 shows that among women who worked there was a trend in mortality with the social class based on the mother's occupation over and above that for the father's occupation.

Table 8.8 Rate per 1000 total births of stillbirth and neonatal death according to whether mother worked during pregnancy, within social class based on husband's occupation

	Husband's social class			
	I and II	III	IV and V	All I-V
Working mothers	31	35	42	36
Mothers not working	25	32	40	32

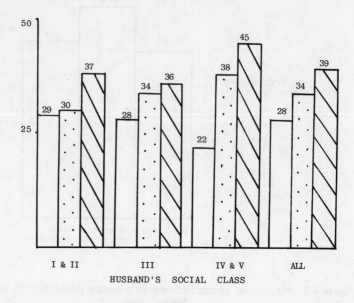

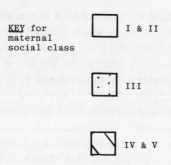

Figure 8.6 Rate per 1000 total births of stillbirth and neonatal death within social class classifications based on husband's occupation and that of mother

Classification into the actual industries is shown in table 8.9. It can be seen that, although several of the numbers are small, in 3 of the 19 groups there were statistically significantly more deaths than expected. These were the chemical industry, the laundry and dry-cleaning industry and the hospital workers. The excess of deaths among the hospital workers was especially associated with the sub-group which included student, assistant and auxiliary workers (48 three-month deaths, 31 in the control population; death rate 125.0 per 1000).

Table 8.9 Occupation at start of pregnancy of women who gave birth to stillbirths or neonatal deaths compared with control week population

Maternal occupation group	No. of deaths	No. of control week births	Estimated death rate[a]
Agriculture, horticulture	37	88	35.0
Food and drink industry	142	292	40.5
Tobacco industry	7	32	18.2
Chemical industry	67	112	49.9[b]
Jute and rope industry	8	18	37.0
Heavy engineering	140	281	41.5
Light and electrical engineering	117	270	36.1
Paper and printing	64	138	38.6
Glass and pottery	27	43	52.3
Woodworkers and furniture manufacturers	24	41	48.8
Textile workers	124	287	36.0
Clothing and furnishing	237	569	34.7
Leather and shoe	38	75	42.2
Hospital workers	140	231	50.5[c]
Laundry, dry cleaning	56	96	48.6[b]
Shop assistants	364	787	38.5
Service industries	473	989	39.9
Miscellaneous	844	2114	33.3
All known	2909	6581	36.8

[a] Per 1000 total births.
[b] $P < 0.05$.
[c] $P < 0.001$.

The data were also examined to assess whether there were any indications of teratogenic effects. Information on the 491 deaths with anencephalus, 254 deaths with spina bifida and 214 deaths with congenital heart disease are given in table 8.10. There is little to indicate that the high perinatal mortality rates in the chemical, laundry and hospital workers resulted from an excess of major malformations. The only industry where there were consistently high death rates from all the three congenital abnormalities was the glass and pottery industry. Among the actual jobs involved within this industry, the finishers, painters and examiners appeared at especially high risk (6 major malformations among three-month deaths, 22 in the control population; death rate 22.7 per 1000). These jobs would involve contact with dyes and glazes.

Among other small sub-groups, the hairdressers were of particular interest. There were 10 major malformations (5 anencephalus, 4 spina bifida and 1 congenital heart disease), giving a death rate of 12.9 — twice as many as expected ($P < 0.05$).

Table 8.10 Death rates (per 1000) from certain major malformations by maternal occupation in pregnancy

Maternal occupation group	Spina bifida	Anencephalus	Congenital heart disease
Agriculture, horticulture	0.9 (1)	1.9 (2)	0.9 (1)
Food and drink industry	2.6 (9)	2.9 (10)	1.5 (5)
Tobacco industry	2.6 (1)	— (0)	— (0)
Chemical industry	2.6 (4)	2.6 (4)	— (0)
Jute and rope industry	— (0)	— (0)	4.6 (1)
Heavy engineering	3.0 (10)	3.0 (10)	1.2 (4)
Light and electrical engineering	3.4 (11)	1.9 (6)	— (0)
Paper and printing	1.2 (2)	2.4 (4)	2.4 (4)
Glass and pottery	7.8 (4)	5.8 (3)	3.9 (2)
Woodworkers and furniture manufacturers	2.0 (1)	2.0 (1)	2.0 (1)
Textile workers	0.6 (2)	6.1 (21)	0.6 (2)
Clothing and furnishings	2.5 (17)	2.6 (18)	0.5 (5)
Leather and shoe	2.2 (2)	1.1 (1)	1.1 (1)
Hospital workers	2.5 (7)	1.4 (4)	1.1 (3)
Laundry, dry cleaning	1.6 (2)	1.6 (2)	1.6 (2)
Shop assistants	1.8 (17)	3.4 (32)	1.2 (11)
Service industry	1.6 (19)	2.3 (27)	1.1 (13)
Miscellaneous	1.9 (48)	2.6 (67)	1.3 (33)
All known	2.0 (157)	2.7 (212)	1.4 (88)

Number of deaths in parentheses.

FOLLOW-UP OF SURVIVORS

Height at 7 years

Peters[13] found that children whose mothers worked during pregnancy had an average height of 48.24 inches, with a standard error of 0.03, compared with 48.02 ± 0.03 inches for those who did not work. In addition, the longer the mother worked during pregnancy, the more likely was the child to be taller:

worked into 3rd trimester	48.32 ± 0.05 inches
stopped in 2nd trimester	48.22 ± 0.06 inches
stopped in 1st trimester	48.08 ± 0.09 inches

There were also differences according to the type of work involved. When the mother had been in non-manual employment, the child's height was 48.55 ± 0.05 inches on average, whereas for manual occupations the mean height was 47.94 ± 0.05 inches.

These differences are highly significant $(P < 0.001)$ for each of the three aspects of maternal employment considered: whether the mother worked or not; if so, for how long; and whether the work was manual or non-manual. Clearly, however, there are many factors relating to the child's background which are associated with his eventual height. Multiple regression was therefore carried out, taking account of the mother's height, age, parity, and smoking during pregnancy, and the child's sex, birth weight, number of surviving younger siblings and social class (from occupation of male head of household when the child was 7). The analysis controlled for all these possible confounding factors by constraining the maternal occupation variables to enter the regression equation after the others.

Maternal occupation during pregnancy was represented in the analysis by two variables. First, the length of the working week and the date at which the mother stopped working were combined to give an approximate measure of the total duration (in hours) worked during pregnancy. Three groups were subsequently obtained from this variable: mother did not work (zero duration); mother worked outside the home for less than a total of 720 hours during pregnancy; mother worked at least 720 hours (correspondong to 30 hours a week for 6 months). Second, the type of job was categorised as either manual or non-manual. In fact, working for long durations during pregnancy was more common among mothers in non-manual employment.

After controlling for the possible confounding factors, and for the manual nature of the work, the association between the duration of the work and the child's height was no longer significant. There was still a significant difference in height between children of mothers in non-manual and manual work, however, although the difference was reduced from an original 0.61 inches to 0.27 ± 0.072 inches $(P < 0.001)$ after multiple regression analysis.

Head circumference

The differences between the mean head circumferences are similar in nature to those between the heights. If the mother had worked during pregnancy, the mean head circumference was 20.46 ± 0.01 inches, compared with 20.43 ± 0.01 inches if she had not worked $(P < 0.01)$. There was no association with the length of time the mother worked, but once again it was found that children of mothers in manual occupations were at a disadvantage:

mother in manual occupation 20.39 ± 0.01 inches
mother in non-manual occupation 20.52 ± 0.02 inches $(P < 0.001)$

After carrying out a similar regression analysis as for height, the difference between children of working and non-working mothers was not significant. Among working mothers, however, there was still a significant advantage for those in non-manual occupations (adjusted mean difference 0.08 ± 0.025 inches).

Problem arithmetic score

There were no differences in the mean scores between the children of mothers who had worked and of those who had not. Nevertheless, for those who worked, there were again strong variations with the manual nature of the work. Among children of manual workers, the mean score was 4.76 ± 0.05; if the mother had been employed in a non-manual job, the mean score was 5.54 ± 0.05 ($P < 0.001$).

The association with manual maternal occupations remained after controlling for father's social class, maternal age and parity, birth weight, sex, maternal smoking, overcrowding, number of younger siblings and region. Adjusted for these factors, the mean difference between children of manually and non-manually employed mothers was 0.52 ± 0.078.

Reading test

For the child's performance on the Southgate reading test there were differences if the mother had been employed, such that children of mothers who had not worked were slightly more likely to score poorly. Among children of mothers who did not work during pregnancy, 8.7 per cent failed to score more than 10 out of 30, compared with 6.5 per cent for children of working mothers ($P < 0.001$). Once again, however, children of mothers in manual occupations were less likely to perform well. The proportion of children who scored poorly ($\leqslant 10$) was 3.1 per cent for mothers in non-manual jobs and 9.7 per cent for manual occupations ($P < 0.001$).

As with the other outcome measures, only the deleterious association for manual jobs remained after all the factors described for the arithmetic score had been taken into account[13]. The adjusted mean difference was 0.37 ± 0.039 ($P < 0.001$).

CONCLUSIONS

Even with the large data set available to us for analysis, it is difficult to conclude that working in pregnancy has a harmful effect on either the mother or the fetus, although there were indications that perinatal death rates were higher in certain industries and among women working in the manual occupations.

The search for teratogenic associations in a sample such as ours would be unlikely to pick up major effects in small industry groups; nevertheless it is interesting that certain associations were of statistical importance, and that these involved occupations where contact with chemicals was involved (hairdressers and workers in the glass and pottery industry). This should only be considered important, however, if repeated in another study.

There is no evidence from the analyses to suggest any differences in long-term development for children of mothers who worked during pregnancy compared with those who did not, or for mothers who worked for different durations during their pregnancy. Among mothers who worked, however, the differences in developmental outcomes between the manual and non-manual maternal occupations remained after controlling for factors such as the social class of the father.

Clearly, further analyses are required to determine whether particular manual occupations of the mother are more likely to have a long-term effect on the growth and intellectual ability of the child. At the moment we feel that rather than observing a causative association, we are merely identifying a factor indicative of social disadvantage over and above the classification based on the father's occupation.

ACKNOWLEDGEMENTS

We are very grateful to the Executive Committees of the National Birthday Trust Fund and the National Child Development Study for permission to use the data of the 1958 British Perinatal Mortality Survey and the seven-year follow-up.

Abstraction and coding of the information on maternal employment was supported by a generous grant from the British Heart Foundation to Jean Golding. The work on long-term outcome was carried out for an MSc dissertation by Tim Peters, while in receipt of an MRC studentship and under the supervision of Dr J. F. Bithell of the Department of Biomathematics, University of Oxford.

We thank Miss Yasmin Iles and Miss Penny Hicks for their invaluable help in the preparation of this chapter.

REFERENCES

1. Ruskin, J. (1851). *Pre-Raphaelitism*
2. McDonald, A. D. (1958). Maternal health and congenital defect. A prospective investigation. *New Engl. J. Med.*, **258**, 767–773
3. Pharoah, P. O. D., Alberman, E., Doyle, P., and Chamberlain, G. (1977). Outcome of pregnancy among women in anaesthetic practice. *Lancet*, i, 34–36
4. Knill-Jones, R. P., Newman, B. J. and Spence, A. A. (1975). Anaesthetic practice and pregnancy: Controlled survey of male anaesthetists in the United Kingdom. *Lancet*, ii, 807–809
5. Meirik, O., Kallen, B., Gauffin, U. and Ericson, A. (1979). Major malformations in infants born of women who worked in laboratories while pregnant. *Lancet*, ii, 91
6. Butler, N. R. and Bonham, D. G. (1963). *Perinatal Mortality: The First Report of the 1958 British Perinatal Mortality Survey*, Livingstone, Edinburgh

7. Butler, N. R. and Alberman, E. D. (1969). *Perinatal Problems: The Second Report of the 1958 British Perinatal Mortality Survey*, Livingstone, Edinburgh, London
8. Davie, R., Butler, N. R. and Goldstein, H. (1972). *From Birth to Seven*, Longman, London
9. Davies, A. M. (1971). *The Geographical Epidemiology of the Toxaemias of Pregnancy*, Thomas, Springfield, Ill.
10. Stewart, A. (1955). A note on the obstetric effects of work during pregnancy. *Br. J. Prevent. Soc. Med.*, 9, 159-161
11. Fedrick, J. and Anderson, A. B. M. (1976). Factors associated with spontaneous pre-term birth. *Br. J. Obstet. Gynaecol.*, 83, 342-350
12. Fedrick, J. and Adelstein, P. (1978). Factors associated with low birthweight of infants delivered at term. *Br. J. Obstet. Gynaecol.*, 85, 1-7
13. Peters, T. J. (1980). A statistical analysis of the mother's employment during pregnancy and the subsequent development of the child. MSc Dissertation, University of Oxford

9

Occupational Fatigue and Preterm Birth

NICOLE MAMELLE and BERNARD LAUMON

Our purpose in this chapter is to try to answer the question whether the way of life and particularly the occupational activity can have a harmful effect on pregnancy.

The mother undergoes certain modifications in order to adapt to the needs of the fetus. These changes modify, in particular, the cardiovascular and respiratory functions, which also undergo variations during physical effort. The result is that a physical effort may cause physio-pathological reactions in pregnant women. These physiological modifications lead us to think that pregnancy has effects on the way of life, and, inversely, working has consequences for pregnancy and the development of the fetus. The consequences for the mother can be determined easily by direct observations during various activities. However, epidemiological studies are needed to determine the consequences for the fetus and to establish a relationship between the way of life and the evolution of pregnancy. For this purpose we have performed research into the elements of the way of life which constitute possible risk factors, and which are evaluated by the perinatal indicators: intrauterine mortality (rate 1 per cent in France), prematurity (rate 7 per cent) and birth weight light for date (rate 5 per cent).

Before listing the elements of the way of life constituting risk factors, we should now like to report our results concerning the socio-cultural and medical factors frequently associated with the way of life: these factors were cited by Berkowitz (1981), Goujard *et al.* (1974), Hoffman *et al.* (1974), Drillien (1957), Kaminski *et al.* (1978), Niswander (1977), Weidinger and Wiest (1976), Fedrick and Anderson (1976) and Masse and Papiernik (1973). The French National Surveys in 1972 and 1976 (Rumeau-Rouquette, 1979) showed the importance of certain socio-cultural factors (i.e. immigrant origin, low socio-economic class, low education level, unmarried mother). Each factor gives rise to a relative risk of about 2 for intrauterine mortality and about 1.5 for prematurity (table 9.1). The same surveys provided the personal and medical risk factors (table 9.2). In comparison the relative risk is about the same for social risk factors or medical risk

Table 9.1 Socio-cultural risk factors

Issue of pregnancy Socio-cultural risk	Average rate	Intrauterine mortality 1%	Prematurity 7%	Lightness for date 5%
Origin: non-immigrant/immigrant		× 2	× 1.5	–
Socio-economic class: I/II/III/IV		× 2–3.5	× 1.5–3.5	–
Education level: sup./second./primary		× 2–5	× 1–2	–
Family status: married/single			× 1.5	× 1.5

Relative risk

Table 9.2 Medical risk factors

Issue of pregnancy Medical risk	Average rate	Intrauterine mortality 1%	Prematurity 7%	Lightness for date 5%
Maternal age: < 20/21–29/> 30		× 1.2–2.5	× 1.5	–
No. of previous pregnancies: < 3/> 3 > 1/=0		× 3	× 1.4 × 1.5	– 1.5
Issue of the last pregnancy: viable infant/stillborn weight > 2500 g/ < 2500 g viable infant/miscarriage		× 5 × 4 × 2	× 1.5 × 2	– × 3
Short interval after last pregnancy: > 6 months/< 6 months			× 1.5	–
Tobacco: 0/1–9/> 10 cig./day				× 1.5–2

Relative risk

factors. Therefore, it is just as important to define social preventive measures as medical preventive measures.

In France every obstetrician uses the pre-term delivery risk, established by Papiernik (1977), which takes into consideration medical, socio-cultural, family and occupational factors.

The next question is: 'Is it possible to explain the relationship between social risk factors and premature births of perinatal deaths by occupational or maternal fatigue?'

THE LYON AND HAGUENAU SURVEY

In order to answer these questions, we carried out a survey in 1977–1978 on 3437 pregnant women in Lyon and Haguenau (a big city and a small town) with respect to their way of life and occupational activity during their pregnancy. The women were interviewed and the questionnaire consisted of 150 questions giving in detail: the personal data, family activity (housekeeping, daily commuting time, holiday transport time, exceptional events, sporting activities), the occupational activity (job category, work on machine, physical load, mental load, temperature, atmospheric pollution, noise, manipulation of toxic substances) and the modifications of activity during pregnancy (change of work station, reduction of weekly working hours, sick leave and antenatal maternity leave) (table 9.3).

By juxtaposing the data records from the routine obstetrical survey and the data from our special questionnaire survey, it was possible to correlate the way

Table 9.3 Structure of the questionnaire used in the Lyon and Haguenau survey

Identification	Professional activity
Personal data	job category
age and personal characteristics	postures
socio-economic and cultural level	work on industrial machine
habitat	physical load
Familial activity	psychological context
housekeeping	temperature
daily commuting time	atmosphere
holiday transport time	noise
exceptional efforts	manipulation of toxic substances
sport	Modifications of activity during pregnancy
	change of work station
	reduction of weekly working hours
	sick leave
	prenatal maternity leave

of life and occupational activity of these women to the evolution of their pregnancy (first report, Mamelle *et al.* (1982)).

Among the parameters used to measure the quality of the pregnancy, we especially took prematurity into consideration, as it is generally held responsible for perinatal death, and also because it is easier to estimate than the latter, owing to its higher frequency. We defined prematurity as delivery before 259 days' or 37 weeks' gestation. The delay was calculated between the first day of the last menses and the day of delivery. This was then checked with the Dubowitz score established by the paediatrician, as a control measure.

The results of the survey are as follows.

The job itself

The fact that a woman works, in itself, cannot be said to be a risk of prematurity, given that, globally speaking, housewives show a higher rate of premature birth: 7.2 per cent as against 5.8 per cent for women who work. These figures coincide with those in national surveys carried out by INSERM in 1976.

It must not be concluded from these apparently contradictory results that there is no relationship between working and prematurity. On the contrary, research should be carried out to determine the distinct factors concerning prematurity risk specific to each of these two categories of women.

Occupational category

Among working women, certain occupational categories are more prone to prematurity, such as shop staff 9.2 per cent, medico-social staff 7.5 per cent, unskilled workers 8.2 per cent, cleaning staff 8.6 per cent, with an average rate as high as 8.3 per cent, whereas other occupational categories do not exceed 3.8 per cent on average — shopkeepers 6.2 per cent, executive staff 4.4 per cent, teachers 3.9 per cent, office staff 3.4 per cent, skilled workers 2.7 per cent. The occupational categories first mentioned involve strenuous working conditions, so that we hypothesise that a strenuous job may have a harmful effect on pregnancy.

In table 9.4 the most important elements of the occupational activity are listed and the prematurity risk is rated according to whether each element is present, together with the relative risk and statistical significance. The work patterns with the greatest effect are those requiring: physical effort, work on a conveyor belt, little attention, and work in a standing position.

Table 9.4   Elements of occupational fatigue and prematurity

	No	Yes	Relative risk	Statistical significance
Standing position $\geqslant$ 3 h	4.6	7.5	1.6	$P < 0.05$
Work on industrial machine	5.6	5.8	1.0	NS
Work on machine with effort	5.4	9.1	1.7	$P < 0.01$
Work on machine with vibration	5.9	5.2	0.9	NS
Work on industrial conveyor belt	5.4	9.7	1.8	$P < 0.01$
Physical effort	4.8	7.4	1.5	$P < 0.05$
Load carrying	5.6	6.4	1.1	NS
Routine work	5.5	7.5	1.4	NS
Job requiring little attention	5.1	10.9	2.1	$P < 0.001$
Cold temperature	5.6	7.9	1.4	$P < 0.05$
Hot temperature	5.6	6.6	1.2	NS
Very wet atmosphere	5.6	10.0	1.8	$P < 0.05$
No. of loud noises	5.5	9.7	1.8	NS
Manipulation of chemical substances	5.4	7.7	1.4	$P < 0.05$
Long daily commuting time	7.7	6.8	0.9	NS

Weekly working hours

Generally speaking, there is a regular increase in premature birth rate as the number of working hours per week increases, from 3.6 per cent for a part-time job to 10.0 per cent for more than 45 hours per week (figure 9.1). This result is not simply the reflection of the occupational category, as the same relationship is obtained, at different levels, from unskilled workers or office staff.

Quantitative analysis of fatigue

We have tried to quantify occupational fatigue in order to detect the women subjected to a more intense fatigue. An analytical breakdown of the job into its diverse components has allowed us to define five indices related to each source of occupational fatigue (table 9.5) – posture, work on machine, physical load, mental load and environment. Each index was defined as an ordered variable and then classified as either low or high according to whether the job presents one of the characteristics listed in the occupational risk chart.

When any one of these indices passes from low to high, there is a significant increase in the occurrence of prematurity, shown in table 9.6. However, no single index must be held responsible for a cause and effect relationship between the source of fatigue and prematurity. Each index constitutes a risk factor which aids in detecting women with high prematurity risk, and it would be an illusion to believe that getting rid of one of the sources of fatigue (for example, making standing women sit down) would also eliminate the prematurity risk.

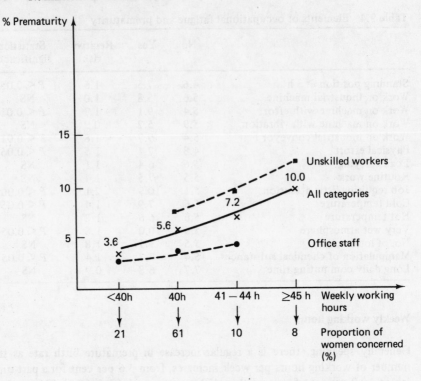

Figure 9.1 Weekly working hours and prematurity

Table 9.5 Prematurity occupational risk chart

Occupational fatigue index	High index if:
Posture	Posture in standing position more than 3 h per day
Work on machine	Work on industrial conveyor belt Independent work on industrial machine with strenuous effort or vibrations
Physical load	Continuous or periodical physical effort Load carrying of more than 10 kg
Mental load	Routine work Varied tasks requiring little attention without stimulation
Environment	At least 2 of the 3 elements { significant noise level cold temperature very wet atmosphere Manipulation of certain chemical substances

Table 9.6 High indices and prematurity

Index	Women with high index (%)	Prematurity		Relative risk	Statistical significance
		Low (%)	High (%)		
Posture	49	4.5	7.2	1.6	$P < 0.05$
Work on machine	7	5.6	8.8	1.6	$P < 0.05$
Physical load	50	4.1	7.5	1.8	$P < 0.01$
Mental load	47	4.0	7.8	2.0	$P < 0.01$
Environment	20	4.9	9.4	1.9	$P < 0.01$

Accumulation of sources of occupational fatigue

The risk of prematurity increases when a woman accumulates two or more sources of occupational fatigue. In this way, we can define a particular job by the number of high fatigue indices and attribute a risk of prematurity. The risk is greater when the number of high indices increases. When this number passes from 0 to 5, the associated rate of premature birth varies from 2.3 per cent to 11.1 per cent. The logistic analysis gives the equation of the curve obtained by plotting the prematurity rate against the number of high indices (figure 9.2).

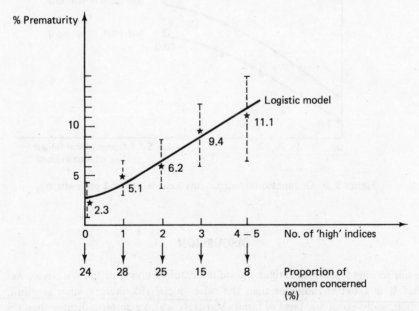

Figure 9.2 Number of high fatigue indices and prematurity: solid, logistic model; dashed, observed rate $\pm 2\sigma$

Our occupational risk chart allows us to define the profiles of women in working conditions which may have a harmful effect on their pregnancy. Twenty-three per cent of the female working population is concerned, and the rate of premature birth is of the order of 10 per cent.

Accumulation of medical factor and occupational fatigue

The idea of a cumulative effect of medical factor and occupational fatigue suggested by Papiernik is confirmed in this survey. Let us define medical factor as the existence of antecedents of prematurity, spontaneous abortion, stillbirth or perinatal death/pathology related or not to prematurity in the first 5 months of pregnancy. Thirty-five per cent of women exhibit such a factor, whereas 65 per cent have a completely normal pregnancy. The presence of such a factor generally leads to a 2 per cent higher risk of prematurity (figure 9.3).

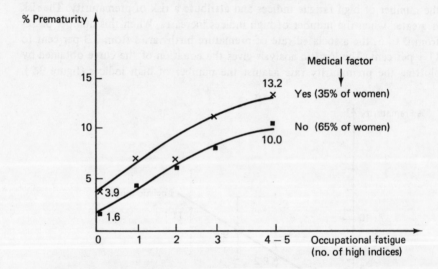

Figure 9.3   Occupational fatigue, medical factor and prematurity

DISCUSSION

Is our scoring system for fatigue a good indicator of prematurity? We can answer that it is a better indicator than the other social risk factors, such as ethnic origin, socio-economic level or family status. It is also a better indicator than the occupational categories themselves.

The results of the multiple logistic analysis are given in table 9.7, where all

Table 9.7 Multiple logistic analysis

Risk factor	Regression coefficient	Statistical significance (t value)
Number of high indices	0.36	4.56[a]
Previous pre-term birth	1.70	4.15[a]
Parity	− 0.50	− 2.59[a]
Socio-economic class	0.23	1.80
Pathology during pregnancy	0.51	1.50
Other previous pathology	0.22	0.79
Family status	0.09	0.23
Ethnic origin	0.03	0.10
Intercept	− 3.91	

[a]Statistically significant.

the medical, social and occupational factors are taken into account. The most indicative factors are the occupational fatigue indicated by the number of high indices, previous pre-term birth and parity (with negative effect). The other social factors (ethnic origin, socio-economic level or family status) do not contribute any new information when fatigue is taken into account.

Furthermore, it is possible to evaluate the proportion of premature births due to the occupational factor (table 9.8). If E is the proportion of the population exposed to occupational risk factors, F_1 is the prematurity rate in the exposed population and F_0 is the prematurity rate in the non-exposed population, then 21 per cent of premature births seem to be due to the occupational risk factor.

It is urgent, therefore, to research into preventive measures in a woman's occupational milieu. Which measures can we propose? A reduction of weekly working hours, some change of work station, periodical leave or extended maternity leave. . .?

Our survey leads us to suggest a reduction of weekly working hours and we were able to evaluate the potential efficiency of such measures retrospectively. We suggest such preventive measures according to occupational fatigue. It seems logical to lighten the load of women whose working conditions may have a harm-

Table 9.8 Proportion of premature births due to the occupational factor

E = proportion of population exposed to occupational risk factors = 0.23

F_1 = prematurity rate in exposed population = 0.10

F_0 = prematurity rate in non-exposed population = 0.045

R_A = attributable risk = $\dfrac{E(F_1 - F_0)}{F_0 + E(F_1 - F_0)}$ = 0.21

21% of premature births are due to occupational risk factor?

ful effect on pregnancy, rather than to apply a preventive system to all pregnant women with the risk of it being inefficient or even harmful to women who are not subjected to occupational fatigue. In this way, if the women exposed to intense occupational fatigue (that is, 20 per cent of them) could benefit from such measures, it would be possible to expect a reduction of premature birth rate by 1 per cent (i.e. 4000 premature births fewer per year in France).

Therefore, the prevention of prematurity can be considered from two parallel aspects: (1) The *traditional aspect* of obstetricians and general practitioners who concentrate on the pregnancy and take into account factors of occupational fatigue (especially in primiparous women and/or women who exhibit a medical factor). (2) The *new aspect* of doctors in factories who analyse a work station in collaboration with the competent services (concerning hygiene, safety, improvement of working conditions and organisation) in order to detect the higher-risk work stations and to define appropriate measures.

A new survey is being carried out at the moment among working women: 50 000 women are being observed in 50 companies in the Rhône Alpes region. The annual rate of pregnancy is 3 per cent − that is to say, we can expect 1500 pregnancies per year. Seven different types of job have been defined to control the occupational fatigue factors. The first year will be a year of observation to determine the percentage of prematurity in each group. The second year we shall reduce the weekly hours in half of the companies and then we shall be able to evaluate the effect of such preventive measures on the rate of prematurity.

REFERENCES

Berkowitz, G. S. (1981). An epidemiologic study of preterm delivery. *Am J. Epidemiol.*, 113, 81−92

Drillien, C. M. (1957). The social and economic factors affecting the incidence of premature birth. *J. Obstet. Gynaecol. Br. Emp.*, 64, 161−184

Fedrick, J. and Anderson, A. B. (1976). Factors associated with spontaneous preterm births. *Br. J. Obst. Gynaecol.*, 83, 342−350

Goujard, J., Hennequin, J. F., Kaminski, M., Marendas, R. and Rumeau-Rouquette, C. (1974). Prévision de la prématurité et du poids de naissance en début de grossesse. *J. Gyn. Obst. Biol. Repr.*, 3, 45−59

Hoffman, H. J., Stark, C. R. and Lundin, F. E. (1974). Analysis of birthweight, gestational age, and foetal viability, United States 1968. *Obstet. Gynec. Surv.*, 29, 651−681

Kaminski, H., Blondel, B. K., Breart, G., Franc, M. and Duhazaubrun, C. (1978). Issue de la grossesse et surveillance prénatale chez les femmes migrantes. *Rev. Epidemiol. Santé Pub.*, 26, 29−46

Mamelle, N., Dreyfus, J., Van Lierde, M. and Renaud, R. (1982) Mode de vie et grossesse. *J. Gyn. Obst. Biol. Repr.*, 11, (1), 55−63

Masse, N. and Papiernik, E. (1973). Conditions de vie et éducation de la femme enceinte. In: *Vers une Grossesse sans Risque − Monaco II*, Nestlé-Guigoz, 211−220

Niswander, K. (1977). Obstetric factors related to prematurity. In Reed, D. M. and Stanley, (Eds.), *The Epidemiology of Prematurity*, Urban and Schwarzenberg, Baltimore, Munich, pp. 249–268

Papiernik, E. (1977). L'accouchement prématuré et sa prévention. *Arch. Fr. Ped.*, **34**, 488–491

Rumeau-Rouquette, C. (1979). *Naitre en France. Enquêtes Nationales sur la Grossesse et l'Accouchement*, INSERM

Wiedinger, H. and Wiest, W. (1976). A comparative study of the epidemiological data of pregnancies with and without tendencies for premature delivery. *J. Perinat. Med.*, **2**, 276–287

10

The Effect of the Mother's Work on the Infant

ANN OAKLEY

There is, at the present time, a renewed interest in what Myrdal and Klein[1] in their classic text dubbed 'women's two roles' — participation in the employment world, on the one hand, and in domestic work, child-bearing and child-rearing, on the other. That there are certain conflicts and problems involved in mixing the two is evidenced by a long history of public debate on the matter. It is important when attempting to make sense of this debate to establish a number of basic points. What is the definition of work used? From whose point of view are the advantages and disadvantages of the dual-role pattern being discussed? (From that of women, men, children or government?) What is the methodological status of any research studies cited? What do we know, and what do we still need to know, and why?

MOTHERS HAVE ALWAYS WORKED

Although the terms of the current debate may be new, there is nothing new about women's work. A tract for domestic servants published in 1743 runs: 'Consider my dear girl that . . . you cannot expect to marry in such a manner as neither of you shall have occasion to work, and none but a fool will take a wife whose bread must be earned solely by his labour and who will contribute nothing towards it herself.'[2] Before the process of industrial development created a division between work and home, productive activity was integrated with family life for both sexes. Men's work did not automatically separate them from their children, and women's work, in agriculture, textiles and community health care particularly, was regarded by everyone as indispensable to the successful functioning of the household and the national economy[3]. This type of work frequently had what economists term use value rather than exchange value: it did not necessarily produce a cash income but rather served household needs directly. Under these circumstances, motherhood was a facet of life imposed onto, rather

117

than determining, the pattern of women's productive activity. For both mothers and fathers, the demands of work and child care could be adjusted so that there was no major conflict of choice.

This same pattern obtains in undeveloped and developing countries today. For example, among the Mbuti pygmies of the African Congo[4], who have a gatherer–hunter economy, motherhood brings no abrupt dislocation to women's work. Infants may either accompany their mothers on the daily search for vegetable foods or stay in the home camp to be cared for by older children or by men and women who are too old for hunting. The criterion determining who works and who does not is not sex or parenthood but age. This is a very common arrangement in pre-industrial societies.

Surveying the available data on 202 such societies held in the Yale University Human Relations Area files, Jimenez and Newton[5] reported that maternal post-partum work was the rule rather than the exception. Table 10.1 shows the

Table 10.1 Length of maternal post-partum breaks from work in different pre-industrial societies

Region	No. of societies	Post-partum days before mother resumes full work duties			
		0–7	8–14	15–42	43 or more
Asia	44	9	7	21	7
Europe	13	3	–	8	2
Africa	22	9	5	4	4
Middle East	16	5	1	8	2
N. America	35	12	6	14	3
S. America	33	18	8	4	3
Oceania	22	6	4	3	9
Russia	10	4	1	4	1
All societies	195	66	32	66	31

Adapted from reference 5, p. 174.

findings for the 195 out of the 202 societies on which the relevant data were available. In slightly more than half of the sample cultures (98/195), women were back at work fully within 14 days of childbirth and 42 days saw 164 of the 195 (84 per cent) women back at work. As Jimenez and Newton note, it is a salient feature of maternal work in such cultural settings that prolonged breast-feeding is both possible and culturally prescribed. On rare occasions when the mother's work does mean separation from the infant, other lactating women may temporarily take over the maternal breast-feeding role[6].

Once societies move from an agricultural to an industrial stage of development, this integration of work with domestic life is disturbed. The advice given in 1743 to the female domestic servant was given at a time when industrialisation in Britain was just beginning to make its impact on the work roles of men and women. The story told by the statistics of labour force composition from the time at which they first began to be reliably collected is one of remarkable stability in women's share of the labour force (figure 10.1). In 1850, 1911 and 1915 alike, 31 per cent of the employed labour force was female. From the late 1940s on, however, in many countries there began a shift towards the greater representation of married women in the labour force. In 1911 1 in 10 married women in Britain had a job; in 1951, 1 in 5; by 1976, 1 in 2. Thus, and as we can see from table 10.2, the proportion of the labour force accounted for by married women stood in 1979 at about the same (25.9 per cent) as that taken up by non-married women (25.7 per cent) in 1921.

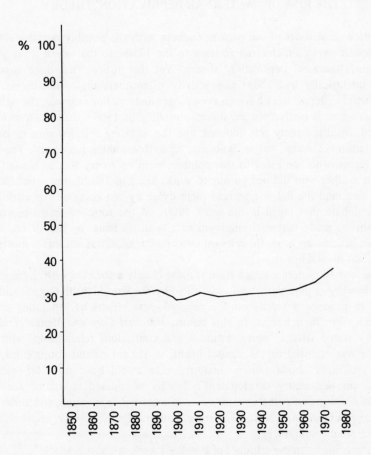

Figure 10.1 Working women as percentage of total labour force, Great Britain, 1851–1976 (after Tilly and Scott[50])

Table 10.2 Composition of the labour force in Britain

	Married women (%)	Non-married women (%)	Men (%)	Total (%)
1921	3.8	25.7	70.5	100
1951	11.8	19.0	69.2	100
1971	23.1	13.5	63.4	100
1979	25.9	13.4	60.6	100

Adapted from reference 20, p. 15.

THE RISE OF 'MATERNAL DEPRIVATION' THEORY

The ideological roots of our present concern with the possibly negative effects of mothers' work on children go back to the 1950s, to the rise of what might be called 'maternal deprivation' theory. Yet this notion, that there is something intrinsically bad about any activity of mothers that takes them away from their children, does have an even longer history. For example, the opinion was stated at a conference on infant mortality in 1906[7] that when mothers worked, child mortality was doubled, and the surviving children were no better than 'anaemic, saucy, vulgar, ignorant, cigarette-smoking hooligans'. The MP, John Burns, who confessed to this opinion, went on to say that he himself had a good mother who did not go out to work. She had 18 children — but half of them died, and she did not prevent them dying by not going out to work. The public debate that raged in the early 1900s on the topic of infant mortality nevertheless made maternal employment a sensitive issue: by the 1950s, when it again became an issue, the relevant outcome measure was not infant mortality but infant mental health.

The idea of maternal deprivation is most closely associated with the name of John Bowlby, a psychiatrist who was asked by the World Health Organization in 1948 to produce a report on the psychological effects of separating young children from their homes. In this report, *Maternal Care and Mental Health*[8], Bowlby stated that a 'warm, intimate and continuous relationship' with the mother was essential to the mental health of the infant and young child, and that *'prolonged deprivation* of maternal care would have grave far-reaching effects on personality development'. Bowlby considered failure of a child's *natural home group* to be a major cause of maternal deprivation, and under this heading put illegitimacy, divorce, chronic maternal illness, poverty, imprisonment and maternal employment.

Many comprehensive critiques of Bowlby's work are now available[9-12], which draw attention to the untested assumptions endemic in his approach and to the need, unrecognised by Bowlby, to specify the many different variables involved in the relationship between child development and maternal (or parental) employment. These are spelt out by Michael Rutter in his *Maternal Deprivation Reassessed*[12] as including the quality of the affectional relationship between the infant and not only her or his mother, but also father, siblings, and other relatives and friends; the need to distinguish short- and long-term effects of separating infants from any of their familiar relationships; the age, sex, temperament and social history of the infant as factors affecting the impact (if any) of any such separation. Also outlined were the modifying effect of the place in which separation occurs, and of the presence or absence of other familiar people; whether overt distress in infants, the usual index taken, is a good measure of the separation/deprivation effect; the length, nature, reason for, and any other (positive or negative) consequences of the separation. Under the quality of the infant's various relationships it appears to be especially important to consider not only the amount of time spent with different individuals and who performs routine caretaking activities, but also the character of the interaction, particularly the extent to which different people provide the infant with social stimulation.

Bowlby in his report was most concerned with the effects on children of residential care in institutions, and, since he wrote, evidence has accumulated to show that many infants and young children do indeed suffer acute distress when admitted to hospital or residential nursery care[13]. Moreover, poor-quality residential care is good for no one and multiple separation experiences in early childhood can sometimes lead to an adult inability to form affectional bonds with others. On the other hand, there is no evidence that adult mental health is dependent on childhood care by one's biological mother, or by any mother: infants have a capacity for multiple attachments, and a capacity for surviving unharmed those discontinuities in relationships that are, in fact, a normal part of life.

In speaking of maternal deprivation as a unitary syndrome, as a single morbidity with a single cause, Bowlby did, however, establish a most fertile ground for subsequent confused argument on such specific issues as maternal employment. As with those other great philosophers on the human condition, Marx and Freud, it is not so much what Bowlby said but what he is said to have said that has profoundly influenced people's thinking on the matter of maternal employment. Soon after the publication of the 1951 Report, it was being hailed as a self-evident truth that no mother should go out to work[14]. Partly in the light of the use made of his work, Bowlby has since published a much more sophisticated account[15] of the role played by maternal care in the development of the infant's capacity for attachment behaviour.

The idea of maternal deprivation, together with its implied corollary of a negative effect on children of maternal employment, gained popularity in Europe and North America in the 1950s and early 1960s. These were years of postwar reconstruction, with a renewed emphasis on the desirability of family life structured around the male breadwinner/female homemaker formula. In addition, analyses of the falling birth rate[16] implicated the emancipation of women in work outside the home as contrary to children's interests. In this sense the issue of the effect on children of their mothers' work is never wholly academic. but must be understood as in part a product of the climate of the times. In the 1980s the subject is coming to the fore again in the context of economic recession, a growing unemployment rate, and cuts in public spending on health and social services, all of which affect both the family roles and the employment roles of women. In addition, international comparisons of crude perinatal mortality rates[17] and a strengthened recognition of the influence of social factors on child-bearing[18] has focused the spotlight on the possibly negative effects of maternal employment.

RESEARCH ON MATERNAL EMPLOYMENT AND CHILDREN

One commentator on the state of the art with respect to the effects of maternal employment on children observed in 1960 that 'one can say almost anything one desires about the children of employed mothers and support the statement by some research study'[19]. As Rimmer and Popay[20] noted in 1982, the situation has not improved since then, and opinions remain far more common than facts. The main methodological inadequacies of existing studies are as follows:

(1) Data collection, measurement and analysis are biased by researchers' assumptions either that there will be effects of maternal employment or that there will not be; if effects are assumed, the direction, positive or negative, also tends to be assumed.

(2) Maternal employment, like maternal deprivation, is usually treated as a unitary phenomenon. Social class, type of employment and sex of child are rarely considered as important differentiating factors.

(3) The typical study plots maternal employment status against child outcome measures (e.g. intelligence test scores or personality inventories), omitting such intervening variables as child-rearing practices, children's and mothers' perceptions of maternal employment and the parental division of labour in the household.

(4) Many studies control insufficiently for such factors as family size and ordinal position known to affect the child characteristics selected as outcome measures.

(5) Most studies ignore the impact of maternal household work on children.

(6) In most studies fathers do not figure at all.

There is a paucity of research on the effects of maternal employment on infants particularly. This would seem to be both because of the difficulty of measuring within the first year of life effects which may be extrapolated to long-term effects, and because it is still relatively uncommon for mothers of infants to be employed. In 1979, according to the *General Household Survey*[21], some 28 per cent of mothers with a child under 5 were in the labour force in Britain, compared with 61 per cent and 72 per cent, respectively, of those whose youngest dependent child was aged 5-9 or 10 years or over. However, only 6 per cent of the 28 per cent with under-5s were employed full-time (16 per cent and 26 per cent of mothers with children aged 5-9 and 10 or over). Table 10.3 gives maternal employment in Britian in 1974-1976 from

Table 10.3 Children of mothers in paid employment by age of child and hours mother works, 1974-1976, Great Britain

Hours per week	Children in age group		
	0-2 (%)	3-4 (%)	5-10 (%)
1-12	37	33	24
13-21	27	32	30
22-30	12	17	23
31+	21	17	24

From reference 45, table 5.
Percentages do not add up to 100, since some mothers
did not state hours.

the child's point of view: it shows the proportion of children of different age groups with mothers in paid employment. The column headed 0-2 shows that more than a third of children in this age group with employed mothers had mothers who worked from 1 to 12 hours per week only.

DOES MATERNAL EMPLOYMENT AFFECT INFANTS?

The answer to the question as to whether maternal employment affects infants, phrased in this very general way, has to be 'yes', simply on the common-sense grounds that maternal employment is unlikely to make no difference to the everyday lives of infants. In attempting to answer the question in a more detailed manner, it is essential to bear in mind the caveats listed above, and also the findings of studies concerned with maternal employment effects on all ages of children. These were presented by Hoffman in her comprehensive analysis[22] of the literature in the following terms:

(1) Maternal employment affects boys and girls differently. Daughters of employed mothers compare positively with daughters of non-employed mothers with respect to independence, achievement-related variables and evaluation of the competence of women: no such effect is apparent for sons.

(2) The mother's satisfaction with her employment status is important. Children of mothers who are satisfied with their employment and experience

a minimum of conflict, guilt and role strain in relation to it are more likely to regard their mothers' employment positively and to have higher adjustment scores themselves on personality tests.

(3) In some cases (and where this has been specifically investigated) maternal employment is accompanied by an alteration in child-rearing practices in the direction of stressing earlier independence, or firmer control, of children, and changes in the parental division of labour in the direction of more participation by the father in child-rearing. Middle class mothers sometimes overcompensate for their employment by taking special trouble to plan time and activities with their children.

(4) There is no evidence that maternal employment *per se* leads to inadequate supervision of children (the latchkey and juvenile delinquency hypotheses).

The importance of these intervening variables probably accounts for the fact that there does not appear to be much of a relationship between maternal employment and one obvious measure of effects on the infant, namely whether or not the mother breast-feeds. A study carried out in 1975–1976 by the British Office of Population Censuses and Surveys[23] did not find that breast-feeding rates were related to maternal employment status in the first 4 post-partum months. This study suggested that the small number of mothers employed during this period fell into two different groups: women who had strong financial reasons for going back to work soon after the birth (for example, unsupported mothers) and who were most likely never even to begin breast-feeding, and professional mothers whose breast-feeding behaviour was no different from that of their non-employed peers (and some of whom made particularly determined efforts to continue employment and breast-feeding).

For some of the hypothesised effects on children of maternal employment, the findings of different studies conflict and no general pattern emerges. This is especially true of academic achievement. For example, in Britain the seven-year follow-up of the National Child Development Study[24] reported an apparent loss in reading age of about 3 months for children of mothers who were employed before the children started school, as against the reading age of those children whose mothers' employment began only after the onset of full-time schooling. There was no such association with arithmetic attainment, and on another measure, that of social adjustment, the children of the mothers who began in employment after their children went to school did less well than any other group. The reading effect was small, compared with the effect of social class, family size and the child's sex. In the USA a study of pre-schoolers[25] found that more of the children of employed mothers fell in the highest quartile on an instrument known as the Peabody Picture Vocabulary Test, and another study[26] analysing various longitudinal data sets found a differential sex effect, with the daughters of employed mothers having higher IQs at 6 than the daughters of their non-employed counterparts, but the relationship going in the opposite direction for boys, with a lower IQ at age 6 in the mother-employed group.

With respect to infancy, Hoffman noted in her review that no data are available on the effect, if any, of maternal employment on mother–infant interaction or the amount of stimulation given to infants by mothers or the impact, if any, of the substitute child care provided on the infant's daily life, development and attachment relationships.

Going beyond the somewhat limited genus of studies plotting maternal employment against this or that measure of child development, a number of broad questions are raised in relation to the growth in, and future of, maternal employment. Some of the most important of these are: What is the effect of children on mothers' work, their domestic as well as their employment work? What is the effect of mothers not being employed on children? How does paternal employment affect children, and how do children affect men's work? Finally, what alternative forms of child care are provided for the children of employed parents, and what is, or should be, the involvement of the State in this area?

DO INFANTS AFFECT WOMEN'S WORK?

The pattern of women's employment is affected by child-bearing and child-rearing in a number of ways.

First, and most obviously, protective labour legislation forbids the employment of women within a specified period following childbirth in many countries – 4 weeks in Britain in factory work. Among the financial benefits available to child-bearing women are some that cover the post-partum period; in Britain there is the *maternity allowance*, introduced in 1948, and payable only to those women who qualify on the basis of their own National Insurance contributions. At present the maternity allowance stands at £25.95 per week and it extends normally until 7 weeks after the birth. There is also *maternity pay*, which is 90 per cent of a woman's basic pay and is available under the 1975 Employment Protection Act to women who have worked for 2 years continuously at the same job and have worked for 16 hours or more a week. (An alternative qualification is 5 or more years' service of from 8 to 15 hours' work a week.) Under these circumstances a woman is also entitled to be given her job back if she notifies her intention to return to work in due time after the birth. Maternity allowance is deducted from maternity pay, irrespective of a woman's eligibility. There is also *child benefit*, now payable to the mother at the rate of £6.50 per child. In general, the maternity rights system is complex and at present appears to operate in a most unsatisfactory way. In a survey of some 2500 British women having babies in 1979, Daniel[27] found that only 54 per cent of the women who had worked during pregnancy satisfied the qualifying requirements of the 1975 Act.

In Daniel's survey 24 per cent of the women employed during pregnancy were employed again within 8 months of childbirth; a further 14 per cent were looking for jobs. Return to employment was greatest among part-time employees and among women who had been homeworkers (doing work for pay at home) when pregnant. Clearly, these types of work were found to be compatible with the demands of infant care. Daniel also reported a phenomenon found by other investigators[28], namely, a tendency for women to move following childbirth into less favoured sectors of employment. Indeed, almost the whole of the increase in the proportion of mothers employed in Britain since 1971 is accounted for by the move into part-time employment[21]. Women with pre-school children are also more likely than other women to be doing evening shift-work[26]. The resulting concentration of women employees in part-time work (40 per cent of employed women work part-time, compared with 4 per cent of men) is a primary factor accounting for the disadvantaged labour market position of women as a group, particularly the continuing 40 per cent gap between the average earnings of women and men[29].

Infants also have an impact on women's household work. According to French time-budget studies[30], one child adds on average 23 hours a week to housework time, two children add 35 hours, and three or more add 41 hours. The demands of infants on mothers are often not timed to fit in with the demands of household work, especially meal-getting, and the resulting conflict may be experienced as inherently frustrating.

IS THERE AN EFFECT ON MOTHERS AND CHILDREN OF NOT BEING EMPLOYED?

The increase in maternal employment has taken place over a period when two incomes have increasingly been required to maintain a family at the same standard of living secured by one 20 years ago[31]. In many cases a family is taken out of poverty by a mother's earnings. In addition, there has been a big increase in single-parent families — a rise of 32 per cent in Britain in the 5 years between 1971 and 1976, for example. About 1 in 8 of all families in Britain are now single-parent families, and 4 out of 5 of these are headed by women[32]. What these figures mean is that, quite irrespective of any other advantages of employment to mothers, it would be financially irresponsible for many mothers not to be in employment.

The literature on why mothers are in employment is considerable and, on the whole, rather uninformative, since there is unlikely to be only one reason for having a paid job, the question as to why fathers work is not asked and the question of maternal employment is still a moral issue in many people's eyes[33], so that the answers to survey questions are liable to be influenced by what mothers are expected to say, rather than accurately to reflect the mothers' own experiences. There is considerable evidence[34-36] suggesting that employment is valued by mothers both for the negative reason of offering escape from captivity in the home and for the positive reason of involving the mother in social relationships.

The positive benefits for mothers and their young children of the mother's employment are also highlighted by research on maternal depression. Brown and Harris[37], in their study of depression in London women, found motherhood to be a risk factor: 42 per cent of working class women with a child under 6 were psychiatrically disturbed. The figure for comparable middle class women was 5 per cent: there were no class differences in the incidence of psychiatric disturbance among women without children. Other studies have yielded similar figures for depression in mothers of young children[38]. In Brown and Harris's study employment outside the home was a factor protecting against maternal depression; that is, mothers without employment (either full- or part-time) were considerably more likely to become depressed in the face of difficulty.

Brown and Harris suggest that the mediating structure here is the effect of employment on a mother's self-esteem. Whatever the explanation, it can hardly be beneficial for infants to have depressed mothers. The incidence of child accidents is raised among depressed mothers[39] and there is also some evidence that depressed mothers treated with Valium are more likely to be violent towards their children[40].

THE INVISIBLE FATHER

In Britain in 1979 41 per cent of employed women were responsible for dependent children, but so were 43 per cent of employed men[21]. Since the debate about the impact of parental employment on children has been entirely concerned with maternal employment, we know almost nothing about the relationship between the employment of fathers and their roles *vis-à-vis* their children.

What we do know from employment statistics indicates that investment in work outside the home is a culturally prescribed feature of fatherhood. The highest economic activity rates are to be found among married fathers, and paternal employment rates show no variation by child's age or number of children, as is the case with mothers. Fathers with a large number of children work on average longer hours than those with few children[20]. Overtime is especially common among fathers — one study[41] showed that fathers under 30 worked four times as much paid overtime as childless husbands of the same age. The employment careers of lone fathers are, perhaps not surprisingly, much more like those of mothers[42].

Obviously, therefore, paternal employment impinges on infants if only by restricting the amount of time available for father–infant interaction. In one study[36] of first-time parenthood in the mid-1970s, a third of fathers saw their 5-month-old infants for an hour or less per day. Different patterns of paternal employment must affect infants in different ways, but this is an unresearched area. Similarly, we know very little about the long-term effects (if any) on child development of parental employment and different levels of paternal participation in child-rearing. A number of studies appear to suggest that relatively higher levels of father participation in child-rearing are associated with educational advancement and a lowered risk of delinquency in children, but the data do not as yet justify firm conclusions[43].

SUBSTITUTE CHILD CARE PROVISION

Last, but certainly not least, the effects of parental employment on infants cannot be considered without taking into account who looks after the children while the parents work.

Table 10.4 is taken from Daniel's study and describes the forms of child care used by the employed mothers of 8-month-old babies. It is striking that more than a third of babies were cared for by their fathers. Even among mothers

Table 10.4   Type of child care used by employed mothers

Type of care	Total (%)	Employed full-time (%)	Employed part-time (%)
Baby's father	35	11	43
Baby's grandmother	23	33	20
Self	17	13	18
Friend	7	9	6
Child minder	6	14	3
Other relative	4	6	3
Nursery	2	3	2
Au pair/paid help at home	2	3	1
Other/not stated	4	8	3
Total	100	100	100

From reference 27, p. 95.

employed full-time, very little use was made of non-family child care, and the major caretaker in this group was the baby's grandmother. It is also interesting that 17 per cent of babies were actually cared for by their mothers during employment work time.

It is not surprising in view of these findings that when the employed mothers in Daniel's survey were asked for their suggestions for change, better and more extensive child care facilities came far and above any other change mentioned. This adds to the evidence of other surveys demonstrating the enormous unmet demand for out-of-home child care provision by mothers (fathers have not been asked). In a 1968 survey[44] the level of demand stood at seven times the number of currently provided places. In 1978 another survey[45] showed that State-provided care was available to only 13 per cent of under-5s with employed mothers in Britain. A consequence of this minimal level of provision is the use of unregistered child-minders: one estimate[46] puts the number of British children cared for by unregistered minders at 1 200 000 per day.

Public policies with respect to the care of children of employed mothers vary a great deal between countries and reflect historical shifts of opinion about the proper role of woman — worker or mother?[47] Whatever the current status of opinion on this matter, maternal employment is likely only to increase, and so long as substitute child care facilities remain inadequate, the situation from both the children's and the parents' point of view will be far from ideal. There are many policy options here — from redefining the problem as one of parental employment, the Swedish solution, to a payment to mothers enabling them to stay at home, as in Hungary, to community and government-run nurseries, the Chinese answer. However, each option requires a political commitment, which has so far been lacking in Britain, to solving the problem.

CONCLUSION

Women's two roles — home and work — are here to stay. So are men's; it is simplistic to view the issue of maternal employment and its impact on infants in isolation from the broader social context of changes in family life and the social position of women, men and children today. There are no grounds for coming to general conclusions about either the good or the bad effects of either maternal or paternal employment on children. What is at issue is, rather, the different opportunity structures for parent–child relations and child development provided by different articulations in men's and women's lives of the domestic and employment domains.

The concentration in research over the last 30 years on maternal deprivation theory has prevented some of the more interesting and relevant questions being asked. For example, there are almost no studies addressing the question of the effects on infants of different substitute child care arrangements, or examining the possible impact on children's personality development of increased paternal involvement in employment during infancy and early childhood.

Aside from the need for research, there are also pressing public policy questions. The most important of these is the need to confront the consequences to children and their parents of a sitting-on-the-fence attitude to the conflict between parenthood and employment. For example, in both Britain and the USA lone mothers and children have emerged as the main population group living in poverty over the period since the 1950s[48], and with increasing rates of marital breakdown this group will increase in size. Low pay is still a major cause of family poverty[49]. The level of State financial support for children has fallen considerably over the last 15 years and many parents are able to take themselves and their children out of poverty only by providing two incomes. The importance, even sanctity, of motherhood and the mother–child relationship is a dominant cultural theme in the industrialised world. What is too often lacking, however, is the practical support needed to underwrite this commitment.

ACKNOWLEDGEMENTS

I should like to thank my colleague at the National Perinatal Epidemiology Unit for their comments and the Department of Health and Social Security for financial support.

REFERENCES

1. Myrdal, A. and Klein, V. (1956). *Women's Two Roles*, Routledge and Kegan Paul, London
2. Quoted in Pinchbeck, I. (1930). *Women Workers and The Industrial Revolution*, Frank Cass, London, reprinted 1969
3. Clark, A. (1919). *The Working Life of Women in the Seventeenth Century*, Frank Cass, London, reprinted 1968
4. Turnbull, C. (1965). *Wayward Servants*, Natural History Press, New York
5. Jimenez, M. H. and Newton, N. N. (1979). Activity and work during pregnancy and the postpartum period: cross-cultural study of 202 societies. *American Journal of Obstetrics and Gynecology*, **135**(2), 171-176
6. Raphael, D. (1973). *The Tender Gift: Breastfeeding*, Prentice-Hall, Englewood Cliffs, N. J.
7. Burns, J. (1906). [Inaugural Address.] *Report of the Proceedings of the National Conference on Infantile Mortality*, P. S. King, London
8. Bowlby, J. (1951). Maternal care and mental health. *Bulletin of the World Health Organization*, **3**, 355-534
9. Ainsworth, M. D., Andry, R. G., Harlow, R. G., Lebovici, S., Mead, M., Pugh, D. G. and Wootton, B. (1966). *Deprivation of Maternal Care: A Reassessment of its Effects*, Schocken Books, New York
10. Clarke, A. M. and Clarke, A. D. B. (1976). *Early Experience: Myth and Evidence*, Open Books, London
11. Morgan, P. (1975). *Child Care: Sense and Fable*, Temple Smith, London
12. Rutter, M. (1972). *Maternal Deprivation Reassessed*, Penguin, Harmondsworth
13. Yarrow, L. J. (1964). Separation from parents during early childhood. In Hoffman, M. L. and Hoffman, L. W. (Eds.), *Review of Child Development Research*, Vol. I, Russell Sage Foundation, New York
14. Baers, M. (1954). Women workers and home responsibilities. *International Labour Review*, **69**, 338-355
15. Bowlby, J. (1974). *Attachment*, Hogarth Press, London
16. Report of the Royal Commission on Population (1949). HMSO, London
17. Chalmers, I. and Macfarlane, A. (1980). Interpretation of perinatal statistics. In Wharton, B. (Ed.), *Topics in Perinatal Medicine*, Pitman Medical, London
18. Oakley, A., Chalmers, I. and Macfarlane, A. (1982). Social class, stress and reproduction. In Rees, A. R. and Purcell, H. (Eds.), *Disease and the Environment*, Wiley, Chichester
19. Stolz, L. (1960). Effects of maternal employment on children: evidence from research. *Child Development*, **31**, 749-782
20. Rimmer, L. and Popay, J. (1982). *Employment Trends and the Family*, Study Commission on the Family, London
21. Office of Population Censuses and Surveys (1981). *General Household Survey 1979*, HMSO, London

22. Hoffman, L. W. (1974). Effects on child. In Hoffman, L. W. and Nye, F. I. (Eds.) *Working Mothers*, Jossey-Bass, San Francisco
23. Martin, J. (1978). *Infant Feeding: Attitudes and Practice in England and Wales* (OPCS), HMSO, London
24. Davie, R., Butler, N. and Goldstein, H. (1972). *From Birth to Seven*, Longman, London
25. Rieber, M. and Womach, M. (1967). The intelligence of pre-school children as related to ethnic and demographic variables. *Exceptional Children*, **34**, 609–614
26. Rees, A. N. and Palmer, F. H. (1970). Factors related to change in mental test performance. *Developmental Psychology Monograph*, **3** (2, Pt 2)
27. Daniel, W. W. (1980). *Maternity Rights*, Policy Studies Institute, London
28. Moss, P. (1980). Parents at work. In Moss, P. and Fonda, N. (Eds.), *Work and the Family*, Temple Smith, London
29. Chiplin, B. and Sloane, P. J. (1982). *Tackling Discrimination at the Workplace*, Cambridge University Press, Cambridge
30. Girard, A. (1958). Le budget – temps de la femme mariée dans les agglomerations urbaines. *Population*, 591–618
31. Hamill, L. (1978). *Wives as Sole and Joint Breadwinners*, Government Economic Service Working Papers, No. 13, HMSO, London
32. Anon. (1980). *Happy Families?*, Study Commission on the Family, London
33. Anon. (1982). *Values and the Changing Family*, Study Commission on the Family, London
34. Lopata, H. (1971). *Occupation Housewife*, Oxford University Press, New York
35. Gavron, H. (1966). *The Captive Wife*, Penguin, Harmondsworth
36. Oakley, A. (1979). *Becoming a Mother*, Martin Robertson, Oxford
37. Brown, G. W. and Harris, T. (1978). *Social Origins of Depression*, Tavistock, London
38. Wolkind, S. N., Zajicek, E. and Ghodsian, M. (1980). Continuities in maternal depression. *International Journal of Family Psychiatry*, **1**, 167–181
39. Brown, G. W. and Davidson, S. (1978). Social class, psychiatric disorder of mothers and accidents to children. *Lancet*,
40. Hyman, C. A. (1978). Non-accidental injury. *Health Visitor*, **51**(5), 168–172
41. National Board for Prices and Incomes, cited in Moss, P. (1980). Parents at work. In Moss, P. and Fonda, N. (Eds.), *Work and the Family*, Temple Smith, London
42. O'Brien, M. (1982). The working father. In Beail, N. and McGuire, J. (Eds.) *Fathers: Psychological Perspectives*, Junction Books, London
43. Lewis, C., Newson, E. and Newson, J. (1982). Father participation through childhood and its relationship with career aspirations and delinquency. In Beail, N. and McGuire, J. (Eds.) *Fathers: Psychological Perspectives*, Junction Books, London
44. Hunt, A. (1968). *A Survey of Women's Employment*, HMSO, London
45. Central Policy Review Staff (1978). *Services for Young Children with Working Mothers*, HMSO, London
46. Jackson, B. (1979). *Childminder*, Routledge and Kegan Paul, London
47. Adams, C. T. and Winston, K. T. (1980). *Mothers at Work*, Longman, New York
48. Ross, H. L. (1976). Women and children last. In Chapman, J. R. (Ed.), *Economic Independence for Women*, Sage, Beverly Hills, Cal.

49. McNay, M. and Pond, C. (1980). *Low Pay and Family Poverty*, Study Commission on the Family, London
50. Tilly, L. A. and Scott, J. W. (1978). *Women, Work and Family*, Holt, Rinehart and Winston, New York

Part 2
Teratology

11

Mechanisms of Teratogenesis: The Extrapolation of the Results of Animal Studies to Man

E. MARSHALL JOHNSON

It is a large assignment to relate mechanisms of teratogenesis to cross-species extrapolations within the context of women in the work place. The task may seem particularly difficult in that:

(1) Teratogenesis is but one of four possible manifestations of perturbed development.

(2) We do not know the exact mechanism by which any chemical substance interferes with development of the products of conception.

(3) Cross-species extrapolations are extremely difficult in view of the remarkable difference in pharmacology and toxicokinetics from one species to another.

(4) Last, this chapter will not address the topic of safety for women, but will concern itself with the work place's third inhabitant – the conceptus.

To attain a level of protection for the conceptus anywhere near that which we provide for ourselves as adults, one must address the definitions of some relevant terms. The word 'teratogenic' has come to be synonymous with invariably dangerous to the embryo. 'Dangerous' in the same singular frame of reference as the term 'carcinogenic', for instance, is used, as if it were a unique and particularly feared property of certain substances. To be non-teratogenic would be to be non-hazardous to the conceptus. Such concepts are incomplete to the point of being inaccurate[1] and actually the mere detection of terata certainly is not our intention when making developmental toxicity safety evaluations. Teratology is the study of the causes, manifestations, mechanisms and pathogenesis of perturbed developmental biology. The production of terata is but one of four possible manifestations of adverse effects on the conceptus. Equally unacceptable for our grandchildren are the other three signs of developmental toxicity: death, decrement of functional ability (whether this be of the CNS or any other organ system is immaterial) and runting (or other dose-related developmental delays directly attributable to a specific chemical substance). Developmental toxicology is the study of outcomes of perturbed development and this is our goal in safety evaluations — that is, to detect substances hazardous to any aspect of development.

Perhaps the largest single impediment to protecting the embryo from adverse effects is extrapolation of the binary concepts and nomenclature of mutagenesis and carcinogenesis into the realm of abnormal developmental biology. There has developed a tendency to phrase questions of developmental toxicology in simple binary form: Is substance X teratogenic? This is not a highly relevant question from the view of developmental toxicology and is misleading and even counter-productive when answered in either the negative or the affirmative.

Setting aside all considerations of dosage for the moment and considering only the developmental biology involved, we can more clearly address the precision of our terminology. Production of terata is but one of the manifestations of developmental toxicity — it is but one of the four outcomes of pregnancy which we do not seek to have any substance achieve. The absence of terata among the offspring of a teratology safety evaluation experiment does not exonerate the test substance from further concern regarding developmental toxicity. The production of dead conceptuses at term, but no terata, has been used to classify substances as embryo-toxic (or feto-toxic) but not teratogenic, as if this distinction were somehow less damning of a chemical's reputation. In addition to being an equally inacceptable pregnancy outcome, such euphemistic designation of effect does not address the more basic question of whether or not the conceptus was normal or abnormal prior to demise.

This topic can be addressed in another way by recalling that during the 1950s a large number of experiments explored the relationship between severity of insult and the duration of its application during organogenesis, to pregnancy outcomes[2,3]. Some of these studies even employed intercurrent serial autopsies and microscopic examination of the conceptus[4,5] to establish that teratogenesis often preceded death of the products (figures 11.1, 11.2). One should review the papers of that decade, for they clearly establish that the currently applied safety evaluations of developmental toxicity are the most severe challenges one can offer to an embryo and, not surprisingly, they result in death of the products more frequently than live terata (table 11.1). This is as it should be, but we need to remember that standard testing protocols do not call for examinations early in gestation and are really chronic exposures in the view of the developmental phenomena characteristic of an embryo. This is not a call for examination of early-stage embryos to find whether they are normal or abnormal, nor is it a plea for multiple experiments of short duration, with each spanning but a few days of the ontogenic period. It is simply to make the point that the designation 'nonteratogenic' does not have much meaning. Should someone still be unconvinced on this point, we could bring forth Karnofsky's law[6], which states to the effect that one cannot term a test chemical nonteratogenic until one has examined all stages of development in all species treated by all available routes

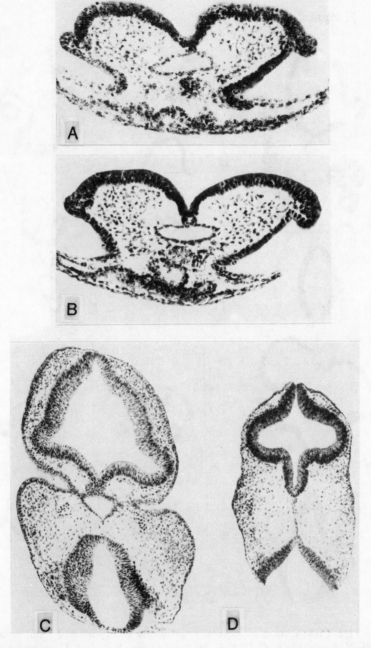

Figure 11.1 Cross-sections of normal control rat embryos and embryos from mothers treated with 9-methyl pteroylglutamic acid (9-MePGA) on days 8 and 9 of pregnancy. A, B: Day 9 1/2 embryos from normal control and 9-MePGA-treated mothers, respectively. Note that they appear to be identical in developmental stage (neural folds) and conformation. C, D: Day 10 embryos from normal control and 9-MePGA-treated mothers, respectively. Note delayed closure of neural tube and reduced size of embryo from treated mother.

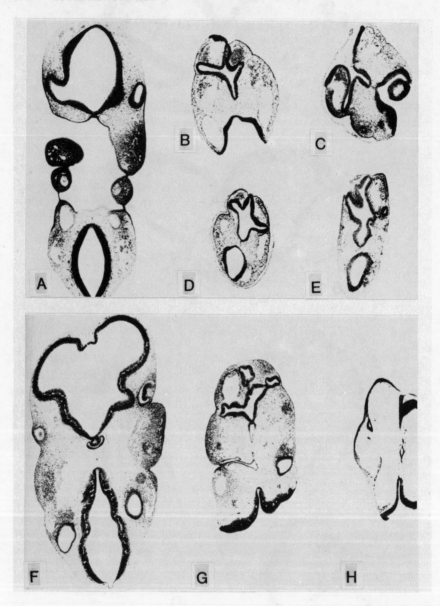

Figure 11.2 Cross-section of normal control rate embryos (A, F) and embryos of 9-MePGA-treated (B, C, D, E; G, H) pregnancies. A–E: Day 11 embryos. Note that those of treated mothers are markedly smaller than controls and have a variety of developmental abnormalities. F–H: Day 12 embryos. Note reduced size and multiple developmental abnormalities in treated embryos. In no instance was a normal-appearing embryo encountered in a treated mother after 10 days of gestation and the only live embryo encountered from among 20 litters examined is present in G.

Table 11.1 Developmental toxicology – determinants of designation[a] (embryo-lethal, teratogenic)

Gestation days of treatment[b]	% Embryos		% Survivors	
	Dead	Alive	Normal	Abnormal
8–10	100	0	0	0
9–11	26	74	1	99
10–12	0	100	22	78
9–12	100	0	0	0
10–13	14	86	0	100
11–14	0	100	30	70
9–21	100	0	0	0
11–21	5	95	5	95
13–21	0	100	70	30

[a] After Nelson, M. M. (1957). *Pediatrics*, **19**, 764–776.
[b] All groups received the same dose level of 9-methylpteroylglutamic acid. Note that: (a) the earlier stages of pregnancy are more severely affected than are later stages, and (b) treatments begun on the same day produced greater toxicity when continued in effect for a longer period and even a 24 hour extension (days 9–11 v. days 9–12) caused a 'teratogen' to become an 'embryo-lethal' substance.

of exposure and at all doses. Obviously this is an insurmountable task, and as will be illustrated, totally unnecessary.

Rephrase the question 'Is substance X teratogenic' to another, 'Can X disrupt development?' This question can be answered. The answer is always 'Yes', and the relevant question then comes to be one of dosage. At this point in our discussion, we will accept that, when given enough of almost any test substance, the embryo will be adversely affected and exhibit one or more of the manifestations of perturbed development and do so in a dose-related manner.

MECHANISMS OF ABNORMAL DEVELOPMENT

It has rightfully been said that by understanding the mechanisms of teratogenesis we will be able to predict more efficiently and accurately, adequately control and effectively regulate exposure of embryos to substances and situations capable of placing them in jeopardy. While this is probably accurate (and we must press ahead to improve our understanding of abnormal developmental biology), protection of the conceptus cannot await our full comprehension. Table 11.2 is an abbreviated list of some of the more salient developmental phenomena required of a zygote in its development into an embryo and then a fetus and

Table 11.2 Some of the developmental phenomena indirectly evaluated by standard developmental toxicity safety evaluation protocols

Pattern formation and its fixation
Directional migrations
Proliferation of specific cells
Regeneration of specific tissues
Production and transmittal of inductive stimuli
Receipt of and response to inductive stimuli
Cellular and tissue morphogenesis
Establishment and regulation of organ fields
Acquisition or loss of inductive competence
Sequential gene expression
Cellular and tissue differentiation
Organogenesis
Attainment of functional ability
Programmed cell death
Recognition and response to spatial orientation
Directional migration

newborn. Most, if not each, of these phenomena must be achieved by the anlagen of each organ and differentiated tissue. Not only must each be achieved in each case, but the developmental events must be correct in their quality (e.g. induction), quantity (e.g. organ field formation), ontogeny (e.g. attainment of polarity), timing (e.g. programmed cell death) and integration (e.g. cell movements). This means that literally thousands of things could go awry and the outcome could be manifest as any one of the four classes of perturbed development. The variety of end-point assays is limited to these four classes of response and furthermore, within a class, responses are remarkably stereotyped. For instance, cleft palate is an easily recognised and relatively simple gross anatomical abnormality. Possible contributing or triggering factors leading to this endpoint (improper formation of palate) are factors as diverse as face shape[7,8], development of sphenoid bone[9-11], elevation of palatine shelves[12], development of motive factors[13,14], failure of timely programmed cell death of medial edge epithelial cells[15] and altered macromolecular synthesis[16].

Any one of a variety of developmental phenomena in a variety of cells, tissues or organs may be perturbed in any one of several ways and the single endpoint assay or manifestation of perturbed development is the single effect — the cleft palate. The potential diversity of effects leading to the same end-point determination explains why we still lack a clear understanding of the mechanism of action of any chemical on development. Pathogenesis of some defects, however, is beginning to be understood to a significant level of reductionistic analysis, and this type of information does provide valuable tools for the analysis of specific developmental abnormalities.

This chapter may not be projecting a markedly optimistic view for contemporary applications, but there is a brighter side and there are items of use here already. It is obvious that by understanding the diversity of potential mechanisms and sites of action, one can appreciate why structure–activity relationships are not of significant predictive value for developmental toxicology and why one-hit models cannot be used for low-dose extrapolations.

CROSS-SPECIES EXTRAPOLATION

Widely studied and reported during the 1950s and 1960s were six general principles of teratology[17] or developmental toxicology: (1) the developmental stage at which an agent acts on an embryo determines the nature of the developmental abnormality; (2) the maternal and embryonic genotypes modulate susceptibility to adverse pregnancy outcomes; (3) there are four manifestations of developmental toxicity (live terata, decrements of function, growth retardation and death of the products of conception); (4) manifestations of perturbed development range from no observed effect levels through 100 per cent lethality as treatment levels are increased; (5) the physicochemical nature of substances influences their access to the placenta and embryo; (6) at a sufficiently high dose or concentration almost any substance is capable of triggering abnormal developmental sequences in the embryo.

The clear statement of each of these principles had a salutary influence and a substantial utility to those studying abnormal developmental biology. It turns out that there is a seventh general principle of developmental toxicology, and data pointing towards this have been available but largely unrecognised since the beginning of the modern era of experimental teratology. Generally understood by all those interested in teratology and developmental toxicology is the fact that there are substances capable of disrupting one or more of the developmental events characteristic of embryos at treatment levels below those producing toxic signs in either adult males or adult females. This concept can serve as the starting point for understanding the seventh general principle of developmental toxicology, which can, in turn, have a significant beneficial effect on our ability to make safety evaluations regarding the *in utero* human population.

The seventh principle of developmental toxicology is: (7) there is a fixed relationship between adult and developmental toxicity independent of species or route of treatment. That this actually exists can be established by anyone with access to a library; and once alerted to the possibility, the task of confirming its existence is an easy one. From the published literature of developmental toxicity studies, one can find data allowing determination of, or at least close estimation of, the developmental minimal effective concentration (MEC), that lowest dose or exposure capable of producing minimal expression of any one of the four manifestations of developmental toxicity. This developmental MEC is usually expressed either as mg or p.p.m. of agent per kg of pregnant female body weight, and it can serve as the denominator of an extremely useful ratio. The ratio's numerator comes from that MEC capable of producing any minimal expression of toxicity in the female. The minimal sign of adult toxicity most frequently reported in the literature is decrement of anticipated maternal weight gain. However, other equally acceptable signs (e.g. altered maternal liver weight) are occasionally reported at the low end of the dose–response curve in the somewhat standardised and state of the art teratology safety evaluations as practised and published throughout the developed world. The ratio adult/ developmental toxicity (A/D ratio) derived in this manner is the first means yet discovered to allow some degree of cross-species extrapolation for detection of hazards to the third population. It makes no difference what end-point manifestation of developmental toxicity the agent produces or its suspected mechanisms of action, the A/D ratio can still be calculated. This is of major and fundamental importance, because developmental biology consists of multiple phenomena, both known and unknown, and disruption of any one or more is potentially capable of disrupting the embryo's development.

A good test of the stability of the A/D ratio is obtained by examining the databases for substances which have been tested in a number of species treated by a variety of routes. Dioxin (or TCDD) is such a substance, and when the published data are sufficiently complete and reported clearly enough for the A/D ratio to be calculated, it is always near unity. The dose or exposure needed to produce the MEC A or the MEC D varies considerably from one species and route of exposure to another, but the ratio does not change markedly, provided that the A and D are both gleaned from studies using the same species, route and general duration of exposure. The bottom line in all these studies is that, regardless of species or route, TCDD will affect the conceptus only in sick mothers. If maternal toxicity is not present, then the chemical will not disrupt development. Stated another way: All one need know is the adult toxic dose and one can calculate the developmentally toxic dose for another species or the same species treated by the same or any other route. The single caution regarding the cross-species stability of the ratio involves substances with totally unique metabolism in one species.

We do not ban substances just because they have been tested in some mammal by an experimental protocol capable of generating structurally abnormal or otherwise damaged offspring – for example, aspirin, vitamin A, lithium or arsenicals. We do ban substances, however, because of their developmental toxicity, when they disrupt development at a small fraction of the adult toxic dose[18]. The A/D ratio for the four substances just mentioned is about 2 regardless of species or route of treatment.That for thalidomide is somewhere between 40 and 100, depending on how solubility problems were dealt with in any particular report. Most substances prove capable of perturbing embryogenesis only at treatment levels exceeding the dam's homeostatic mechanism (A/D ratio near unity), but a complete spectrum of developmental toxicity potential is present, as evidenced by the A/D ratios.

Application of the A/D ratio calculation – that is, determination of the teratogenic hazard index — allows us to cross species boundaries but so crudely that one may logically wonder — so what? The ratio is quite crude and largely ignores considerations of pharmacology and toxicokinetics. Also, data on which to make a reliable calculation of the A/D ratio still require large numbers of pregnant mammals, although there have been some worth-while recent attempts to reduce the number of animals[19] and the complexity[20] involved in detection of end-point assays.

Thus far in our discussion, we have made but little advance in the effort to identify work places safe for women of child-bearing potential, and it would seem as though it still requires $30 000–50 000 (approx. £20 000–32 000) per chemical to calculate the A/D ratio. This is accurate, because studies in the common laboratory species are the time-honoured and generally accepted means for detecting substances hazardous to the conceptus (high A/D ratio). They are also the standard means for determining the no observed effect level (NOEL) in a sensitive species, so that a safety factor can be established prior to setting acceptable levels of pregnant human exposure. What is needed is a simpler means for determining the A/D ratio of otherwise untested chemicals, so that a mammalian NOEL need be determined only for substances actually needing detailed evaluation for effects in embryology.

Just as discovery of the first six general principles of developmental toxicology fostered new types of studies, so, too, does elucidation of the seventh. Once phrased, the seventh can have far-reaching practical application. Serving as a unifying principle for developmental toxicology, it permits development of predictive *in vitro* safety evaluation systems for developmental biology. All such a system need achieve is a simple standard endpoint for adult toxicity A and, in an ontogenic system encompassing as much of the known and unknown phenomena of basic developmental biology as possible, a simple standard endpoint for developmental toxicity D. These two end-points can then be manipulated until they become predictive of pre-existing data from studies in pregnant mammals.

AN ALTERNATIVE TO PREGNANT MAMMALS FOR DETECTING HAZARDS TO THE CONCEPTUS

Hydra attenuata is a fresh-water coelenterate species uncomplicated by symbiotic algae or other such confounding factors. It is a unique animal in that it represents the lowest form of animal life composed of complex cells, tissues and organs on the one hand, while, on the other, it is the highest form of animal life capable of total whole-body regeneration. These tiny animals have been studied intensively by developmental biologists for over 200 years. By studies reported this century it has been established that, during regeneration, *Hydra* achieves all of the developmental events or phenomena known to be characteristic of developing systems in general — for example, induction, pattern formation and formation of organ fields, etc.[21].

Adults are readily grown in the laboratory, where, under controlled conditions, they reproduce by asexual budding[22]. Obviously, one can find some concentation of almost any substance which is capable of producing toxicity in adult hydra — the A of the A/D ratio (figure 11.3). One can also dissociate

RESPONSE OF ADULT HYDRA ATTENUATA
TO NOXIOUS STIMULI

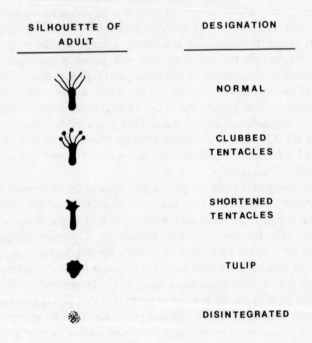

SILHOUETTE OF ADULT	DESIGNATION
	NORMAL
	CLUBBED TENTACLES
	SHORTENED TENTACLES
	TULIP
	DISINTEGRATED

Figure 11.3 Schematic depiction of adult hydra and their toxicological responses to an increasing concentration or a longer treatment period of any test chemical. The minimal effective adult-toxic (A) concentration for calculation of the A/D ratio is the tulip stage or the organisms' disintegration which immediately follows this stage. (After reference 25)

adult hydra and randomly reaggregate their cells into pellets. When several hundred adult hydra are placed into a hypertonic solution, their cells become less adherent and may be separated from one another by gentle repeated pipetting. These dissociated cells can then be drawn into 0.5 mm i.d. plastics tubing and packed into pellets of randomly reaggregated cells by gentle centrifugation. These sausage-like pellets are expelled from the tubing into glass dishes containing the test chemical. They are termed artificial embryos because they will totally regenerate new hydra in about 90 hours after having undergone an elaborate development entailing events such as spatial orientation and pattern formation, achieved by previously differentiated cells, and induction and organ field formation, achieved by previously undifferentiated cells[23,24]. Obviously, one can also determine a concentration of any test substance capable of preventing development of this artificial embryo — the D of the A/D ratio (figure 11.4).

How does one establish whether or not such a system can be used prospectively on previously untested substances and be relied upon to direct correctly our attention to the developmental hazards (higher A/D ratio) while giving a green light to those not posing a potential hazard to the conceptus (lower A/D ratio)? Validity is established by examining pre-existing literature and finding

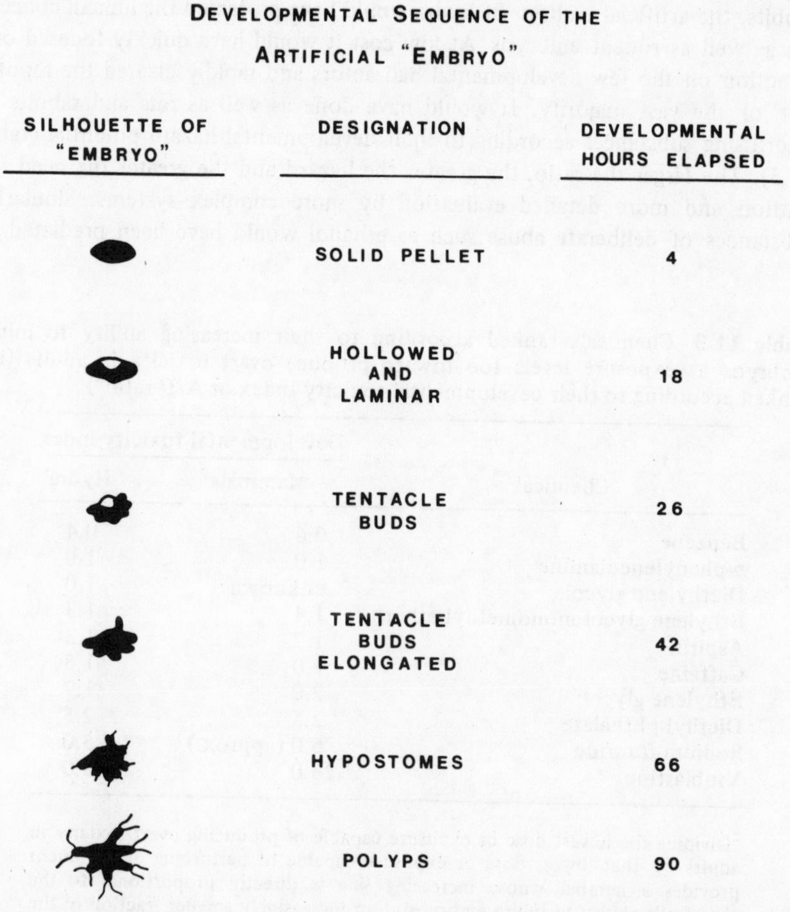

DEVELOPMENTAL SEQUENCE OF THE ARTIFICIAL "EMBRYO"

SILHOUETTE OF "EMBRYO"	DESIGNATION	DEVELOPMENTAL HOURS ELAPSED
	SOLID PELLET	4
	HOLLOWED AND LAMINAR	18
	TENTACLE BUDS	26
	TENTACLE BUDS ELONGATED	42
	HYPOSTOMES	66
	POLYPS	90

Figure 11.4 Sequential developmental stages of artificial 'embryos' constructed of randomly reaggregated adult hydra cells. The lowest concentration of a test chemical preventing the normal ontogeny of this preparation and resulting in its disintegration is taken as the 'D' for calculation of the A/D ratio. (After reference 25)

as diverse a group of substances as possible in which one can determine the mammalian A/D ratio with confidence[25]. Over 100 such substances exist, and we have tested over 60[26]. In each instance the hydra assay's A/D ratio has been within 0.1 of a log of the mammalian A/D ratio. In other words, the seventh principle of developmental toxicology applies not only to mammals, but also to the extreme end of the animal kingdom artificially forced to self-regulate, differentiate and develop. Just as in mammals, the A/D ratios generated by the hydra test form a continuum of the developmental hazard potential of substances. Most have ratios near unity and only a few have ratios larger than 10. If the substances tested to date in hydra had never been tested in rats, mice and rabbits, the artificial embryo of hydra would have protected the human conceptus as well as rodent embryos. At low cost it would have quickly focused our attention on the few developmental bad actors and rapidly cleared the reputation of the vast majority. It would have done as well as rats and rabbits in prioritising substances according to their developmental hazard potential (table 11.3). The larger the ratio, the greater the hazard and the greater the need for caution and more detailed evaluation by more complex systems. Similarly, substances of deliberate abuse such as ethanol would have been predicted as

Table 11.3 Chemicals ranked according to their increasing ability to injure embryos at exposure levels too low to produce overt toxicity in adults (i.e. ranked according to their developmental toxicity index or A/D ratio[a])

	Developmental toxicity index	
Chemical	Mammals[b]	Hydra[c]
Benzene	0.6	0.4
p-phenylenediamine	1.0	1.0
Diethylene glycol	unknown	1.0
Ethylene glycol monomethyl ether	1.4	1.3
Aspirin	1.7	1.3
Caffeine	1.0	1.5
Ethylene glycol	2.0	1.7
Diethyl phthalate	2.5	2.5
Sodium fluoride	6.0 (approx.)	5.0
Vinblastine	26.0	45.0

[a]Dividing the lowest dose or exposure capable of producing overt toxicity in adults by that lowest dose or exposure capable of perturbing development provides a number whose increasing size is directly proportional to the chemical's ability to injure embryos at an increasingly smaller fraction of the dose necessary to injure an adult of the same species treated by the same route of exposure. It must be noted that even a substance with a low A/D ratio will injure the conceptus if used to the level of adult toxicity — for example, ethyl alcohol.
[b]The A/D ratio as calculated from published reports of effects in rodents and rabbits.
[c]The A/D ratio as calculated from the hydra assay.

capable of disrupting development if their mothers chose to use the chemical at their own toxic level. This is as true for the A/D ratio of hydra as it is for that of rodents and humans. It should be noted that the hydra assay can rank substances according to their relative abilities to disrupt development. The doses or exposure levels employed in hydra, however, do not appear relevant to mammals, and for this type of data a test such as the Chernoff–Karlock test using mice may be considered.

DETERMINATION OF A WORK PLACE SAFE FOR THE CONCEPTUS

Whether or not a particular work place is safe for the conceptus can be determined by using the concepts assembled and outlined here in conjunction with the seventh principle of developmental toxicology. If data are available from a standard developmental toxicology safety evaluation made in groups of pregnant rodents, one can calculate the A/D ratio according to the end-point assays of adult and developmental toxicity characteristic of such studies. A requirement[27] of such a test is that the test substance be examined for adverse effects at an exposure sufficiently high to produce some sign of overt toxicity in the dams. (Another requirement is that the test substance be examined at a dose level sufficiently low to produce no observed effect on either the adult or the conceptus.) The most frequently reported indication of effect on the adult is decrement of anticipated maternal weight gain (with careful avoidance of a spurious determination due to reductions of fetal size or number). This exposure level is the A of the A/D ratio. The D is determined by ascertaining the minimal effective concentration of the test substance producing manifestations of any of the four types of developmental toxicity. This is most frequently reported as delay of fetal skeletal development or as minor variations in skeleto-genesis.

Our experience is that the vast majority of chemicals have A/D ratios near 1 or 2. The combination of dose selection, the crudeness of the maternal end-point assays of toxic signs and biologic variation precludes exact precision, and an A/D ratio of 1 or 2 must be considered as the same number and not be considered as indicative of a hazard to the conceptus. That is, although a substance with a low ratio certainly will perturb development if the exposure is high enough, the dose needed for this is also the dose which will be toxic to the female. This means that the conceptus needs no special protection or safety factor to provide it with the same degree of protection provided for the adult. Whether the size of this safety factor be 0.1 or 0.01 of the adult toxic dose, it will provide both mother and conceptus with the same margin of protection. As the developmental toxicity index (A/D ratio) increases, the safety factor must increase proportionally if the conceptus is to be equally protected from adverse effects of each chemical, regardless of the magnitude of its individual propensity for disrupting developmental biology in the presence or the absence of adult toxicity.

Although the A/D ratio does not vary markedly from species to species, the actual amount of a test substance needed to attain A and D varies not only according to species, but also according to route of administration, rate of absorption and metabolism. Outlining of such considerations is not possible in the limited space for this chapter, but they are of paramount importance, because the actual acceptable exposure level must be calculated on the basis of the most sensitive species and one that pharmacologically and toxicologically is most similar to humans.

CONCLUSIONS

Application of the hydra assay can markedly reduce both the time and expense of determining the A/D ratio of previously untested substances. If the A/D ratio is near 1 or 2 and there is no suspicion that the chemical is toxic to adults in the range of anticipated human exposure or use, the hydra assay provides sufficient data for one to conclude that women of child-bearing potential need not be excluded from that chemical work place. Furthermore, larger A/D ratios as determined in hydra allow quantification directly proportioned to the increased size of the safety factor needed in order to assure a uniform level of protection for the conceptus, while still not calling for the exclusion of women of child-bearing potential.

In the total absence of data on adult toxicity, the A/D ratio cannot be used by itself, but when available from hydra, it obviates the need for routine testing in pregnant animals. Closer attention can, therefore, be focused on determining the A in the most sensitive species when exposed by the route most relevant to the anticipated human exposure.

The hydra assay should be part of the pre-manufacturing notification for new chemicals being released into our environment. Currently, some countries require no definitive biological tests, while others call for at least an Ames test for mutagens and the mouse LD_{50} for acute toxicity to provide a degree of safety for us – the adults[28]. Addition of hydra would provide at least a similar degree of protection for the unborn also.

Hydra can serve as an alternative to elaborate testing in large groups of pregnant mammals for substances with a low A/D ratio. For instance, benzene has a mammalian A/D ratio of 0.6; in hydra the ratio is 0.4. In other words, the conceptus is less vulnerable to adverse effects due to this substance than is the adult. The adult protects the conceptus from any adverse developmental toxicological effects of benzene. Once this is established and understood, there is no longer a justification for testing benzene in any more pregnant rats and rabbits. Substances with larger A/D ratios (10 and higher) will still need to be tested in pregnant mammals in order to determine the no observed effect level.

The hydra assay allows one to predict accurately the A/D ratio as it will occur in mammals. It does as well as laboratory mammals in indicating which substances need exposure controls only on the basis of adult toxic levels. It also tells us which substances are uniquely hazardous to development in mammals and are, therefore, in need of an extra safety factor of exposure to protect the conceptus. It even allows objective determination of the safety factor's magnitude. Thus far, the hydra assay proves incapable of consistently estimating the actual adult and developmentally toxic doses in any mammal. Therefore, it must not be considered as a valid means for risk estimation; it is only a system for detecting hazards and ranking them according to their developmental toxicity potential. As such, it also (1) eliminates the need for testing many substances in pregnant mammals, (2) focuses attention on substances meriting close examination for developmental toxicity, (3) provides the industrial toxicologist with a reliable and objective means for advising management regarding the developmental hazard posed by each of a series of acceptable alternatives or substitution forms and (4) can identify work places safe for women of child-bearing age because of its ability to screen large numbers of chemicals, quickly and at low cost.

ACKNOWLEDGEMENT

This research was aided by Reproductive Hazards in the Workplace Research grant No. 15-19 from the March of Dimes Birth Defects Foundation.

REFERENCES

1. Johnson, E. M. (1980). Screening for teratogenic potential: are we asking the proper question? *Teratology*, **21**, 259
2. Nelson, M. M. (1955). Mammalian fetal development and antimetabolites. In *Antimetabolites and Cancer*, American Association for the Advancement of Science, New York, pp. 107-128
3. Kalter, H. and Warkany, J. (1959). Experimental production of congenital malformations by metabolic procedure. *Physiol. Rev.*, **39**, 69-115
4. Johnson, E. M. and Nelson, M. M. (1959). Morphological changes in embryonic development resulting from transitory pteroylglutamic acid (PGA) deficiency early in pregnancy. *Anat. Rec.*, **133**, 294
5. Johnson, E. M., Nelson, M. M. and Monie, I. W. (1963). Effects of transitory pteroylglutamic acid (PGA) deficiency on embryonic and placental development in the rat. *Anat. Rec.*, **146**, 215-224
6. Karnofsky, D. A. (1965). Mechanisms of action of certain growth-inhibiting drugs. In Wilson, J. E. and Warkany, J. (Eds.), *Teratology: Principles and Techniques*, University of Chicago Press, Chicago, pp. 185-213
7. Ross, R. B. and Johnson, M. C. (1972). Isolated cleft palate-embryogenesis, epidemiology and etiology. In *Cleft Lip and Palate*, Williams and Wilkins, Baltimore, pp. 47-67

8. Fraser, F. C. (1968). Workshop on embryology of cleft lip and cleft palate. *Teratology*, 1, 353–358

9. Taylor, R. G. (1978). Craniofacial growth during closure of the secondary palate in the hamster. *J. Anat.*, 125, 361–370

10. Long, S. Y., Larsson, K. S. and Lohmander, S. (1973). Cell proliferation in the cranial base of A/J mice with 6-AN-induced cleft palate. *Teratology*, 8, 137–138

11. Brinkley, L. L. and Vickerman, M. M. (1979). Elevation of lesioned palatal shelves *in vitro. J. Embryol. Exp. Morphol.*, 54, 229–240

12. Greene, R. M. and Pratt, R. M. (1976). Developmental aspects of secondary palate formation. *J. Embryol. Exp. Morphol.*, 36, 225–245

13. Wee, E. L. and Zimmerman, E. F. (1980). Palate morphogenesis. II. Contraction of cytoplasmic processes in ATP-induced palate rotation in glycerinated mouse heads. *Teratology*, 21, 15–27

14. Zimmerman, E. F., Wee, E. L., Phillips, N. and Roberts, N. (1981). Presence of serotonin in the palate just prior to shelf elevation. *J. Embryol. Exp. Morphol.*, 64, 233–250

15. Pratt, R. M. and Greene, R. M. (1976). Inhibition of palatal epithelial cell death by altered protein synthesis. *Dev. Biol.*, 54, 135–145

16. Pratt, R. M. Figueroa, A. A., Greene, R. M. and Salomon, D. S. (1979). Alterations in macromolecular synthesis and function during abnormal palatal development. In Persaud, T. V. N. (Ed.), *Advances in the Study of Birth Defects*, Vol. 3, *Abnormal Embryogenesis: Cellular and Molecular Aspects*, MTP Press, Lancaster, pp. 161–176

17. Wilson, J. G. (1973). *Environment and Birth Defects*, Academic Press, New York

18. Fabro, S. (1981). The biochemical basis of thalidomide teratogenicity. In Juchau, M. R. (Ed.), *The Biochemical Basis of Chemical Teratogenesis*, Elsevier/North-Holland, New York, pp. 159–178

19. Chernoff, N. and Kavlock, R. J. (1982). An *in vivo* teratology screen utilizing pregnant mice. *J. Toxicol. Environ. Hlth.*, 10, 541–550

20. Chernoff, N. and Kavlock, R. J. (1983). A teratology test system which utilizes postnatal growth and viability in the mouse. In Waters, M. D., Sandu, S. S., Lewtas, J., Claston, L., Chernoff, N. and Nesnow, S. (Eds.), *Short-term Bioassays in the Analysis of Complex Environmental Mixtures*, Vol. III, Plenum, New York, pp. 417–427

21. Johnson, E. M. (1981). Screening for teratogenic hazards: nature of the problems. *Ann. Rev. Pharmacol. Toxicol.*, 21, 417–429

22. Johnson, E. M., Gorman, R. M., Gabel, B. E. G. and George, M. E. (1982). The *Hydra attenuata* system for detection of teratogenic hazards. *Teratogen. Carcinogen. Mutagen.*, 2, 263–276

23. Chun, Y. H., Johnson, E. M. and Gabel, B. E. G. (1983a). Relationship of developmental stage to effects of vinblastine on the artificial 'embryo' of hydra. *Teratology*, 27, 95–100

24. Chun, Y. H., Johnson, E. M., Gabel, B. E. G. and Cadogan, A. S. A. (1983b). Regeneration of dissociated adult hydra cells: a histologic study. *Teratology*, 27, 81–87

25. Johnson, E. M. and Gabel, B. E. G. (1982). Application of the hydra assay for rapid detection of developmental hazards. *J. Am. Col. Toxicol.*, 1, 57–71

26. Johnson, E. M. and Gabel, B. E. G. (1983). An artificial 'embryo' for detection of abnormal developmental biology. *Fund. Appl. Toxicol.*, 3, 243–249.

27. OECD, Paris (1981). *OECD Guidelines for Testing of Chemicals*
28. Arcos, J. C. (1983). Comparative requirements for premarketing/premanufacture notifications in EC Countries and the USA, with special reference to risk assessment in the framework of the US Toxic Substances Control Act (TSCA). *J. Am. Col. Toxicol.*, **2**, 131–145

12

What Evidence is Required to Identify a Chemical as a Reproductive Hazard?

DONALD R. MATTISON

Existing social data suggest that men and women generally do not alter their life styles, personal habits, jobs or hobbies prior to or during pregnancy. Therefore, to identify and understand the site and mechanism of action of a reproductive toxin, it is necessary to consider the influence of xenobiotic exposures on pre-, peri- and post-conception events.

Fortunately, our ability to identify the sites and mechanisms of action of reproductive toxins is increasing[1]. If this volume had been prepared 2 years ago, there would have been only a few references available: (1) *Guidelines on Pregnancy and Work*, compiled by the American College of Obstetricians and Gynecologists[2]; (2) *Proceedings* of a *Conference on Women and the Workplace*, sponsored by the Society for Occupational and Environmental Health[3]; and (3) the NIEHS *Target Organ Toxicity* conference proceedings devoted to gonadal and endocrine toxicity[4,5].

During recent years there has been a flurry of publications reflecting increased interest in reproductive toxicology. These new publications include: *Work and the Health of Women*, by Hunt[6]; *Guidelines for Studies of Human Populations Exposed to Mutagenic and Reproductive Hazards*, by Bloom, prepared in response to the Love Canal tragedy[7]; *Health Effects of Environmental Chemicals on the Adult Human Reproductive System*, an annotated bibliography prepared by the National Library of Medicine[8]; *Reproductive Hazards of Industrial Chemicals*, by Barlow and Sullivan, a critical and exhaustive review of the reproductive and mutagenic effects of 48 commonly used industrial chemicals[9]; and *Reproductive Toxicology*, an overview of the diverse sciences which make up reproductive toxicology and consideration of epidemiological and social issues[10]. There are several sources addressing specific issues in reproductive toxicology, including: *Pregnant and Mining: A Handbook for Pregnant Miners*[11]; and *Reproductive Toxicology, A Medical Letter on Environmental Hazards to Reproduction*[12]. Several additional resources will also be published in the coming year: the World Health Organization, through the Scientific Group on

153

Methodologies for the Safety Evaluation of Chemicals sponsored a meeting on the effects of xenobiotics on reproduction in Ispra, Italy in the spring of 1981[13]; the Finnish Institutes of Occupational Health held a meeting on *Occupational Hazards and Reproduction* at Kaupunkiopisto, outside Helsinki, in the summer of 1981[14]; and the University of Rochester and the Permanent Commission on the Occupational Hazards of Metals held a conference on *The Reproductive and Developmental Toxicity of Metals* in the summer of 1982[15]. In addition, there are more than a dozen similar volumes in pre-publication stages.

REPRODUCTIVE TOXICOLOGY

Reproductive toxicology is unique for several reasons: (1) it is a young science, as attested by the rapid growth of publications; (2) it is at the interface of several established sciences (figure 12.1), each with its own language and methodology; and (3) it deals with sexual medicine[16]. These aspects of the subject require that we use bias-free language understood by the diverse sciences which make up reproductive toxicology. To foster this interaction it is useful to begin by defining

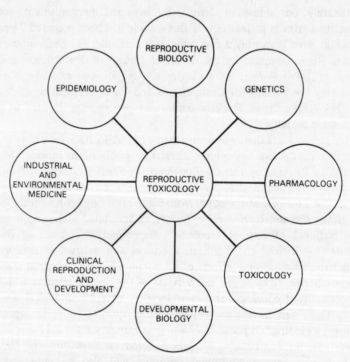

Figure 12.1 The hybrid nature of reproductive toxicology, at the interface between several established sciences, is emphasised in this figure

successful reproduction, then reproductive failure. Using those definitions, it will be possible to define the criteria necessary for identification of the site and mechanism of action of reproductive toxins.

Successful reproduction

A simplistic definition of successful reproduction is the production of a healthy offspring. Unfortunately for many organisms, including humans, this definition is inadequate, because reproduction is not without cost in terms of time, energy and resources of the parental organisms or family unit. This suggests that not only does the offspring have to be healthy, but also it must be delivered during the appropriate season, or time in the life cycle of the parental organisms. A more complete definition of successful reproduction may be the production of healthy offspring at the appropriate time in the life cycle of the parents.

Reproductive toxin

Using this definition of successful reproduction, a reproductive toxin is any xenobiotic or biotic compound which can alter the timely expression of reproduction, either by blocking the production of healthy offspring when fertility is desired or by stimulating fertility when contraception is desired.

Enhanced fertility

Although our main focus is on exposures which impair fertility or alter the production of healthy offspring, it is important to recognise that there are xenobiotics which can alter the effectiveness of oral contraceptives. There are a diverse group of compounds which act to induce hepatic and extrahepatic microsomal cytochrome P45-dependent mono-oxygenase, a group of enzymes important in oxidative metabolism of many endogenous and exogenous compounds[17]. These mono-oxygenases play an important role in the clearance of steroid hormones. Patients taking the currently recommended low-dose oral contraceptives who are treated with, or exposed to, compounds which increase hepatic clearance of the contraceptive steroids can have the effectiveness of their contraceptives impaired or abolished. In clinical settings this has been reported for several drugs[18,19]. This form of reproductive toxicity, enhanced fertility when contraception is desired, has not been explored to my knowledge in an occupational setting.

Another interesting interaction which has not been investigated is the effect of cigarette smoking, known to induce several hepatic mono-oxygenases, and oral contraceptive effectiveness[20]. Enhanced fertility, or contraceptive failure, is not a trivial issue; for example, a patient taking anticonvulsants may be using contraceptives to avoid pregnancy, with its associated risk of fetal hydantoin syndrome. Alternatively, the patient may be using another drug known or suspected to be teratogenic. Contraceptive failure, especially among those who do not accept abortion, can be enormously stressful for the woman, her family and her physician.

HUMAN REPRODUCTIVE TOXINS

Having established a working definition of successful reproduction and reproductive toxicity, it is appropriate to consider identification of reproductive toxins in humans. One source for exploring suspected reproductive toxins is the annotated bibliography published by the National Library of Medicine, which collects the approximately 270 articles published between 1963 and 1981 dealing with effects of xenobiotics on human reproduction[8]. Slightly less than half of these articles dealt with effects on the male, and the rest with effects on the female, reproductive system. These data emphasise that it is important to consider the effects of xenobiotics on reproductive end-points mediated through the male, such as spermatogenesis, libido, spontaneous abortion or congenital malformation.

Since our focus is on female reproduction, it is useful to dissect the reproductive events reported altered (table 12.1). About 45 per cent of the reports dealt with adverse effects associated with miscarriage or pregnancy toxicity — that is, compounds suspected to be embryotoxins, fetotoxins, placental toxins or teratogens.

Table 12.1 Adverse effects of xenobiotics on female reproductive function

Adverse effect	Site of toxicity[a]	Reported (%)
Miscarriage	E, F, P, O, U, C	23
Pregnancy	E, F, P, O, U, C	21
Menstruation	H, Pi, O, U	18
Genitalia	S	10
Fertility	H, Pi, O, U, T	8
Ovary	H, Pi, O	7
Hormones	H, Pi, O	5
Uterus	U	4
Cervix	C	3
Vagina	S	1
Libido	CNS, H, Pi, O	1

[a]Key for site of toxicity: E = embryo, F = fetus, P = placenta, H = hypothalamus, Pi = pituitary; O = ovary, S = skin, C = cervix, U = uterus, CNS = central nervous system, T = fallopian tube.

Spontaneous abortion

It is instructive to explore a small sub-set of this topic relating to spontaneous abortion[21]. Several studies have suggested a relationship between occupational exposures and recognised spontaneous abortion[22]. A recent study by Hemminki *et al.* focused on spontaneous abortion in a Finnish mining community[23]. These authors made two fascinating observations suggesting: (1) seasonal variations in spontaneous abortions and (2) work-related increases in the frequency of spontaneous abortion. The lowest rate in spontaneous abortions was observed in the summer months, May–August, and the highest rate was observed in the late winter and early spring, January–April. The other interesting observation concerned the effect of work status on spontaneous abortion. Among women employed outside the home, the rate of spontaneous abortion was about twice the rate observed in women who did not work outside the home.

Two important factors must be considered with respect to these observations.

First, these are recognised, hospital-treated, spontaneous abortions obtained by linkage of hospital discharge data with census data. In the USA a study like this would be difficult to conduct because of the inability to link databases. Additionally, incomplete ascertainment may also impair such a study. For example, it has been estimated that 40 per cent of recognised first trimester spontaneous abortions in New York City do not seek medical care[7]. With decreasing proportions of women seeking prenatal care, our ability to monitor xenobiotic influences on recognised spontaneous abortion may be diminishing.

Second, it is important to recognise that this study deals with recognised spontaneous abortions, a category which may only reflect half of the total spontaneous abortion rate. Using sensitive radioimmunoassays for the β-subunit of HCG, it is possible to monitor populations attempting pregnancy and ascertain the frequency of recognised and unrecognised spontaneous abortion, two events which may represent different sites and mechanisms of reproductive impairment[21].

In one study 207 cycles were monitored; of those cycles, 198 were ovulatory and 118 had elevated HCG, but only 51 had clinically recognised pregnancies, 6 with recognised spontaneous abortions[24]. If the individuals with elevated HCG are normalised, about 45 per cent of the pregnant women had clinically recognisable pregnancies and about 50 per cent had unrecognised spontaneous abortions. These data suggest that it is necessary to take a very critical look at the effects of xenobiotics on both recognised and unrecognised (or clinical and sub-clinical) spontaneous abortion rates.

Ovarian function

I should now like to explore an area of female reproductive function which may contribute to recognised and unrecognised spontaneous abortions – that of functional ovarian competence. The second-largest category of adverse reproductive effects reported in the NLM bibliography involved toxicity to menstruation, fertility, ovarian function and hormone metabolism, all suggesting toxicity along the hypothalamic–pituitary–ovarian (HPO) axis (table 12.1).

In a sexually mature female successful reproduction requires integrated function of the HPO axis. The hypothalamus functions in a permissive role, releasing pulses of GnRH which reach the pituitary through a portal system[25]. In the pituitary GnRH acts to allow pituitary response to ovarian or extraovarian steroids, producing both long- and short-term variations in the release of the gonadotrophins FSH and LH[26]. The controlling element of the primate reproductive cycle is through the dominant follicle complex[27,28]. The follicle complex, composed of oocyte, granulosa cells, basement membrane and surrounding thecal cells, is the basic functional unit of the ovary.

Xenobiotics which alter the hormonal interactions along the HPO axis, or alter hypothalamic, pituitary, ovarian or endometrial function, may impair fertility. In my laboratory and among my patients at the National Institutes of Health I have been exploring the site and mechanisms of action of reproductive toxins which may contribute to unexplained infertility or spontaneous abortion. We have followed this line of research, combining common exposures with measures of reproductive function. Two major focal points for this research have been effects of smoking or of xenobiotics on ovarian function and fertility in women, non-human primates and rodents, and they illustrate one procedure which may be used to identify the site and mechanism of action of a reproductive toxin.

Ovarian toxicity

One common exposure is cigarette smoking, reported to increase the frequency of recognised spontaneous abortions of chromosomally normal conceptuses[7,20]. Interestingly, cigarette smoking has also been reported to increase infertility. In a retrospective study by Tokuhato the incidence of infertility, defined as never being pregnant throughout the total reproductive life of the woman, was about 12 per cent among white non-smokers, while among the white smokers it was 18 per cent[29]. Approximately 19 per cent of the non-white non-smokers were infertile, while among smokers 28 per cent were infertile. While we know that smoking has pleiotropic effects on the female reproductive system, our particular interest has focused on smoking effects on the follicular complex, because it may explain the increased frequency of spontaneous abortion and infertility among smokers.

The upper portion of figure 12.2 summarises circulating levels of FSH, LH, oestradiol and progesterone in a normal ovarian cycle. The cycle is defined as

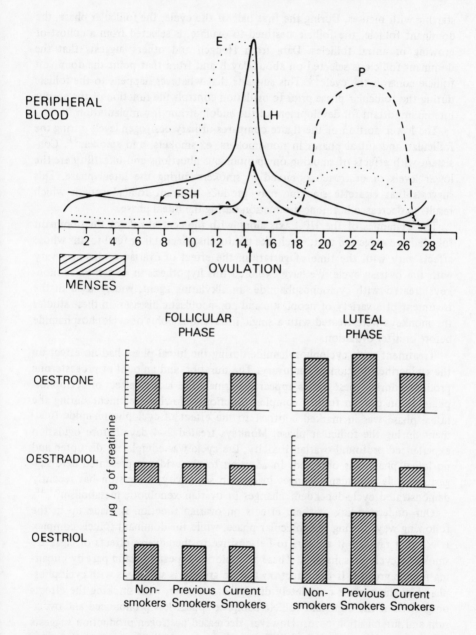

Figure 12.2 Circulating levels of FSH, LH, oestradiol and progesterone in a typical menstrual cycle are demonstrated in the upper portion of this figure. Underneath the cycle are bar graphs indicating the urinary levels of oestrone (E_1), oestradiol (E_2) and oestriol (E_3) in the luteal and proliferative phases of the menstrual cycle. Data from reference 31

starting with menses. During the first half of the cycle, the follicular phase, the dominant follicle, the follicle destined to ovulate, is selected from a cohort of growing or antral follicles. Data from Hodgen and others suggests that the dominant follicle is selected on about day 8 and from that point the dominant follicle controls the cycle[28]. This suggests that whatever happens to the follicle during the follicular phase prior to ovulation controls the function of the corpus luteum important for development of the endometrium for implantation[30].

The lower portion of the figure compares urinary oestrogen levels during the follicular and luteal phases in non-smokers, ex-smokers, and smokers[31]. Consistent with effects of smoking on spontaneous abortions and infertility are the lower levels of oestrogen observed in smokers during the luteal phase. This suggests that cigarette smoking may produce aberrant folliculogenesis which results in decreased hormone production during the luteal phase.

The dynamics of the HPO axis along with the central role of the dominant follicle have suggested that, much like teratogens, placental or fetal toxins whose effects vary with the time of gestation, the effect of ovarian toxins may vary with the ovarian cycle. We have explored this hypothesis in *Cynomolgus* monkeys treated with cyclophosphamide, an alkylating agent, widely used in the treatment of a variety of neoplastic and non-neoplastic diseases. In these studies the monkeys were treated with a single intravenous bolus of cyclophosphamide before or after ovulation.

Treatment with cyclophosphamide during the luteal phase had no effect on the endocrine function of the ovary. The duration and amount of progesterone produced during these cycles appeared normal. The lack of effect of cyclophosphamide on ovarian follicle complex function following treatment during the luteal phase was in marked contrast to the effect of cyclophosphamide treatment during the follicular phase. Monkeys treated 2–4 days before ovulation experienced profound ovarian toxicity, the cycle was completely disrupted and no luteal phase was observed. In addition to the evidence presented here suggesting cycle-dependent changes in ovarian sensitivity, Bengtsson has recently demonstrated cycle-dependent changes in ovarian xenobiotic metabolism[37,38].

Our understanding of these effects on ovarian function is made up in the following way. During the follicular phase, while the dominant follicle complex is growing rapidly, it appears to be sensitive to the adverse effects of cigarette smoke or cyclophosphamide. These xenobiotics appear to act in part by impairing follicle growth. If the effect on follicle growth is severe, as with cyclophosphamide, the cycle is completely disrupted. However, with smoking the effects on growth of the dominant follicle complex appear less pronounced and ovulation and luteinisation occur. However, decreased oestrogen production suggests that full development of the follicle complex is impaired. The amount of progesterone produced during the luteal phase may be decreased in smokers. With decreased luteal function endometrial development may be impaired, and an increase in the frequency of spontaneous abortion of chromosomally normal conceptuses occurs.

Age of menopause

Interestingly, the effect of smoking on luteal function and fertility is not the only adverse effect observed on ovarian function. One prominent effect of smoking is a decrease in the age of spontaneous menopause[20]. Data collected by Jick[32] from women in the USA and Europe demonstrate the effect of smoking on the age of menopause. The median age of menopause was over 50 in non-smokers in both populations, and was decreased by 2 years in the women smoking one or more packs of cigarettes per day. Those smoking half a pack per day had their median age of menopause moved back 1 year. Other studies have confirmed this observation, with some suggesting an even greater effect on the age of menopause. For example, one study has suggested as much as 4 years' decrease in age of menopause per pack of cigarettes smoked[33].

We have been exploring the mechanism of this effect on the age of menopause using experimental studies with ovarian toxins in rodents and computer models of the functional lifespan of the ovary. The rodent studies have been complex and comprehensive, exploring effects of benzo(a)pyrene (BP), a cigarette smoke component, on follicle complex destruction and subsequent effects on fertility[34]. The rodent studies demonstrate that BP, a polycyclic aromatic hydrocarbon, is an indirect ovarian toxin, requiring metabolism before producing follicle destruction[1,34]. Dose–response curves following intraperitoneal treatment with BP derivatives suggests that one pathway to an ultimate follicle toxin was through the formation of the 7,8-diol (figure 12.3). Subsequent studies using intraovarian treatment with BP and BP metabolites have confirmed the intraperitoneal data and suggest that the 7,8-diol-9,10-epoxide is an ultimate follicle toxin.

Our present understanding is that follicle destruction produced by BP requires formation of the 7,8-oxide, hydration to the 7,8-diol and recycling of the diol through the mono-oxygenases to form the diol-epoxide which is the reactive species responsible for follicle destruction.

The computer model, based on human data collected by Block[35,36], is a simple one with two parameters: oocyte number at birth and rate of atresia from birth. Using this model, we have explored the effect of alterations in oocyte number or rate of atresia on the age of menopause. The model suggests a direct relationship between the rate of atresia and the age of menopause. In contrast, variations in oocyte number have a weak effect on the age of menopause. This suggests that factors governing the rate of atresia are more important in determining the age of menopause than factors governing oocyte number.

In summary, we think we have identified the site and mechanism of reproductive toxicity produced by BP, a prototype ovarian toxin. BP and presumably other ovarian toxins can act by three pathways: (1) distribution to the ovary and metabolic activation by ovarian enzymes; (2) metabolic activation by extraovarian (hepatic) enzymes with distribution of reactive metabolites to the ovary; (3) metabolic co-operation between extraovarian and ovarian enzymes. The site

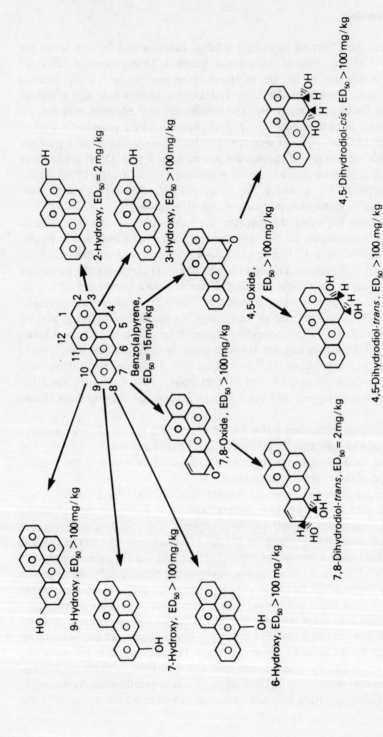

Figure 12.3 Oocyte destruction following intraperitoneal treatment with BP or indicated derivative. C57BL/6N mice were treated with doses ranging from 1 to 100 mg/kg and were sacrificed 14 days later, and oocyte destruction was determined for calculation of estimated dose which destroys 50 per cent of the oocytes (ED₅₀)

2-Hydroxy, ED₅₀ = 2 mg/kg

3-Hydroxy, ED₅₀ > 100 mg/kg

Benzo(a)pyrene, ED₅₀ = 15 mg/kg

4,5-Oxide, ED₅₀ > 100 mg/kg

4,5-Dihydrodiol-*cis*, ED₅₀ > 100 mg/kg

4,5-Dihydrodiol-*trans*, ED₅₀ > 100 mg/kg

7,8-Oxide, ED₅₀ > 100 mg/kg

7,8-Dihydrodiol-*trans*, ED₅₀ = 2 mg/kg

9-Hydroxy, ED₅₀ > 100 mg/kg

7-Hydroxy, ED₅₀ > 100 mg/kg

6-Hydroxy, ED₅₀ > 100 mg/kg

of action appears to be within the ovary, where the toxic metabolite (7,8-diol-9, 10-epoxide) acts on the follicle, destroying either the oocyte directly or the oocyte–granulosa cell interactions necessary for support of the oocyte.

CONCLUSIONS

The ovary is sensitive to the adverse effects of xenobiotic compounds which can alter the gamete or endocrine functions of the ovary. Toxic effects which impair follicular development and alter the endocrine function of the ovary may act to increase the frequency of spontaneous abortions. The sensitivity of the ovary to endocrine and perhaps gamete toxicity is not consistent but varies during the cycle. The most sensitive phase of the ovarian cycle appears to be after selection of the dominant follicle and before ovulation. Gamete toxicity has also been demonstrated in rodents, non-human primates and women. Gamete toxicity may act simply to destroy oocytes; the role of ovotoxicity and congenital malformation remains to be explored.

REFERENCES

1. Mattison, D. R. (1983). The mechanisms of action of reproductive toxins. In D. R. Mattison (Ed.), *Reproductive Toxicology*, Alan R. Liss, New York, pp. 65–79
2. American College of Obstetricians and Gynecologists (1978). *Guidelines on Pregnancy and Work*, Contract #210-76-0159, DHEW (NIOSH) Publication, Rockville, Maryland, 78–118
3. Bingham, E. (Ed.) (1977). *Proceedings Conference on Women and the Workplace*, Society for Occupational and Environmental Health, 364
4. Dixon, R. L. (1978). Symposium on Target Organ Toxicity: Gonads (reproductive and genetic toxicity). *Environ. Hlth Perspect.*, **24**, 1–128
5. Korach, K. S., Thomas, J. A. and McLachlan, J. A. (1981). Target organ toxicity: endocrine system. *Environ. Hlth Perspect.*, **38**, 1–146
6. Hunt, V. R. (1978). *Work and the Health of Women*, CRC Press, Florida, 236
7. Bloom, A. D. (1981). *Guidelines for Studies of Human Populations Exposed to Mutagenic and Reproductive Hazards*, March of Dimes Birth Defects Foundation, New York, 163
8. Pruett, J. G. and Winslow, S. G. (1982). *Health Effects of Environmental Chemicals on Human Reproduction. A Selected Bibliography with Abstracts, 1963–1981*, NLM/TIRC-82/1, Bethesda, Maryland
9. Barlow, S. M. and Sullivan, F. M. (1982). *Reproductive Hazards of Industrial Chemicals*, Academic Press
10. Mattison, D. R. (Ed.) (1983). *Reproductive Toxicology*, Alan R. Liss, New York

11. Bell, B. and Rostan, J. (1982). *Pregnant and Mining: A Handbook for Pregnant Miners*, Coal Employment Project and Coal Mining Womens Support Team, Oak Ridge, Tennessee, 38
12. Fabro, S., Brown, N. A. and Scialli, A. R. (Eds.). *Reproductive Toxicology, A Medical Letter on Environmental Hazards to Reproduction*, Reproductive Toxicology Center, Columbia Hospital for Women, Washington, D. C. (published bimonthly)
13. Vouk, V. B. and Sheehan, P. J. (Eds.) (1983). *Methods for Assessing the Effects of Chemicals on Reproductive Functions*, Wiley, New York
14. Hemminki, K. (Ed) (1983). *Occupational Hazards and Reproduction*, Hemisphere, New York
15. Clarkson, T. and Nordberg, G. (Eds.) (1983). *The Reproductive and Developmental Toxicity of Metals*, Plenum, New York
16. Kolodiny, R. C., Masters, W. H. and Johnson, V. E. (1979). *Textbook of Sexual Medicine*, Little, Brown, Boston
17. Conney, A. H. (1982). Induction of microsomal enzymes by foreign chemicals and carcinogenesis by polycyclic aromatic hydrocarbons. *Cancer Res.*, **42**, 4875–4917
18. Mattison, D. R., Nightingale, M. S. and Shiromizu, K. (1983). Effects of toxic substances on female reproduction. *Environ. Hlth Perspect.*, **48**, 42–52
19. Aronson, J. K. and Grahame-Smith, D. G. (1981). Clinical pharmacology, adverse drug interactions. *Br. Med. J.*, **282**, 288–291
20. Mattison, D. R. (1982). The effects of smoking on fertility from gametogenesis to implantation. *Environ. Res.*, **28**, 410–433
21. Wilcox, A. J. (1983). Surveillance of pregnancy loss in human populations. In D. R. Mattison (Ed.), *Reproductive Toxicology*, Liss, New York, 285–292
22. Hemminki, K., Axelson, O., Niemi, M.-L. and Ahlborg, G. (1983). Assessment of methods and results of reproductive occupational epidemiology: spontaneous abortions and malformations in the offspring of working women. In D. R. Mattison (Ed.), *Reproductive Toxicology*, Alan R. Liss, New York, pp. 293–307
23. Hemminki, K., Kyyronen, P., Niemi, M.-L., Koskinen, K., Sallmen, M. and Vainio, H. (1983). Spontaneous abortions in an industrialized community in Finland. *Am. J. Publ. Hlth*, **73**, 32–37
24. Edmonds, D. K., Lindsay, K. S., Miller, J. F., Williamson, E. and Wood, P. J. (1982). Early embryonic mortality in women. *Fertil. Steril.*, **38**, 447–453
25. Takizawa, K. and Mattison, D. R. (1983). Female reproduction. In D. R. Mattison (Ed.), *Reproductive Toxicology*, Alan R. Liss, New York, pp. 17–30
26. Knobil, E. (1980). The neuroendocrine control of gonadotropin secretion in the rhesus monkey. *Recent Prog. Horm. Res.*, **36**, 53–58
27. Mattison, D. R. and Ross, G. T. (1984). Laboratory methods for evaluating and predicting specific reproductive dysfunctions: oogenesis and ovulation. In V. B. Vouk and P. J. Sheehan (Eds.), *Methods for Assessing the Effects of Chemicals on Reproductive Functions* (in press)
28. Hodgen, G. D. (1982). The dominant ovarian follicle. *Fertil. Steril.*, **38**, 281–300
29. Tokuhatu, G. M. (1968). Smoking in relation to infertility and fetal loss. *Arch. Environ. Hlth*, **17**, 353–359
30. diZerega, G. S. and Hodgen, G. D. (1981). Luteal phase dysfunction infertility: a sequel to aberrant folliculogenesis. *Fertil. Steril.*, **35**, 489–499

31. MacMahon, B., Trichopoulos, D., Cole, P. and Brown, J. (1982). Cigarette smoking and urinary estrogens. *New Engl. J. Med.*, **307**, 1062–1065
32. Jick, H., Porter, J. and Morrison, A. S. (1977). Relation between smoking and age of natural menopause. *Lancet*, **1**, 1354–1355
33. Daniell, H. W. (1976). Osteoporosis and the slender smoker. *Arch. Intern. Med.*, **136**, 298–304
34. Mattison, D. R., Shiromizu, K. and Nightingale, M. S. (1983). Oocyte destruction by polycyclic aromatic hydrocarbons. In D. R. Mattison (Ed.), *Reproductive Toxicology*, Alan R. Liss, New York, pp. 191–202
35. Block, E. (1951). Quantitative morphological investigations of the follicular system in women. Methods of quantitative determinations. *Acta Anat. Scand.*, **12**, 267–285
36. Block, E. (1952). Quantitative morphological investigations of the follicular system in women. Variations at different ages. *Acta Anat. Scand.*, **14**, 108–123
37. Bengtsson, M. and Rydstrom, J. (1983). Regulation of carcinogen metabolism in the rat ovary by the estrous cycle and gonadotropin. *Science, N.Y.*, **219**, 1437–1438
38. Bengtsson, M., Montelius, J., Mankowitz, L. and Rydstrom, J. (1983). Metabolism of polycyclic aromatic hydrocarbons in the rat ovary. Comparison with metabolism in adrenal and liver tissues. *Biochem. Pharmacol.*, **32**, 129–136

13

Animal and Human Studies in Genetic Toxicology

M. S. LEGATOR and J. B. WARD, JR.

Although a great deal of justified attention has been focused on the vulnerability of the fetus following *in utero* exposure to toxic chemicals, recent scientific evidence would suggest the importance of chemically induced genetic lesions during spermatogenesis and their possible adverse health outcome. Rather than discussing the hazards of chemicals to pregnant women at work, it may be more appropriate to discuss the risk to the fetus from parental exposure, recognising the role of both male and female exposure in transmission of deleterious health outcomes. These effects to the fetus should be viewed as a continuum from pre-zygotic chemical exposure to chemical effects during *in utero* exposure, and effects that may not be apparent for several generations. Tables 13.1-13.3 describe possible adverse health outcomes to female reproductive function, to male reproductive health outcomes and to the fetus following exposure to chemical or physical agents[1].

Several procedures exist in animals for identifying transmissible genetic abnormalities, including such procedures as the dominant lethal test, heritable

Table 13.1 Possible adverse effects of occupational exposure to chemical or physical agents on female reproductive function

---

Ovulation disorders
Oligomenorrhoea
Amenorrhoea
Dysfunctional uterine bleeding
Premature ovarian failure
Inhibited sexual desire
Hyperprolactinaemia
Impaired fertility
Spontaneous abortion
Premature labour
Chromosomal abnormalities

Table 13.2   Possible adverse effects of occupational exposure to chemical or physical agents on male reproductive function

Abnormal sperm production
Oligospermia or azoospermia
Abnormal sperm morphology
Decreased sperm motility
Abnormal sperm function
Decreased ability to penetrate oocyte
Abnormal sexual function
Inhibited sexual function
Impotence
Ejaculatory disorders
Abnormal sperm transport
Chromosomal abnormalities

Table 13.3   Possible adverse effects of occupational exposure to chemical or physical agents on the fetus

Spontaneous abortion
Chromosomal abnormalities
Congenital malformations
Fetal growth retardation
Altered sex ratio
Pre- or intrapartum fetal distress (low Apgar score)
Fetal demise
Neonatal death
Developmental disabilities
Behaviour disorders
Childhood illness
Childhood malignancies

translocation and specific locus test. Many of the commonly used procedures, however, do not detect final adverse health outcomes but detect the early steps in a process that may lead to the final expression of a disease. Adduct formation, alkaline elution, repair induction, metaphase analysis, sister chromatid exchange, unscheduled DNA synthesis and sperm morphology studies are all procedures in animals that measure early, and in some cases indirect, events in a process that may eventually lead to genetic abnormalities and cancer. Table 13.4 is a summary of reproductive effects associated with parental exposure, with the few chemicals that have been studied in human subjects[1]. The largest database in humans has to do with indirect short-term indicators for phenotypic expression of adverse health outcomes.

With our limited ability to ascertain actual transmissible disease risk after chemical exposure with many procedures in animals and in almost all cases in man, we shall describe briefly some exciting new developments linking

Table 13.4 Adverse reproductive effects associated with parental exposure

Effect	Altered fertility	Spontaneous abortion	Low birth weight	Developmental disability	Birth defects	Childhood cancer	Mental disorders	Decreased libido
Paternal exposure								
Anaesthetic gases	+	+	+					
Vinyl chloride	+	+						
Irradiation	+							
Chloroprene		+			+		+	
Lead	+	+			+	+		
Hydrocarbons	+					+[a]		
Solvents	+							
trichloroethylene	+	+[a]					+	
EDB	+	+					+	
DBCP	+	+	+					
carbon disulphide	+		+					
Kepone	+	+						
Oral contraceptives	+							
Microwaves	+							
Maternal exposure								
Anaesthetic gases		+	+		+			
Irradiation			+		+			
Methyl mercury				+	+			
Lead	+	+	+		+		+	
PCBs					+			
Formaldehyde		+			+			
2,4,5-T		+						
Oral contraceptives	+							

[a] Positive but questionable data.
Modified from reference 1.

behavioural anomalies and cancer to parental exposure to chemicals. We shall review the role of available short-term animal and human monitoring procedures for predicting disease outcomes, specifically the link between cytogenetic damage and cancer, as well as the genetic basis for teratogenic responses. We shall then consider our present ability to monitor high-risk populations by a battery of short-term tests and suggest that these procedures may be the optimum approach for detecting chemicals that have the potential to induce reproductive problems in addition to cancer.

PARENTAL TRANSMISSION OF BEHAVIOURAL ANOMALIES AND CANCER

A series of recent investigations may well add a new dimension in our ability to evaluate chemicals for the induction of transmissible genetic damage and, if we can extrapolate from animal data, alert us to the profound importance of genetic effects produced by chemicals in man. With human subjects there are numerous examples of the association between mental retardation and autosomal chromosomal syndromes as well as between inborn errors of metabolism and mental retardation. Several studies at the University of Texas Medical Branch in Galveston reported behavioural anomalies in F_1 progeny of rats following treatment of the male parent with the known alkylating agent cyclophosphamide[2-5]. These studies would indicate a specific genetic lesion induced during post-meiotic stages of spermatogenesis which resulted in a significant increase in behavioural anomalies in the progeny. Similar results were reported by Schroeder, who found behavioural effects in mice progeny following parental exposure to radiation and chemicals[6]. The work of Brady *et al.* also described a gametotoxic effect in rats treated with lead which includes behavioural anomalies in the F_1[7]. These studies may indicate that the behavioural end-point is polygenic and a general consequence of potential exposure to genotoxic agents. In addition to behavioural anomalies, Tomatis *et al.*[8] found that transmission via germ cells induced an increase in brain cancer in F_1 progeny of mice following paternal exposure to ethylnitrosourea. Together these studies suggest that genetic lesions during spermatogenesis may play a role in the transmission of behavioural changes as well as cancer to the offspring of the treated male. These findings may have profound significance in implicating the role of chemically induced transmissible genetic damage in man and could also serve as a valuable approach for detecting mutagenic agents in animals. Our ability to detect these effects in human studies, as is the case with all reproductive and chronic effects, is limited.

EPIDEMIOLOGY AND REPRODUCTIVE OUTCOMES

We may consider well-designed classical epidemiological studies as the primary tool for identifying hazardous chemicals in the work place. The advantages of human epidemiology studies include:

(1) The data are directly relevant to man.

(2) A well-conducted study with statistically significant positive results is the strongest possible evidence of reproductive activity in man.

(3) The data are the most reliable for risk assessment.

(4) The data are most readily accepted by the public and institutions responsible for control.

Unfortunately, in the area of reproductive effect and chronic studies epidemiology is a very limited, time-consuming tool. The following are some of the problems associated with this technique:

(1) Difficulty in identifying suitable study populations
      adequate size
      unreliability of death or birth medical records
      lack of good incidence data

(2) Latency period in onset of effects (excluding *in utero* exposure for major anomalies)
      complicates data collection
      prevents detection of effects of new exposures
      assessment of current risks based on much earlier exposures

(3) Lack of sensitivity
      normal incidence of specific diseases can obscure increased rates
      multiple exposures confound attempts to establish cause–effect relationship
      difficult to detect effects of ubiquitous exposure
      large populations required to detect common effects

(4) Allows substantial population exposure to agent prior to detection
      dilution of exposed population
      failure to consider power (β error) of study

The frustrations of epidemiology studies related to reproductive hazards can be perceived from the introduction to a study by Erickson[9] where the following statement appears: 'If we are lucky we may catch some real associations, but most are likely to get away. Further, because of the small numbers involved, this sort of exploration can do virtually nothing to help us in pronouncing an occupation or industry safe for reproducing humans. On the other hand, utmost caution in the interpretation of those associations which do appear is in order. Due to the large number of comparisons made, many associations might be expected to result from chance alone. Our approach is less than ideal but does represent a start in a rather barren field.'

The acknowledgement of the present and projected limitation of epidemiological studies to detect chemical carcinogens–mutagens by industry can be further perceived from a recent survey conducted by Karstadt and Bobal[10]. Manufacturers of 75 known International Agency for Research on Cancer (IARC) animal carcinogens were asked about the status of epidemiological studies with these chemicals. Of the 75 chemicals, epidemiological data were available for only 8, and studies with 5 other chemicals were reported in progress. With 62 of the 75 chemicals, no epidemiological data were available, nor do the manufacturers contemplate future studies. Of the 75 IARC animal carcinogens, 18 were reported to have volumes greater than 10^6 lb/year and epidemiological data were not available or anticipated for 10 of these 18 high-volume chemicals. In many respects, detection of carcinogens in man is less difficult than reproductive hazards. In all probability extensive epidemiological studies for either cancer or reproductive problems will not identify hazardous chemicals, to any great extent, in the immediate future.

CORRELATION BETWEEN CARCINOGENESIS AND MUTAGENESIS

A great deal of evidence exists at present establishing the correlation between carcinogens and mutagens, especially at the chromosomal level. Most mutagenic and, therefore, carcinogenic agents can be detected by cytogenetic studies in either animal or man. While the association remains unresolved, numerous observations implicate the relationship between instability in the structure and number of chromosomes and carcinogenesis and have been discussed in detail elsewhere. These observations can be summarised as follows:

(1) Marker chromosomes which are derived from normal chromosomes through breakage and rearrangement can be identified in some clones of cancer cells. In fact, the consistency of marker chromosomes in cancer cells of a given host provides one of the main bodies of evidence supporting a clonal origin of cancer. While most marker chromosomes are unique to that one clone of cancer cells, at least two human cancers consistently have the same chromosome abnormality: the Philadelphia chromosome in as many as 90 per cent of the cases of chronic granulocytic leukaemia; and an extra band on the long arm of chromosome 14 in cells from Burkitt's tumours and in cell lines derived from these tumours.

(2) In general, progression from simple chromosomal anomalies to more complex ones is associated with increasing malignancy of a cancer.

(3) Aneuploidy is a common finding in cancer cells. By comparison, certain

aneuploid states in man have higher incidences of certain cancers: leukaemia in Down's syndrome; breast cancer in Klinefelter's syndrome; cancers of neural crest origin in Turner's syndrome; and gonadoblastoma in the dysgenetic gonad having a Y chromosome cell line. Furthermore, *in vitro* irradiation with X-rays induces a greater frequency of chromosomal aberrations in lymphocytes cultured from individuals with Down's syndrome as well as other trisomic (but not monosomic) disorders than in cells cultured from normal diploid donors.

(4) *De novo* chromosomal aberrations are observed in lymphocytes cultured from individuals at increased risk of developing cancer because of their inheritance of certain genetic diseases: ataxia telangiectasia, Bloom's syndrome and Fanconi's anaemia are examples. Lymphocytes cultured from these afflicted individuals also show a heightened radiosensitivity as measured by an increased frequency of X-ray-induced chromosomal aberrations. In like manner, fibroblasts cultured from individuals to develop skin cancer are more sensitive to the cell-killing and chromosome-breaking effects of ultraviolet irradiation and some chemical agents.

(5) *De novo* chromosomal aberrations are observed in cells cultured from individuals at increased risk of developing cancer because of their exposure to ionising radiation and certain chemical carcinogens (e.g. benzene, cyclophosphamide and vinyl chloride).

Many of these observations can have different interpretations. For example, marker chromosomes and worsening karyotype could just be features that are temporally but not causally associated with cancer induction; they may, indeed, contribute causally to the progression of a cancer that was initiated by some other preceding events. Further, patients with aneuploidy and rare genes for chromosome instability suffer from many afflictions, including immunological disorders, which could also account for their predisposition to cancer development. However, the argument that some known human carcinogens cause chromosome damage is not as easily refuted. All carcinogens that have been thoroughly tested have been found to induce some kind of chromosomal rearrangement[11].

Our understanding of the neoplastic process indicates that chromosomal rearrangement is a step in the neoplastic process. Current information indicates that carcinogens can act to induce chromosomal rearrangements by inducing or exposing sites on DNA for recombination, or by inducing or activating cellular systems, resulting in stimulation of recombination. Chromosomal rearrangment may affect carcinogenesis by altering gene expression, perhaps by allowing the activation of cellular cancer genes. Estimates of the life span of human lymphocytes vary widely but are of the order of at least a few years[12-15]. The observation of unstable aberrations in mitogen-stimulated lymphocytes, years after radiation exposure[16], suggests that certain types of genetic damage can persist for long periods in non-replicating cells. Because the lymphocyte is long-lived and tolerant of some types of genetic damage, when not proliferating, it is a very suitable target cell in which to look for cumulative damage resulting from long periods of exposure. The technique for culturing lymphocytes and analysing for chromosome aberrations are now well established[17].

From available information and theoretical considerations the detection of chromosome abnormalities in man induced by chemical exposure indicates that the chemical is in all likelihood a human carcinogen–mutagen, and lymphocytes are suitable cells for analysis.

RELATIONSHIP BETWEEN MUTAGENS AND TERATOGENS

Even though mutagenesis and teratogenesis are distinctly different biological phenomena, many similar agents are capable of inducing both events. Indeed, the best-understood mode of action for teratogens is through a genetic mechanism. As we consider the largest category of chemicals known to induce genetic lesions, the alkylating agents, the properties of these chemicals suggest how they may function as teratogens as well as carcinogens and mutagens. Common biological properties of these chemicals include their ability to depress DNA synthesis, inhibit cell division and induce extensive genetic damage, rendering cells non-viable. Extensive cell damage leading to cell death in many instances may be visualised by detecting those cells which exhibit extensive chromosomal anomalies. There is a great deal of information about the role played by cytotoxicity, depression of DNA synthesis and cell death in the occurrence of birth defects. Depressed proliferative activity may contribute to teratogenicity by reducing the number of cells available for formation of an organ rudiment. The single most positive correlate with dysmorphogenesis is cell death which accompanies inhibition of DNA synthesis. Numerous teratological investigations have shown that chemicals administered through the embryo produce signs of cell death in tissues which eventually become malformed. Teratogenesis is likely to occur when more cells are removed from a population of cells destined to form an organ rudiment than can be replaced by restorative hyperplasia within a critical period of organogenesis.

The common effects of alkylating agents, including depression of DNA synthesis, inhibition of cell division and cell death due to gross genetic lesions (or to more subtle genetic damage), can lead to developmental errors. In mammals a sequence of biochemical changes underlies morphogenesis and normal development. The activation and repression of structural genes leads to different protein constitution and metabolic capacities in differentiated cells, which can lead to abnormal development. Selectively induced chemical mutations, therefore, could play a major role in abnormal development[18].

Although the final manifestation of a teratogenic agent may be highly diverse, depending upon the species or the organ affected, the molecular basis of action, with chemicals that induce genetic lesions, may be quite similar. Clearly, many teratogenic agents do not act through genetic mechanism. Future studies may well indicate, however, that a significant number of mutagenic and carcinogenic agents are also teratogenic. One of the more exciting developments in animal testing is the procedure whereby cytogenetic abnormalities in the fetus are detected following *in utero* e xposure to chemicals, thus combining fetal abnormalities with a cytogenetic end-point[19].

SHORT-TERM PROCEDURES FOR DETECTING ADVERSE GENETIC EFFECTS

In humand monitoring, short-term procedures are used to detect compounds that induce genetic lesions that may cause reproductive abnormalities and cancer. This approach is needed primarily because of the limitations of classical epidemiological studies in detecting reproductive hazards and our inability to detect an effect at a time when remedial action may be possible. The correlation between mutagenesis, carcinogenesis and teratogenesis, and the fact that effects seen in genetic monitoring can be detected at an early stage in a process which may lead to an adverse health outcome with a minimum population, suggest that these procedures may be an ideal approach to this complex public health problem.

To summarise the preceding sections, the justification and advantages of short-term procedures for detecting a spectrum of potential genetic outcomes in human subjects include:

(1) Known mechanisms and documented correlation between chemicals that are mutagenic, carcinogenic and, with certain classes of chemicals, teratogenic.

(2) The limitations of classical epidemiological procedures as a practical tool for detecting chemicals that induce genetic damage.

(3) Studies conducted in an early phase of the disease process, where remedial action can be taken.

(4) The minimal number of individuals needed for study.

(5) Data are available in a comparatively short period of time.

The following is a brief description of some of the available procedures.

Cytogenetic analysis

The premier procedure for evaluating adverse effects of chemicals in a human population is cytogenetic analysis. The technique is probably the most powerful tool available for evaluating high-risk groups provided that it is used with a sufficient number of cells and sufficient numbers of subjects in exposed and control groups. In a recent presentation a summary of the assessment of cancer risks by the International Agency for Research on Cancer was correlated with cytogenetic studies. Of the 442 chemicals evaluated by IARC since it began providing information on chemical carcinogens in 1968, sufficient evidence of carcinogenicity in animals had been accumulated in 112, but only 53 chemicals had been tested in human studies. These 53 chemicals are categorised as: chemicals carcinogenic for humans (17), chemicals probably carcinogenic for humans (18) and chemicals for which data are insufficient (18). Of the 17 chemicals or chemical processes classified as carcinogenic for humans, 4 have been tested for cytogenetic aberrations in humans and were found to be positive: arsenic compounds, benzene, bis-ether and technical-grade methyl ether and vinyl chloride. Of the 18 chemicals and chemical processes classified as probably carcinogenic for humans, 3 have been tested for production of cytogenetic aberrations in humans and results were positive: cyclophosphamide, epichlorohydrin and thiotepa. Of the 18 chemicals and chemical processes that could not be shown to be carcinogenic for humans, although data from animal studies would indicate their potential carcinogenic activity, 4 were found to be positive for cytogenetic aberrations: chloroprene, ethylene oxide, lead and lead compounds, and styrene. Each of these agents is a cancer suspect, and in every case where human cytogenetics studies have been reported, the results indicate significant chromosomal damage[20].

The evaluation of an exposed and a non-exposed group for chromosomal abnormalities is a comparatively simple procedure; it requires a trained cytogeneticist, a light microscope and several millilitres of blood. At present two types of analysis can be performed. The traditional method is to determine chromosome aberrations in metaphase cells. In this study the identification and classification of chromatid and chromosome abnormalities are carried out and both numerical and structural changes are identified[21].

The development of the bromodesoxyuridine (BudR/Hoechst 33258) staining technique for visualising sister chromatids has facilitated the development of assays for induced DNA damage resulting in sister chromatid exchanges (SCE)[22]. The refinement of the technique using Giemsa staining eliminates the need for observation by fluorescence microscopy and simplifies scoring. A wide variety of chemical mutagens have been shown to induce SCE in several types of mammalian cells, including human lymphocytes[23]. Several studies of SCE in human lymphocytes from individuals with environmental exposures to mutagens have been reported[24-28]. An analysis of factors influencing baseline variation has been recently reported[29].

Haemoglobin alkylation

Most mutagenic and carcinogenic chemicals are electrophilic agents *in vivo*. Alkylating agents react with nucleophilic centres in DNA (e.g. guanine-N-7, guanine-O-6 and adenine-N-3) but also react with nucleophilic centres in proteins such as cysteine-S and -N-1 or -N-3 of the imidazole ring of histidine. Ehrenberg and his colleagues have developed techniques and principles for the determination of the degree of alkylation of specific nucleophilic sites in macromolecules and calculation of the tissue-specific dose of an agent in an exposed animal[30]. Techniques using radiolabelled compounds have been used in animals to determine the degree of alkylation of amino acids of haemoglobin in erythrocytes. The dose (time integral of the concentration of the free agent) in the erythrocyte can be calculated from the degree of alkylation[31,32]. By comparing agents of varying stabilities, it has been possible to estimate the relationships between the dose in the erythrocytes and other tissues, including the gonads[33]. More recently, non-isotopic techniques have been developed for measuring the degree of haemoglobin alkylation in man[34]. A major value of haemoglobin alkylation as a monitor of human exposure is that the time integral exposure to an agent over a period equal to the life length of the erythrocyte (4 months in man) can be measured. In addition, the technique is relatively insensitive to confounding influences of incidental exposures or biological effects not related to the exposure of primary interest. This is because the end-point measured is the formation of a specific adduct of the target amino acid. Consequently, the determination of haemoglobin alkylation can be a powerful technique for evaluating chronic occupational exposures to specific chemicals.

Sperm analysis

A semen sample is an important source of information in any evaluation of the mutagenic impact of a human exposure. Sperm in a semen specimen is the one germinal cell type available in large number and without the use of any invasive procedures. Several different observations can be made on sperm which may reveal the impact of mutagenic activity on their development. The detection of events related to mutation in sperm has direct implications for the reproductive status of the individual and for the transmission of genetic damage to his offspring.

Over the last few years two assays have been developed which detect abnormalities in human sperm which have been associated with exposure to mutagenic agents.

One procedure detects Y chromosome non-disjunction in sperm[35]. It is based on the observation in quinacrine-banded human chromosomes that the Y chromosome absorbs a substantial amount of dye. In human sperm stained with quinacrine hydrochloride the Y chromosome is sufficiently bright to be observed through the cell membrane. In good preparations about 40–50 per cent of sperm heads are observed to contain a Y fluorescent (YF) body as expected on genetic grounds. Sperm containing two fluorescent bodies (YFF) have been observed in about 0.7 per cent of sperm from donors with no known chemical exposures. Furthermore, frequencies of YFF in unexposed individuals are usually quite stable over time[36]. The presence of two YF bodies indicates the occurrence of non-disjunction of the Y chromosome in meiotic anaphase II. The fact that YFF sperm survive and are sometimes capable of fertilisation is shown by the existence of XYY individuals (one per thousand male births)[37]. Exposures to several known mutagenic agents, including adiramycin, X-irradiation and the nematocide dibromochloropropane (DBCP), have produced increases in YFF frequency. DBCP which produced aspermia and oligospermia in exposed males was shown to produce a mean YFF frequency of 3.8 per cent (range 2.0–5.3 per cent) in 18 exposed individuals, as compared with a frequency of 1.2 per cent (range 0.8–1.8 per cent) in a matched control group[38].

The second assay detects agents which increase the frequency of sperm with abnormal morphologies[39]. The normal human sperm head shape is distinctive and changes are easily recognised. In mice several lines of evidence indicate that sperm head shaping is under rigorous genetic control. Studies of strains with different head shapes and hybrids among them indicate that about 10 genetic regions on the X and Y chromosomes as well as autosomes control sperm morphology. In addition, sperm head abnormalities are induced in mice by X-rays and several clinical mutagens. Spermatocytes and late spermatogonia are the most sensitive cell types. The F_1 generation of treated males also have increased rates of abnormality, which suggests that induced abnormalities are heritable. Sperm abnormalities do not correlate with the presence of chromosome abnormalities such as translocations, which indicates that point mutations may be responsible for the occurrences[40].

Urine analysis

The analysis of urine for excreted mutagens using various microbial indicator organisms is a widely used technique[41-44]. A number of studies in humans have also evaluated the urinary excretion of mutagens following exposures to various drugs (e.g. metranidazol)[45-47]. The appearance of mutagens usually occurs rapidly following exposure to mutagens and the technique is sensitive provided that an indicator organism is chosen which is responsive to the agent to be monitored[48]. Body fluid analysis is a simple and rapid process appropriate for general screening purposes. It can be used to screen for continued or repeated exposures or to evaluate the magnitude of isolated acute exposures.

Although urine has been the most frequently studied body fluid, there may be distinct advantages to evaluating blood. The presence of active chemicals in the circulatory system may be more significant than detecting mutagens in a excretory product such as urine.

DNA filter elution

The technique of alkaline elution of DNA from filters was developed originally by Kohn *et al.*[49], for examining size distribution of strands during DNA replication. It has subsequently been modified by several groups and adapted for detection of chemical and radiation damage to DNA[50]. Alkaline filter elution relies on the fact that alkaline denaturing and unwinding of double-stranded DNA and the release of single strands occurs at a rate inversely proportional to single strand size[51]. In practice, then, DNA from mutagen-damaged cells is eluted through a polyvinyl chloride filter under alkaline conditions over a period of many hours. The total eluate of 20–25 ml is collected in 1 ml fractions; the DNA distribution over these fractions compared with control is indicative of the occurrence of a degree of DNA damage resulting in single-stranded breaks.

Alkaline elution has been used successfully to detect carcinogens in whole animal studies. Swenberg *et al.*[52] have shown that results of such studies in mammalian cells treated with various non-carcinogens, procarcinogens and direct-acting carcinogens correlate well with the *in vivo* activity of those compounds. Parodi *et al.*[50] recently adapted the alkaline elution technique for use with the method of Kissane and Robins[53] for microfluorometric quantification of extremely small amounts of DNA. The nature of the alkaline elution technique suggests that it may also, from the same sample, be possible to determine the degree of DNA interstrand linkage and DNA–protein linkage caused by a test agent[54]. Because the alkaline elution technique can now be employed with mammalian cells whose DNA has not been labelled by incorporation of isotopic precursors, the technique appears to be ideally suited to the monitoring of human populations for exposure to genetically active agents.

Point mutation in human lymphocytes

A promising but new and relatively untried technique determines the frequency of 6-thioguanine (6-TG)-resistant lymphocytes in peripheral blood[55]. The resistance to 6-thioguanine presumably occurs because of the inactivation of the gene for hypoxanthine-guanine phosphoribosyl transferase (HGPRT) through mutation. The technique for identifying 6-TG-resistant cells has been developed using reconstruction experiments with lymphocytes from Lesch–Nyhan syndrome patients who are genetically deficient in HGPRT as a result of mutation of the X-chromosome-linked gene. The frequency of 6-TG-resistant cells has been shown to increase in patients on cytotoxic cancer chemotherapy drugs or X-rays or psoriatic patients treated with 8-methoxypsoral with ultraviolet light[56,57]. Early studies were plagued with excessively high frequencies of 6-TH-resistant cells in both normal and exposed individuals, which suggested that phenocopies were being observed; however, this technique problem appears to be better controlled in more recent work[55]. The remaining problem with the technique is the direct confirmation that 6-TG-resistant cells are genuine HGPRT-deficient mutants. This is the most promising currently available technique for development into a somatic mutation assay in man.

RATIONALE FOR CO-ORDINATED TESTING IN MAN AND ANIMALS

By using several of the methods described above, a battery of tests can be developed for the investigation of human exposures to mutagenic environments. Careful test selection would allow the efficient observation of several types of genetic end-point. Both somatic and germinal cells could be observed, and genetic damage at the chromosome level and at the molecular level could be detected. The sensitivity and interpretability of the human test battery could be further strengthened in many instances by co-ordinating specific studies in animals with human monitoring.

Unless the chemical nature of the human environment is well described and the principal agents have been previously well studied, it might not be possible to predict in advance which tests are most appropriate for detecting exposure. Preliminary studies of individual agents or environmental samples in animals could greatly improve the selection of tests for human monitoring. Even when the major environmental agents have been identified, human monitoring alone might not identify the component most responsible for mutagenic activity. Animal or *in vitro* studies could be used to evaluate the activities of individual agents. One of the primary reasons for conducting animal tests in co-ordination with human monitoring is to establish the dose response for specific end-points in the animal. The magnitude of effects in human subjects could be related to responses in animals in order to estimate the exposure level when it could not be determined accurately by environmental measurements. In addition, comparison of human and animal effects might provide an indication of degree of risk posed by the human exposure.

For some tests which must be modified to detect the effects of specific agents, animal or *in vitro* studies might be necessary to establish methods and conditions for conducting human studies. For example, urine testing for the presence of mutagens might require the use of extraction or concentration procedures. Animal or *in vivo* studies might be needed to validate these procedures and may facilitate the identification of active metabolites. Haemoglobin alkylation monitoring in man requires that a specific adduct be identified and that techniques for its isolation and measurement be established. Preliminary studies *in vitro* in animals are necessary to accomplish these objectives.

CONCLUSIONS

One of the most promising areas in the field of genetic toxicology is the use of a series of non-invasive tests to detect hazardous chemicals directly in human studies. These procedures form a bridge between animal studies and the classical epidemiological approach.

The ultimate objective of genetic monitoring is to protect individuals from disease. The ideal approach for accomplishing this goal would be to continuously monitor high-risk populations so that corrective measures could be taken soon after a positive response was detected by suitable techniques. At the present time, however, those studies that have been carried out utilising short-term procedures were initiated only after the presence of mutagenic–carcinogenic chemicals or processes was already suspected of being present. These studies were usually carried out after prolonged exposure had already occurred. The utilisation of these tests on a routine basis in high-risk populations should offer the optimum approach to worker protection.

In interpreting results from these tests several points should be kept in mind. Interindividual and temporal variation, as well as confounding environmental factors, make interpretation on a individual basis unjustifiable.

These tests are advanced warning procedures which indicate that the individuals are exposed to hazardous substances. The distinct advantage of this approach is that remedial action can be taken in the hope of preventing the final disease outcome. A positive finding in all likelihood signifies an early stage in a multistage process, a process that we would like to abort. These techniques should be considered analogous to a radiation film badge capable of providing an early indication that a particular environment contains a genetically hazardous agent.

The remedial action to be taken following a positive finding in short-term procedures should be directed at, if possible, eliminating or at least minimising risk of exposure with irreplaceable products. Improved ventilation and exhausting of toxic chemicals as well as use of protective clothing may be considered. Ashford *et al.*[58] have described the problems associated by the movement of individuals into and out of places where toxic chemicals are used (worker rotation policy). Depending on the shape of the dose–response curve to the toxic agent, the number of people affected would change if a fixed total amount of toxic chemical were spread among populations of various sizes. Figure 13.1 represents an increased dose on the X axis and number of people exposed on the Y axis. For the A convex curve, the number of people expected to be at risk will increase as the total population exposed is increased. In the case of the B curve, spreading the fixed total dosage among a larger population would have no effect on the number of people affected. In the case of the C curve, the number of people affected will decrease as the total exposed population is increased. In the case of curve A or B, rotating populations out of an area of toxic chemicals

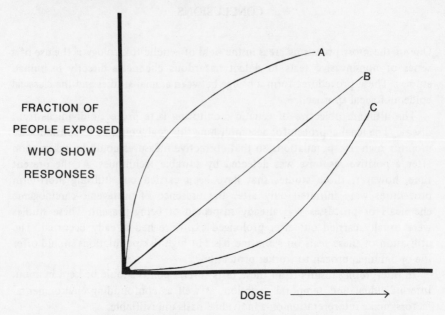

FRACTION OF
PEOPLE EXPOSED
WHO SHOW
RESPONSES

DOSE ⟶

Figure 13.1 Response as a function of dose

would either be of no value (curve B) or actually spread the risk to a larger population (curve A). In terms of mutagenic–carcinogenic agents, assuming a non-threshold, linear response, curve B would be the most typical response.

Confounding factors, including seasonal variation, age, sex, smoking, viral infection and various medications, have been listed as factors which may invalidate the results. These confounding factors, however, are present in many human studies and are not a problem specifically associated with these procedures. Proper experimental design should take into account these factors and neutralise the problems associated with these possible sources of error.

Individual variation may also be a source of error. It should be borne in mind that there is a considerable variation in the way individuals metabolise different chemicals, and this variation will be reflected in all human studies measuring a chemically induced response. Table 13.5 illustrates differences in individual response to antipyrine half-life and clearance, to cytochrome P450 and benzo(a)pyrene binding[59]. Chemical studies will reflect these inherent individual variabilities. Suitable experimental techniques where appropriate numbers of subjects are included should compensate for expected individual variability.

The sensitivities of the various tests to human exposures to mutagens are not well established. In fact, enlarging baseline data are major objectives of investigations in this area. We do know that some tests such as cytogenetics have been successfully used in several circumstances to detect human exposure to carcinogens. A statistical analysis by Whorton *et al.*[60] indicates that a 1 per cent increase

Table 13.5 Examples of the variability of xenobiotic metabolism in human beings

Experimental system (number of individuals)	Parameter measured	Variability (fold)
Unselected patients (200)	antipyrine half-life	25
	antipyrine clearance	41
liver biopsies (200)	cytochrome P450	65
liver biopsies (27)	aryl hydroxylase	30
Bronchus explants (37)	benzo(a)pyrene binding	75
Bladder explants (16)	benzo(a)pyrene binding	34
Colon explants (15)	benzo(a)pyrene binding	31
Oesophageal explants (15)	benzo(a)pyrene binding	31

Modified from reference 6.

in chromosome aberration rate over a background rate of 2 per cent could be detected with 80 per cent certainty with an error rate of 5 per cent in a population of less than 50 exposed and 50 control individuals ($P < 0.05$). The sperm morphology and YFF tests need additional work for validation in man and to define the relationship between observed effect and genetic damage more thoroughly.

Validation may be required for some of the techniques in the battery; other procedures, however, should be viewed as suitable for use. Validation of assays (i.e. when is an assay an acceptable means of testing compounds in industrial populations, as opposed to a research technique?) poses a difficult problem. In a report from the United Kingdom Environmental Mutagen Society on guides to mutagenicity testing the validation of assays is discussed[62]. It is suggested that the decision about when a technique is sufficiently validated for routine application depends to a great extent on the nature of the assay, the purpose for which it will be used and the interpretation placed on the word 'validation'. If one wished to validate an *in vitro* test as indicating a chemical that induces genetic damage in a animal, one would test by an *in vitro* system a series of chemicals known to be either active or inactive in animals. A positive genetic response in animals would need no further validation to indicate a chemical that induces genetic damage. If a chemical causes chromosome damage in man, then the compound is a human clastogen and further testing would be superfluous. We have already established that the assay is valid for indicating chromosome damage in the target species—namely man. Given the number of human carcinogens that cause chromosome aberrations and the theoretical basis linking chromosome aberration to cancer, it is logical to conclude that a positive response has indicated an exposure to a carcinogenic-mutagenic agent. The other procedures in the battery of tests that can be used for human monitoring should be viewed in a similar manner.

Although there may be procedural problems that would restrict the use of these methods for monitoring industrial populations, certainly there is no compelling scientific reason for not proceeding to monitor higher-risk populations. These non-invasive tests are short-term, are comparatively inexpensive and allow remedial action to be taken shortly after exposure. The results obtained with these procedures to date are indeed impressive.

It may be appropriate to summarise the accomplishment of the field of genetic toxicology and put into perspective human monitoring, with probable future development in this area[11]. Based on the work in the mid-1960s and early 1970s with dimethylnitrosamine and polycyclic hydrocarbons, the concept of proximate carcinogens was developed. This realisation that mammalian cells can metabolise chemically unreactive compounds to electrophiles, which could react with intracellular nucleophiles, including DNA, provided a logical nexus for the long-sought relationship between carcinogenesis and mutagenesis. The twin concept of proximate mutagens naturally followed, and led to the development of microbial and mammalian cell mutagenicity assays, which employ cellular homogenates of mammalian livers, or fractions thereof, to simulate *in vitro* the metabolic activation of the test chemical. The early success of this experimental approach is clearly epitomised by the near-90 per cent correlation between chemical carcinogenesis and mutagenesis that was soon being quoted by many by the mid-1970s. These results were so impressive that they generated a high level of optimism that these *in vitro* assays would suffice in themselves as an efficient means to identify potential genotoxins.

However, by the late 1970s, it became apparent that *in vitro* systems have critical shortcomings that detract from their efficiency as general screening assays. First, the understood activation of some chemicals to electrophiles is more complex than just one or two P450-mediated oxidations, and this complexity does not lend itself easily to stimulation *in vitro*. Second, with regard to the popular microbial systems, their phylogenetic lack of similarity to mammalian organisms poses at least two other problems: their inability to detect the entire spectrum of mutational events and differences in passage of some chemicals across microbial versus mammalian cell membranes. Consequently, the 1970s closed with the growing consensus that a battery of *in vitro* and *in vivo* systems would be the best strategy in screening for genotoxic chemicals.

In the 1980s one can expect that this renewed emphasis on *in vivo* studies will continue and will result in new levels of sophistication in testing. Increasing emphasis will be placed on two areas: animal studies that measure both specific genetic alterations and their accompanying phenotypic manifestations (e.g. histocompatibility changes, behavioural effects), and new procedures for monitoring certain genetic as well as clinical and industrial populations for chemical mutagenesis. Ideologically, there will also be a shift in the perception of the magnitude of the problem of gametic mutagenesis in the human community as a whole. This will be in response to further and further identifications of such human mutagens—for example, as evidenced by dominant lethal effects in exposed males and expressed as increased spontaneous abortions in their unexposed wives. By the end of the 1980s it may very well be that there will be international committees verifying examples of chemically induced genetic diseases and thereby developing an operational listing of human mutagens. In such an atmosphere chemical mutagenesis will assume an importance equalling, if not excelling, that of chemical carcinogenesis and chemical teratogenesis with regard to the study and prevention of these toxicities.

REFERENCES

1. Bang, K. M., Lockey, J. E. and Keye, W. (1983). Reproductive hazards in the workplace. *Fam. Commun. Hlth*, May, 44–56
2. Adams, P. M., Fabricant, J. D. and Legator, M. (1981). Cyclophosphamide induced spermatogenic effects detected in the f_1 generation by behavioral testing. *Science, N.Y.*, **211**, 20–82
3. Adams, P. M., Fabricant, J. D. and Legator, M. S. (1982). Active avoidance behavior in the f_1 progeny of rats exposed to cyclophosphamide prior to fertilization. *Neurobehav. Toxicol. Teratol.*, **4**, 531–534
4. Fabricant, J. D., Legator, M. S. and Adams, P. M. (1983). Post meiotic cell mediation of behavior in progeny of male rats treated with cyclophosphamide. *Mutation Res.*, **119**, 185–190
5. Adams, P., Shabrawy, O. and Legator, M. S. (1982). Male transmitted developmental and neurobehavioral deficits. In *Environmental Influences on Fertility, Pregnancy and Development: Directions for Future Research*. Meeting sponsored by The University of Texas Medical Branch, Galveston; The University of Cincinnati Medical Center, Department of Environmental Health, Cincinnati; the Centers for Disease Control, National Institute for Occupational Safety and Health, and the March of Dimes Birth Defects Foundation (May 24–25)
6. Schroeder, J. H. (1979). Hereditary changes of male aggressiveness after gamma irradiation of mouse spermatozoa with 600 R. *Ber. Nat.-Med. Ver.*, **66**, 131–137
7. Brady, K., Herrera, Y. and Zenick, H. (1975). Influence of parental lead exposure on subsequent learning ability of offspring. *Pharmacol. Biochem. Behav.*, **3**, 561–565
8. Tomatis, L., Cabral, J. R. P., Likhachev, A. J. and Ponomarkov, V. (1981). Increased cancer incidence in the progeny of male rats exposed to ethylnitrosourea before mating. *Int. J. Cancer*, **27**, 475–478
9. Erickson, D. (1979). Contribution to Epidemiology in Biostatistics. *Prenatal Occupation in Birth Defects Report*, vol. 1, 107–117
10. Karstadt, M. and Bobal, R. (1982). Availability of epidemiological data on humans exposed to animal carcinogens. II. Chemical uses and production volume. *Teratogen. Carcinogen. Mutagen.*, 2, 151–168
11. Legator, M. S. and Rinkus, S. J. (1981). Mutagenicity testing: problems in application. In Stich, H. F. and Sau, R. H. C. (Eds.), *Short-Term Tests for Chemical Carcinogens*, Springer, Berlin, pp. 483–504
12. Radman, M., Jeggo, P. and Wagner, R. (1982). Chromosomal rearrangement and carcinogenesis. *Mutation Res.*, **98**, 249–264
13. Norman, A., Sasaki, M. S. and Ohoman, R. E. (1966). Elimination of chromosome aberrations from human lymphocytes. *Blood*, **27**, 706–714

14. Buckton, K. E., Smith, P. G. and Court-Brown, W. M. (1967). Estimation of lifespan from studies on males treated with X-rays for ankylosing spondylitis. In Evans, H. J., Court-Brown, W. and McLean, A. S. (Eds.), *Human Cytogenetics*, North-Holland, Amsterdam, pp. 106-114

15. Dolphin, G. W., Lloyd, D. C. and Purrot, R. J. (1973). Chromosome aberratio analysis as a dosimetric technique in radiological protection. *Hlth Phys.*, **25**, 7-15

16. Nowell, P. C. (1965). Unstable chromosome changes in tuberculin-stimulated leukocyte cultures from irradiated patients. Evidence for immunologically committed, long-lived lymphocytes in human blood. *Blood*, **26**, 798-804

17. Bloom, A. D., Neriishi, S., Kamada, N., Iseki, T. and Hehha, R. J. (1966). Cytogenetic investigation of survivors of the atomic bombings of Hiroshima and Nagasaki. *Lancet*, **ii**, 672-674

18. Manson, J. M. (1981). Developmental toxicity of alkylating agents; mechanism of action. In Juchan, M. R. (ed.), *The Biochemical Basis of Chemical Teratogenesis*, Elsevier, Amsterdam, pp. 95-135

19. Adler, I. D. (1984). New approaches to mutagenicity studies in animals for carcinogenic and mutagenic agents. *Teratogen. Carcinogen. Mutagen.* (in press)

20. International Agency for Research on Cancer (1979). *IARC Monographs on the Evaluation of the Carcinogenic Risk of Chemicals to Humans*, **19**, 131-156

21. Evans, H. J. and O'Riordan, M. L. (1977). Human peripheral blood lymphocytes for the analysis of chromosome aberrations in mutagens tests. In Kilbey, B. J., Legator, M. S., Nichols, W. and Ramel, C. (Eds.), *Handbook of Mutagenicity Test Procedures*, Elsevier, Amsterdam, New York, Oxford, pp. 261-274

22. Latt, S. A. (1974). Localization of sister chromatid exchanges in human chromosomes. *Science, N. Y.*, **185**, 74-76

23. Latt, S. A., Allen, J. W., Rogers, W. E. and Jeurgens, L. A. (1977). *In vitro* and *in vivo* analysis of sister chromatid exchange formation. In Kilbey, B. J., Legator, M. S., Nichols, W. and Ramel, C. (Eds.), *Handbook of Mutagenicity Test Procedures*, Elsevier, Amsterdam, New York, Oxford, pp. 275-291

24. Raposa, T. (1978). Sister chromatid exchange studies for monitoring DNA damage and repair capacity after cytostatics *in vitro* and in lymphocytes of leukemic patients under cytostatic therapy. *Mutation Res.*, **57**, 241-251

25. Crossen, P. E., Morgan, W. F., Horan, J. J. and Stewart, J. (1978). Cytogenetic studies of pesticide and herbicide sprayers. *New Zealand Med. J.*, **88**, 192

26. Nevstad, N. P. (1978). Sister chromatid exchanges and chromosomal aberrations induced in human lymphocytes by the cytostatic drug adriamycin *in vivo* and *in vitro*. *Mutation Res.*, **57**, 253-258

27. Lambert, B., Ringborg, U., Harper, E. and Lindbald, A. (1978). Sister chromatid exchanges in lymphocyte cultures of patients receiving chemotherapy for malignant disorders. *Cancer Treat. Repts*, **62**, 1413

28. Musilova, J., Michalova, K. and Urban, J. (1979). Sister chromatid exchanges and chromosomal breakage in patients treated with cytostatics. *Mutation Res.*, **67**, 289

29. Carrano, A. V., Minkler, J. L., Stetka, D. G. and Morre, D. H., II (1980). Variation in the baseline sister chromatid exchange frequency in human lymphocytes. *Environ. Mutagen.*, **2**, 325-337

30. Ehrenberg, L. and Osterman-Golkar, S. (1980). Alkylation of macromole-

cules for detecting mutagenic agents. *Teratogen. Carcinogen. Mutagen.*, **1**, 105–127

31. Osterman-Golkar, S., Ehrenberg, L., Segerback, D. and Hallstrom, I. (1976). Evaluation of genetic risks of alkylating agents. II. Hemoglobin as a dose monitor. *Mutation Res.*, **34**, 1–10

32. Osterman-Golkar, S., Hultmark, D., Segerback, D., Calleman, C. J., Goethe, R., Ehrenberg, L. and Wachtmeister, C. A. (1977). Alkylation of DNA and proteins in mice exposed to vinyl chloride. *Biochem. Biophys. Res. Commun.*, **76**, 259–266

33. Segerback, D., Calleman, C. J., Ehrenberg, L., Lofroth, G. and Osterman-Golkar, S. (1978). Evaluation of genetic risks of alkylating agents. IV. Quantitative determination of alkylated amino acids in hemoglobin as a measure of the dose after treatment of mice with methyl methanesulfonate. *Mutation Res.*, **49**, 71–82

34. Calleman, C. J., Ehrenberg, L., Jansson, B., Osterman-Golkar, S., Segerback, D., Svennson, K. and Wachtmeister, C. A. (1979). Monitoring and risk assessment by means of alkyl groups in hemoglobin in persons occupationally exposed to ethylene oxide. *J. Environ. Pathol. Toxicol.*, **2**, 427–442

35. Kapp, R. W., Jr. and Jacobson, C. B. (1980). Analysis of spermatozoa for Y chromosome non-disjunction. *Teratogen. Carcinogen. Mutagen.*, **1**, 193–212

36. Zeck, L. (1969). Investigation of metaphase chromosomes with DNA binding fluorochromes. *Exp. Cell Res.*, **58**, 463

37. Barlow, P. and Vosa, D. G. (1970). The Y chromosome in human spermatozoa. *Nature (London)*, **226**, 961–962

38. Kapp, R. W., Jr., Picciano, D. J. and Jacobson, C. B. (1979). Y chromosomal nondisjunction in dibromochloropropane exposed workmen. *Mutation Res.*, **64**, 47–51

39. Wyrobek, A. J. and Bruce, W. R. (1978). The induction of spermshape abnormalities in mice and humans. In Hollaender, A. and deSerres, F. J. (Eds.), *Chemical Mutagens: Principles and Methods for Their Detection*, Vol. 5, Plenum Press, New York, London, pp. 257–285

40. Wyrobek, A. J. (1979). Changes in mammalian sperm morphology after X-ray and chemical exposures. *Genetics*, **92**, 104–119

41. Gabridge, D. A., Denuzio, A. and Legator, M. S. (1969). Microbial mutagenicity of streptozotocin in animal-mediated assays. *Nature, Lond.*, **221**, 68–70

42. Durston, W. and Ames, B. N. A. (1974). Simple method for the detection of mutagens in urine: studies with the carcinogen 2-acetylaminofluorene. *Proc. Natl Acad. Sci. USA*, **71**, 737–741

43. Commoner, B. A., Vithayathil, A. and Henry, J. L. (1974). Detection of metabolic carcinogen intermediates in urine of carcinogen-fed rats by means of bacterial mutagenesis. *Nature, Lond.*, **249**, 850–852

44. Siebert, D. and Simon, A. (1973). Genetic activity of metabolites in the ascitic fluid and in the urine of a human patient treated with cyclophosphamide: Induction of mitotic gene conversion in *Saccharomyces cerevisiae*. *Mutation Res.*, **21**, 257–262

45. Minnich, V., Smith, M. E., Thompson, D. and Kornfield, S. (1976). Detection of mutagenic activity in human urine using mutant strains of *Salmonella typhimurium*. *Cancer*, **38**, 1253–1258

46. Legator, M. S., Connor, T. H. and Stoeckel, M. (1975). Detection of mutagenic activity of metronidazole and niridazole in body fluids of humans and mice. *Science, N.Y.*, **188**, 1118–1119

47. Connor, T. H., Stoeckel, M., Evrard, J. and Legator, M. S. (1977). The contribution of metronidazole and two metabolites to the mutagenic activity detected in urine of treated humans and mice. *Cancer Res.*, **37**, 629–633
48. Kohn, K. W., Erickson, L. C., Ewig, R. A. G. and Friedman, C. A. (1976). Fractionation of DNA from mammalian cells by alkaline elution. *Biochemistry*, **15**, 4629–4637
49. Kohn, K. W., Friedman, C. A., Ewig, R. A. G. and Iqbal, Z. (1974). DNA chain growth during replication of asynchronous L1210 cells alkaline elution of large DNA segments from cells lysed on filters. *Biochemistry*, **13**, 4134–4139
50. Parodi, S., Taningher, M., Santi, L., Cavanna, M., Sciaba, L., Maura, A. and Brambilla, G. (1978). A practical procedure for testing DNA damage *in vivo*, proposed for a pre-screening of chemical carcinogens. *Mutation Res.*, **54**, 39–46
51. Petzold, G. L. and Svenberg, J. A. (1978). Detection of DNA damage induced *in vivo* following exposure of rats to carcinogens. *Cancer Res.*, **38**, 1589–1594
52. Swenberg, J. A., Petzold, G. L. and Harback, P. R. (1976). *In vitro* DNA damage/elution assay for predicting carcinogenic potential. *Biochem. Biophys. Res.*, **72**, 732–738
53. Kissane, J. M. and Robins, E. (1958). The fluorometric measurements of deoxyribonucleic acid in animal tissues with special reference to the central nervous system. *J. Biol. Chem.*, **233**, 184–188
54. Ross, W. E. and Shipley, N. (1980). Relationship between DNA damage and survival in formaldehyde treated mouse cells. *Mutation Res.*, **79**, 277–283
55. Strauss, R. and Albertini, R. J. (1979). Enumeration of 6-thioguanine resistant peripheral blood lymphocytes in man as a potential test for somatic cell mutations arising *in vivo Mutation Res.*, **61**, 353–379
56. Albertini, R. J. (1980). Drug-resistant lymphocytes in man as indicators of somatic cell mutation. *Teratogen. Carcinogen. Mutagen.*, **1**, 25–48
57. Albertini, R. J., Allen, E. F., Quinn, A. S. and Albertini, M. R. (1980). Human somatic cell mutation: *in vivo* variant lymphocyte frequencies as determined by 6-thioguanine resistance. In Hood, E. B. and Porter, I. H. (Eds.), *Birth Defects Institute Symposium XI*, Academic Press, New York
58. Ashford, N. A., Hattis, D., Heaton, G. R., Katz, J. I., Preist, W. C. and Zolt, E. M. (1983). Evaluating chemical regulations: trade-off analysis and impact assessment for environmental decision-making (personal communications)
59. Pelkonen, O., Sotaniemi, E. O. and Karki, N. T. (1982). Interindividual variation in sensitivity to mutagens. In Sorsa, M. and Vairo, H. (Eds.), *Mutagens in Our Environment*, Alan R. Liss, New York, pp. 61–74
60. Whorton, E. B., Jr., Bee, D. B. and Kilian, D. J. (1979). Variations in the proportion of abnormal cells and required sample sizes for human cytogenetic studies. *Mutation Res.*, **64**, 79–86
61. Dean, B., Bridges, B., Kirkland, D., Parry, J. and Taylor, N. (1983). Framework of supplementary testing procedures. In: *Report of the UKEMS Subcommittee on Guidelines for Mutagenicity Testing. Part 1: Basic Test Battery; Minimal Criteria; Professional Standards; Interpretation; Selection of Supplementary Assays*, United Kingdom Environmental Mutagen Society, pp. 175–176

Part 3
Responses

14

A Trade Union View of Reproductive Health

SHEILA McKECHNIE

INTRODUCTION

The involvement of trade unions in reproductive health is relatively new. A number of factors are involved.

An increase in the number of working women

Women now constitute approximately 40 per cent of the work force. Since 1975 women have had the right to 6 weeks' maternity pay and to return to work within 29 weeks of the birth. Their changing pattern of employment is reflected in the growth in female membership of trade unions. In the last 20 years nearly two-thirds of all new recruits to trade unions have been women. It would be surprising if this had not resulted in an increasing concern for issues which directly concern women. Motions passed at recent trade union conferences indicate concern for both the care of pregnant women at work and the effects of work on reproductive health[1].

Protective legislation

The publication in 1979 of the Equal Opportunities Commission (EOC) Report *Health and Safety Legislation; should we distinguish between men and women?* caused considerable concern in the trade union movement[2]. The report contains the only public statement made by the Health and Safety Commission (HSC) on their attitude to the different treatment of men and women in relation to the protection of reproductive capacity. The HSC took the view that every woman must be considered of reproductive capacity unless she provides a doctor's

191

certificate that she is incapable of bearing a child. The EOC took a more liberal view that this should be interpreted as women unlikely to become pregnant. The argument was unresolved by the Lead Code of Practice, which left the decision up to the appointed doctor.

Neither the EOC nor the HSC approach is acceptable to women for the following reasons: it ignores the issue of mutagenicity and concentrates solely on teratogenicity, and by ignoring general male and female reproductive health deals only with part of the problem. The effect of lead on male reproduction is a case in point.

To say, as the EOC does, that men and women should be treated equally except that there should be special provision for women of reproductive capacity avoids the problem that we are actually trying to deal with. The HSC definition, on the other hand, is so ridiculous that the handful of women who get through the net hardly affects the discriminatory impact. Both definitions put women in the position of choosing between work and potential damage to the fetus.

The proposed Ionizing Radiation Regulations define women of reproductive capacity in accordance with the HSC definition. The impact of this definition on women's employment is impossible to estimate but will certainly be greater than that of the Lead Code.

The fears are that women will simply be excluded from certain jobs or, worse, that they will be forced out of economic necessity to be sterilised in order to keep their jobs. The spectre of the women at Cyanamid in the USA and the General Motors case in Canada haunts the whole debate[3].

Occupational health issues

The trade unions' involvement in the issue of reproductive health also results from a more general awareness of the problems of perinatal mortality and occupational health *per se*. The impact of the Short Report on perinatal mortality has been considerable in the trade union movement[4]. The TUC has been encouraging unions to participate in campaigns directed at the provision of NHS maternity and obstetric services[5]. Work place projects for pregnant women have been seized on enthusiastically by trade union activists but it is impossible to estimate how extensive these now are. For a full review of trade union activities in the field of working parents, a number of useful TUC documents can be consulted[6]. The growing concern about healthy reproduction is also paradoxically a result of women's ability to control fertility. The belief in the right to have healthy children becomes more important as the right *not* to have children becomes more generally accepted. These factors, combined with a growing awareness about occupationally related ill-health, mean that reproductive health is now being discussed in the trade union movement.

In November 1980 the General and Municipal Workers Union (now General Municipal Boilermakers and Allied Trades Union) and the Association of

Scientific, Technical and Managerial Staffs held a meeting at Guy's Hospital to discuss the general issue of reproductive health. It was agreed that there was a need for a small conference to allow researchers and trade unionists to exchange views on the problem. This conference took place on 30 March 1981[7]. Since that date both unions have continued collecting information on reproductive hazards and both propose to issue reviews and policy statements later.

The title of this conference, 'Pregnant Women at Work', reflects only one aspect of the problem. The content of the programme reflects the wider issues of reproductive health, and this chapter concentrates on the latter. This is not, it must be emphasised, because one is considered to be more important than the other, but rather that while we are in a position to identify the main requirements of a policy for the care of pregnant women at work, this is certainly not the case in respect of other aspects of healthy reproduction.

At present there are two aspects to the problem of the effects of occupation on reproductive health. First, how big a problem have we got? Does the occupation of male and female workers affect their ability to have healthy children, and if so, *how* does it affect them? What scientific problems are involved in reproductive toxicology and reproductive epidemiology? Are there special problems in setting standards for chemical and physical reproductive hazards which protect all workers? As we are currently considering these aspects, much of what follows is necessarily tentative. The second aspect of the problem concerns social policy and reproductive health. Why have both employers and legislators adopted policies which seem incapable of responding in a way that does not sacrifice the reproductive health of men or the employment prospects of women in the name of protecting the fetus?

THE SCIENTIFIC ISSUES

The size of the problem

It would be nonsense to attempt to quantify the effect of occupation on reproductive health. As many commentators have remarked, this is difficult enough in respect of cancer, where there is only one end-point to look for — that is, the existence of the disease. It is much more difficult where the effects range through infertility, spontaneous abortion, stillbirths, birth abnormalities and deformities. Many factors other than occupation may be involved, and our difficulties are compounded by the lack of background rates for reproductive problems. Total embryonic and fetal loss, in most cases associated with chromosomal or genetic abnormalities, is estimated to happen for as many as 30–80 per cent of pregnancies[8]. Even where there is a positive outcome to the pregnancy, estimates of congenital malformations vary widely, although this may reflect problems of definition more than real differences. However, effects which emerge later in life or in later generations pose particular problems. For those with the inclination to apportion genetic and environmental factors as if they were independent, this latter effect may cause considerable methodological difficulties.

These difficulties with causal factors and reproductive health have not deterred the intrepid. Wilson in 1973 made the oft-quoted estimate of 4–6 per cent malformations being due to environmental chemicals, of which drugs were the major factor[9]. A more recent estimate by Kalter and Warkany considers 5 per cent due to environmental factors, including chemicals, drugs and infectious agents, but, in addition, another 20 per cent may be due to multi-factorial causes of genetic and environmental interaction[10]. (Environment in the context of these estimates does not mean the working environment but the general environment, including work.) To put these figures in perspective, it must be noted that both authors, 10 years apart, ascribe some 60 per cent or more malformations to unknown aetiology! A common response of industry spokespersons to these data is that the problem is small. A number of factors, however, do indicate that the problem is not quite as insignificant as these estimates suggest.

National data

Evidence from national data shows an unmistakable social class gradient, with semi-skilled and unskilled workers' children being worse off for perinatal mortality, many congenital malformations (especially those of the central nervous system), spontaneous abortions and low birth weights. Factors produced by poverty are clearly dominant, but occupation may play a part[11,12]. The data from the Scandinavian, US and British registries on pregnancy outcome, while not substantiating occupational causal factors, have produced evidence of occupational differences affecting men and women and raised the possibility that male and female occupational exposure may act synergistically[13–15]. (Unfortunately for British researchers, occupational analyses have had to be based largely on fathers' occupations alone. Most routine data ignore the occupations of ately for British researchers, occupational analyses have had to be based largely Canada – suggest that environmental factors may outweigh genetic factors for some congenital malformations. These factors comprise mainly work and home environments and nutrition[16].

Reproductive toxicology

In the field of animal toxicology, more and more substances are being identified as fetotoxic or teratogenic. The results of the review by Drs Barlow and Sullivan of 48 important industrial chemicals is significant in this respect[17]. Much of the toxicity testing was restricted to exposure of the pregnant females rather than the 2 or 3 generation tests which provide more comprehensive data, and few chemicals were tested on males. For example, of the 48 chemicals, all but a handful underwent some kind of test on pregnant animals, yet barely half had been tested on male animals for reproductive effects.

The interpretation of toxicological data is itself very controversial, as is their extrapolation to human exposures. However, there is already animal evidence suggesting that many permitted levels of exposure will have to be revised. Comparing the teratologically toxic doses of various chemicals with doses expected at threshold-limit-value (TLV) exposures indicates that the TLVs are potentially hazardous to the fetus. These chemicals include acrylonitrile, methacrylate esters, styrene, carbon disulphide, chloroform, methylene chloride, toluene and xylene[18].

Some of the controversies mirror the debate on the causes of cancer. Many commentators have remarked on the similarity between the understanding of reproductive health and ill-health now and cancer a decade or two ago, yet the analogy extends still further. For many years the dominant view among cancer researchers and most doctors was that a threshold limit existed in the typical dose–response relationship to a carcinogenic substance. Now only a rump retain that view, the majority accepting the view that at low doses the dose–response relationship is broadly linear.

'Unlike carcinogens for which no threshold is assumed to exist, the majority of teratologists believe that thresholds do exist for teratogens', comment Barlow and Sullivan[17]. This, they argue, is because of various theoretical reasons such as the ability of embryonic tissues to repair or substitute damaged cells, as well as frequent findings in animal studies of a level below which there is no apparent effect. Similar justifications were put forward in favour of thresholds for carcinogens. However, the support for thresholds existing is not so universal. White *et al.*, in a review of dose–response data in animal teratology studies, concluded 'the apparent thresholds of nonlinear dose response data could be products of experiments which used too few animals, insufficient dose ranges and/or monitored only a few specific endpoints'[19].

While some chemicals may well exhibit thresholds (and a sound understanding of the relevant biochemistry could support such a conclusion), others may not. The current practice of using as few as 20 animals per dose level is usually insufficient to resolve whether or not a threshold exists. Given these uncertainties, we remember the cancer debate and remain sceptical of claims of thresholds being widespread if not universal in the dose–response relationships of reproductive hazards.

There are many other aspects of scientific controversy in the field of reproductive toxicity. Lack of resources for developing agreed international standards for such testing is a problem. However, I strongly suspect we are in for quite a few years during which those opposed to regulation will have few scruples about making the scientific problems more unsurmountable than they actually are. I await with interest statements such as 'all chemicals are reproductive hazards in large enough quantities' or 'the dose, if administered to a human being, constituted 50 times body weight', or other such red herrings.

Epidemiological data

The problems with reproductive epidemiology are extensive, not least being the intrusive nature of many of the questions that have to be asked. While I do not wish to attempt a comprehensive summary of the epidemiology that suggests a link between occupation and adverse effects of reproduction, the evidence is accumulating. Substances for which evidence exists that the exposure of male workers is important include lead, chloroprene, manganese, mercury, toluene di-isocyanate, vinyl chloride, various pesticides and pharmaceuticals, anaesthetic gases, ionising and non-ionising radiation and hydrocarbons. Substances that may directly affect female fertility or fetal development include mercury, lead, arsenic, beryllium, various solvents, anaesthetic gases, pesticides and pharmaceuticals, ionising and non-ionising radiation[8,17].

Work and pregnancy

Another area which has received wider publicity in recent months is the thorny question of whether any evidence exists that, aside from particular risks, work itself is hazardous to pregnancy. Paid work, that is, because no one suggests that women of reproductive capacity should give up domestic work, averaging some 59 hours a week[20]. This research is particularly hard to interpret, as was the case in the analysis of births just after the last census[21]. The results initially seemed to imply that work during pregnancy increased perinatal mortality but on closer examination the results were more equivocal.

Taking an overview, research results have found positive, negative or no associations with adverse pregnancy outcomes[22]. More detailed analysis points to specific reasons for these various results. Long hours, heavy physical work, prolonged standing, toxic exposures and stress, especially if very late into pregnancy, all prejudice the outcome of pregnancy. Research results indicating that work is beneficial to pregnancy suggest that this may be in part due to the improved standard of living and improved take-up of prenatal medical and advisory services[23].

So, we conclude, if certain accepted risk factors are avoided, and adequate rest, time off for consultation and adequate pregnancy leave are given, then work will most likely improve pregnancy outcome. It is indefensible to pose women with the choice between a healthy pregnancy or no job.

POLICY ISSUES

Trade union concerns

Some of the concerns that trade unions have over policy issues have already been discussed in the previous section, but are illustrated below by reference to two important examples of toxic materials with known reproductive effects: lead and anaesthetic gases. These case studies also illustrate the conservative response of both government and medical authorities to evidence of risk.

Lead

The current Code of Practice requires women to be suspended when the concentration of lead in blood level reaches $40\,\mu g/100$ ml[24]. The level for men is $80\,\mu g/100$ ml, the difference being justified on the grounds of protecting the fetus. There is considerable evidence that $80\,\mu g/100$ ml is far too high to protect against effects on the nervous system and the renal system and a decrease in haemoglobin levels[25]. Evidence of adverse male reproductive effects has been established at the $40\,\mu g/100$ ml level[26]. The standard, therefore, discriminates against women, who may have no desire to have children, and it also discriminates against men, who are permitted exposure with a wide range of possible toxic effects, including their ability to father healthy children.

The effects of lead on the fetus are associated with the central nervous system, the development of which is spread over the full term of pregnancy, not just the embryonic period. A standard of $40\,\mu g/100$ ml for both sexes and allowance for removal from exposure in unplanned pregnancies would offer some assurance that risk of damage is reduced to insignificant levels. Neither is such a perspective utopian. Both the USA and Sweden have set permissible blood lead levels regardless of sex at $50\,\mu g/100$ ml.

Lead is perhaps an easier target for criticism than certain other materials, as effects in men and women are apparent at similar levels and the teratogenic risk may be reduced to acceptable levels by removal as soon as pregnancy is diagnosed.

Anaesthetic gases

After the 1967 Russian paper by Vaisman[27], which reported an incidence of miscarriage among pregnant anaesthetists in excess of 50 per cent, several large surveys were conducted. By the mid-1970s studies had found significantly elevated miscarriage rates associated with maternal exposure to anaesthetic gases together with some weaker evidence of congenital malformations and low birth weight. There was also evidence of increased spontaneous abortion and congenital malformation rates in the partners of exposed anaesthetists and dentists. This latter result, based on two studies, was more speculative. However, it has been confirmed by subsequent work[28]. Many of the studies can be criticised as being subject to some response bias in questioning parents where miscarriages have happened and about past exposures to anaesthetic gases. However, not all are vulnerable to this criticism and it is the consistency of the results which is significant, not any single study considered in isolation.

It should be remembered that epidemiological studies rarely produce perfect information for reasons which are well documented.

It took until 1976 for the DHSS to respond to the growing evidence and issue a circular on the introduction of scavenging equipment into operating theatres[29]. The response of Health Authorities has been varied, and many have failed to provide hospitals with the financial resources to introduce this equipment. They have, unfortunately, been encouraged in this attitude by the Royal College of Obstetricians and Gynaecologists (RCOG), who have stated that 'there is no direct evidence that atmospheric pollution with anaesthetic gases causes any hazard in human beings'[30]. One is tempted to ask what evidence *would* have to be produced to show such a 'direct' effect and would such evidence in practice be obtainable?

The RCOG advice continued: 'Normal healthy psychologically well-balanced women might be reassured that there is every chance that they will have a normal pregnancy and confinement and that the risks suggested are unproven.' The memorandum then asserts anxiety as the only real risk factor: 'Patients who are very anxious, particularly if this is because of the DHSS information, or who have an adverse obstetric history, might be advised on general obstetric grounds to consider changing their employment to a more restful occupation during pregnancy.'

Since that time, a large American study of dentists has established the risk to pregnancies in partners of exposed dentists[31].

This episode has various important lessons. The medical profession, as evidenced by not only DHSS attitudes, but also the RCOG, seems to maintain the attitude of viewing reproductive hazards as issues of pregnancy alone, compounding it with the patronising view that women themselves by unnecessary anxiety are really their own worst enemies. The case of anaesthetic gases does, in fact, raise the most difficult question of all in respect of policy formation. To demand evidence of damage, which is essentially unobtainable, is merely another way of delaying policy decisions. It is at this point that most policies say: 'consult a medical practitioner'. This permits most policy makers to avoid the social, political and economic implications of regulating exposure to chemicals, while allowing themselves the luxury of moral rectitude by passing the problem to the doctor, who, unfortunately, in most cases shows an unscientific willingness to receive it. Most policies in the field of occupational health have to be based on incomplete information. The social implications of particular policies have to take into account cost, but there are few instances of major social advances where a conventional cost-benefit analysis would have produced a socially desirable policy.

It is against the current political background that many trade unionists fear the consequences of discriminatory regulation. A return to Victorian values — that women should remain at home — fits well with the emphasis on protecting women's reproductive health.

Employers' policies

Only one company in the UK to my knowledge has issued a policy on an aspect of reproductive hazards to employee representatives. Ciba-Geigy's policy has been reviewed at length[32]. Other British companies have obviously considered the issue and their spokespersons have made a number of observations. The Chemical Industries Association is currently preparing guidelines, but these were not available at the time of writing. It is worth noting that at no time have the trades unions been consulted in the development of these policies. A number of papers have been published by American company physicians and it must be presumed that these companies would take a similar approach in their British subsidiaries.

These policies have a number of features in common. They almost exclusively concentrate on the teratogenic effect of chemicals and ignore the mutagenic effects on both male and female reproductive capacity. They concentrate on the problems that the issue presents to management, which are defined as follows:

(1) If management decides to remove or bar all women of child-bearing age from a particular job or work site, the company may be faced with discrimination litigation.

(2) If a pregnant female is allowed to stay on a particular job without warning, and aborts or delivers a damaged child, the company may be open to very costly medical claims.

(3) If management attempts to change a process or procedure, they may alter the economic feasibility of producing the product.

(4) If management establishes a policy of transferring women to other jobs at no pay loss, they may be opening a Pandora's box for other workers who seek the same arrangement for different reasons[33].

Such defensive policies may be possible, if not desirable, for employers in some areas of the private sector because of the existing patterns of male and female employment. They are impossible to consider in the public sector, particularly the NHS, where large numbers of women are employed. This raises the possibility of the kind of hypocrisy that has allowed women's hours to be regulated in factories while health care workers, contract cleaners and all other women workers not actually employed in factories, can work without such protection.

The inevitable consequence of allowing employers to develop and implement policies in this field, with or without union agreement, is a recipe for not only discrimination between men and women, but also different standards depending on the bargaining power of groups of women workers or the paternalistic benevolence of their employers.

The immediate need is for employers to make available information on materials and substances used at the work place and to help in the development of more detailed protocols and short-term tests for reproductive toxicity. If our experience in respect of carcinogens is a precedent, we cannot be optimistic about their likely co-operation.

Future action

We will be seeking to remove health and safety policies which systematically discriminate on the grounds of sex, both at a national legislative level and in negotiated agreements with companies. For pregnant women we will seek to maximise the benefits in terms of paid maternity (and paternity) leave, transfer from risky or physically arduous work with no loss of pay, and facilities for prenatal care. Where there is evidence of any risk, transfer to alternative employment for both men and women may be indicated *before* conception, although the organisational aspects of this approach present numerous difficulties.

At present, as the Employment Appeal Tribunal decision on Mrs Page has indicated, an actual change in the Health and Safety at Work Act and/or the Equal Opportunities Act may be required to ensure that less discriminatory health and safety policies are developed[34].

Three recent American legal cases have resulted in decisions that to exclude women, but not men, from jobs with reproductive hazards constitutes sex discrimination[35]. This indicates that unless our legislation is changed, we may find ourselves going down a discriminatory path which few other countries will be prepared to follow.

In terms of standards for work place hazardous exposures, we shall be seeking the establishment of control limits and guidance limits which are stringent enough to protect all workers whether male or female, and to ensure that more information is generally available to employees. Because the whole range of reproductive hazards has been under-emphasised, we shall be providing information and advice to our members, but it is the responsibility of the HSC to provide information and guidance to employers, workers and the medical profession.

A great deal of work is going on at the present time to produce a new set of regulations for the control of substances hazardous to health. Reproductive health is only one aspect of the entire problem of occupational health. Prevention of adverse effects is the only viable long-term strategy. It is to be hoped that this conference can be taken as an indication that the matter is now being taken seriously and that we can hope in the near future for a resolution of some of the scientific problems. In the meantime, those concerned with the policy aspects should exercise great care in an attempt to avoid discrimination against women while ensuring healthy reproduction.

ACKNOWLEDGEMENT

This chapter was prepared with the help of Tony Fletcher, an epidemiologist currently working in the ASTMS Health and Safety Office.

REFERENCES

1. TUC (1980). *Women Workers: 1980*, A report of the TUC Women's Advisory Committee 1979–80 and report of the 50th TUC Women's Conference March 1980, TUC, London
2. Equal Opportunities Commission (1979). *Health and Safety Legislation: Should we Distinguish between Men and Women?*, Equal Opportunities Commission, London
3. Chenier, N. M. (1982). Reproductive hazards at work, Canadian Advisory Council on the Status of Women, Ottawa
4. House of Commons Social Services Committee (1980). Second Report: *Perinatal and Neonatal Mortality*, Vol. 1, HMSO, London
5. TUC (1981). *Women's Health at Risk*, TUC, London
6. TUC (1982). *Collective Bargaining Agreements: Assistance for Working Parents*, Policy document available from the TUC on request
7. McKechnie, S. (1981). Reproductive hazards in employment. *ASTMS Medical World*, June
   Sullivan, F. (1981). Work and sex. *ASTMS Medical World*, September/October
   Barlow, S. (1981). Work and sex. *ASTMS Medical World*, November/December
   Papers presented at *GMBATU/ASTMS Seminar on Reproductive Hazards at Work*, Guys Hospital Medical School, 30 March 1981
8. Council on Environmental Quality, USA (1981). *Chemical Hazards to Reproduction*
9. Wilson, J. G. (1973). *Environment and Birth Defects*, Academic Press, New York
10. Kalter, H. and Warkany, J. (1983). Congenital malformations: aetiological factors and their role in prevention. *New Engl. J. Med.*, **308**, 424–431, 491–497
11. Townsend, P. and Davidson, N. (1982). *Inequalities in Health*, Pelican, Harmondsworth
12. Hemminki, K., *et al.* (1980). Spontaneous abortions by occupation and social class in Finland. *Int. J. Epidemiol.*, **9**, 149–153
13. Office of Population Censuses and Surveys (1982). *Congenital Malformations and Parents' Occupation*, OPCS Monitor MB3 82/1

14. Erickson, J. D., *et al.* (1979). Parental occupation and birth defects: a preliminary report. *Contrib. Epidemiol. Biostat.*, **1**, 107–117
15. Hemminki, K., *et al.* (1983). Spontaneous abortions in an industrialised community in Finland. *Am. J. Publ. Hlth*, **73**, 32–37
16. Elwood, J. M. and Elwood, J. H. (1982). International variation in the prevalence at birth of anencephalus in relation to maternal factors. *Int. J. Epidemiol.*, **11**, 132–137
17. Barlow, S. and Sullivan, F. (1982). *Reproductive Hazards of Industrial Chemicals*, Academic Press, London
18. Hemminki, K. (1980). Occupational chemicals tested for teratogenicity. *Int. Arch. Occup. Environ. Hlth*, **47**, 191–207
19. White, C. G., *et al.* (1981). *Extrapolation Models in Teratogenesis* (Final Report for Experiment 281), NCTR, Jefferson, Ark.
20. Vanek, J. (1974). Time spent in housework. *Sci. Am.*, **231**, 116–120
21. McDowall, M., *et al.* (1981). Employment during pregnancy and infant mortality. *Pop. Trends*, **26**, 12–15
22. Chamberlain, G. and Garcia, J. (1983). Pregnant women at work. *Lancet*, **1**, 228–230
23. Saurel, M. J. and Kaminski, M. (1983). Pregnant women at work (Letter). *Lancet*, i, 475
24. Health and Safety Commission (1980). *Control of Lead at Work: Approved Code of Practice*, HMSO, London
25. US Department of Labor Occupational Safety and Health Administration (1978). Occupational exposure to lead. *Fed. Reg.*, **43**, 52952–53014
26. Lacranjan, I., *et al.* (1975). Reproductive ability of workmen occupationally exposed to lead. *Arch. Environ. Hlth*, **30**, 396–401.
27. Vaisman, A. I. (1967). Working conditions in surgery and their effect on the health of anaesthetists. *Exp. Khir. Anesthesiol.*, **3**, 44–49
28. Edling, C. (1980). Anaesthetic gases as an occupational hazard — a review. *Scand. J. Work Environ. Hlth*, **6**, 85–93
29. Department of Health and Social Security (1976). *Pollution of Operating Departments, etc., by Anaesthetic Gases*, HC (76) 38, DHSS, London
30. Anon. (1978). Counselling on the hazards of pregnancy in operating theatre staff. *Anaesthesia*, **33**, 96–97
31. Cohen, E. N., Brown, B. W., *et al.* (1980). Occupational disease in dentistry and chronic exposure to trace anaesthetic gases. *J. Am. Dent. Assoc.*, **101**, 21–31
32. Anon. (1981). *Protecting the Unborn Child — A Precautionary Policy at Ciba-Geigy* (Health and Safety Information Bulletin No. 66), Industrial Relations Review and Report, p. 3
33. Krausse, L. A. (1979). [Director of Environmental Hygiene and Toxicology, Olin Corporation]. In *National Safety News*, February
34. Page, V. (1981). Freight Hire (Tank Haulage) Ltd, Health and Safety Information Bulletin No. 62, Industrial Relations Review and Report
35. *Women's Occupational Health Resource Centre News*, **5**, No. 1, February/ March (1983)

15

A Management View of Reproductive Health

J. PLAUT

I approach this subject as one trained in engineering and law who has worked in industry, and earlier in US regulatory agencies. Although my responsibility is to manage industry environmental (that is, pollution control), occupational health and safety activities, I hope I will bring to you some different perspectives.

Britain was the birth-place of the Industrial Revolution, which historically was the culmination of the Renaissance. The Industrial Revolution began with the British cottage industries and women in that period served the dual, and what we think now is the modern, role of industrial worker and housewife. Unfortunately, we have few data from that time.

I intend to divide my chapter into three sections. First, some generalisations about industry performance and public perception and pressures. Second, a discussion of enlightened health and business management in the plant. Third, based on the two first sections, some actual industry guidelines. Some of this chapter will be quite specific; at other times it will be intentionally philosophical. What management needs to do should be clear by the time I conclude.

INDUSTRY PERFORMANCE AND PUBLIC PRESSURES

First, in a defence of industry I think we should understand the present state of environmental and health affairs as compared with two decades ago. We should not underestimate the very real gains in protection made in the 1970s or the costs involved in making those gains. Responsible industry in the USA is proud to be a part of what has been accomplished. Our rivers are cleaner. Many varieties of fish, such as Atlantic salmon in the Maine lakes or local varieties of fish in Lake Erie, have returned. The air we breathe in many urban areas is markedly improved. A visit to Pittsburgh or Los Angeles for one who has been away for two decades would be a pleasant surprise. Worker health and safety has never received such attention. My company has shown continued improvement in the safety of its workers (including the female workers) through programmes of safety excellence which use systems and tools of hazard control and account-ability. We are proud of this record.

With the growth in analytical science, toxicology, testing and monitoring programmes, industry has greatly improved its knowledge of the materials it handles and its products. Problems and challenges will continue to exist and new ones will be uncovered. Some great issues face us: acid rain, waste disposal, testing of chemicals, smoking and drug abuse, to mention a few. Nevertheless, we have made real progress, even if at a significant short-term price.

One of the important areas of concern which has emerged is what is called *women in the work place* and seemingly competing health and equal employ-ment demands. Individuals in a society and institutions such as companies are part of a group to which they are responsible. They have obligations as a part of a social contract, and compliance with government regulation and exemplary health protection are basic industry obligations. Sometimes, however, different sets of regulations responsive to different concerns and pressure groups seem to require conflicting programmes of compliance — for example, women in the work place. Very rigid self-interest and advocacy in such situations makes constructive give-and-take and solution-finding difficult.

Can women be treated as equals with men in terms of hazard control and systems of protection? The most honest answer is — almost always. But before elaborating we should step back from the problem to develop some background and make some initial generalisations.

Dr Ben Eisenman, professor of surgery at the University of Colorado, a noted medical scholar and teacher, wrote in his challenging book *What Are My Chances*[1] : 'In this century, life expectancy has almost doubled. In 1900, a new-born child had an average life span of about forty years. Now it is over seventy and climbing. In short, we are the first generation with a reasonable chance to live until we wear out rather than having our lives cut short by acute illness . . . modern man [has an] almost childish confidence in the power of science. In America, in particular, we feel that if sufficient personal resources and money are devoted to a problem, it can be solved. [note the man on the moon accom-plishment] . . . No disease can withstand knowledge, energy and money — so goes the false but generally accepted premise . . . Throughout the century we have stam-peded toward a riskless society . . .' Political and social scientist Aaron Wildavsky of the University of California wrote in 1979 in the *American Scientist*[2] : 'The future won't be allowed to make mistakes because the present will use up its excess resources in prevention . . . . How extraordinary! The richest, longest-lived, best-protected, most resourceful civilisation, with the highest degree of insight into its own technology, is on its way to becoming the most frightened. Chicken Little is alive and well in America.'

Johns Hopkins University recently published troubling data showing the primary deteriorating effect of loss of jobs and income on indices of health protection[3].

Health protection and job opportunity may soon seem like antithetical goals, if in order to achieve zero risk by costly overkill, one abandons an array of methods to control hazards.

Zero risk philosophy often moves the advocate towards fanatical approaches to eliminate risk, as by overengineering − no matter how excessively costly or infeasible − rather than effective control of risk through a rational selection of alternatives which include engineering but also personal protection, good hygiene, medical monitoring or job rotation, for example. A zero risk approach without a paramount concept of control leads to excess usually without affording increased health protection or even eroding confidence in the possibility of such protection. Have you seen the cynical bumper sticker EVERYTHING CAUSES CANCER?

Deep concern about misapplication of resources without accomplishing increased health protection is compounded because we live under the threat of zero sum economics. Simply stated: without growth you must often take from someone or something existing to pay for some new, competing demand. As the eminent MIT economist Lester Thurow has said in his book, *The Zero Sum Society*[4]: 'Our political and economic structure simply isn't able to cope . . . . The gains and losses are not allocated to the same individuals or groups . . . . Each group wants government to use its power to protect it and to force others to do what [it perceives] is in the general interest.'

In a sense, the social contract has gone beserk. Everyone is taking but no one giving! Rational solution to competing demands suffers when zero sum resource allocation is added to zero risk fanaticism.

The Lysenko effect is a third concern. We all know the story of the Russian bureaucrat Lysenko, and the disastrous effects on Russian agriculture resulting from establishment of what Lysenko considered acceptable scientific dogma in the genetics of wheat crop improvement. Certainly, ever since Galileo's struggle with the Church of his time, we in Western society have been wary of those who would, by doctrine, establish unchallengeable scientific dogma. Born in careless, too politically sensitive, or corrupt institutions, the reactionary approach which dictates scientific truth destroys rationality as an approach to a health concern. The experiences of Lysenko and Galileo may be behind us, but there is still danger that the institutional corroding of science and health protection of the past may indeed be prologue. We must not allow uncertain science to give way to destructive dogma, nor let those who seek political or social ends misuse that science to weaken the long-term goal of public health protection.

Allow me to illustrate with the Love Canal debacle. The panel appointed by the Governor of New York, to review the evidence of chronic health risks involving supposed devastating chromosome damage to Love Canal residents, chaired by Dr Lewis Thomas of Sloan-Kettering Memorial Cancer Center, found 'an astonishing amount of scientific and managerial incompetence in several key [governmental] studies of the affair'. One study was 'so poorly designed' it should never have been undertaken. Another could not be taken seriously and had the 'impact of polemic'. The *New York Times*[5], faulting the Environmental Protection Agency (EPA), commented in an editorial: 'When the returns are all in, years from now, it may well turn out that the public suffered less from the chemicals there than from the hysteria generated by flimsy research, irresponsibly handled.'

The original EPA study at Love Canal concluded that there was possibility for wide-spread chromosome damage and birth defects for the residents in the area. The result was understandable hysteria on the part of the local public, which incidentally was all painfully witnessed on the nightly television news. The later, more detailed study concluded that there was hazard, but not of the hysteria-producing degree earlier reported. As a matter of fact, the study conducted by the Center for Disease Control in Atlanta contradicted the earlier disputed EPA study and reported 'no increase in abnormalities' among 46 residents or former residents of the area surrounding the canal, compared with 50 residents of a control area. 'This suggests that no specific relationship existed between exposure to chemical agents in the Love Canal area and increased frequency of chromosome damage,' the Center for Disease Control in Atlanta concluded[6].

This is not to assert that there is not cause for concern about hazard, and the need for control techniques according to the best technology, but those in government and science communities, or in industry, who misuse science to obtain their objectives — their ears should be burning! In this case politics or emotionalism seemed to have just simply pushed aside good science.

An isolated incident? Probably not, and we should all consider whether the necessity for gaining funding for a research or test grant may not, in truth, be a rigidifying force similar to what Galileo faced or Lysenko imposed. The results can stifle creative scientific inquiry. The almost inconceivably large government programmes for medical and toxicological research may determine what is scientifically *acceptable*.

The Lysenkos of the world take advantage of blind prejudice born of lack of understanding and fear. I wonder whether men and women often are reacting to immediate, seemingly unresolvable and frightening health problems and concerns with unreasonable hysteria and stridency, born out of ignorance. Susan Sontag, the American social philosopher with a far-ranging mind and pen, has written a challenging book called *Illness as Metaphor*[7]. Ms Sontag traces the myths that were developed in other centuries by societies to deal with their own ignorance about contemporary scourges such as the plague, and diseases communicated by man and organisms such as syphilis and tuberculosis. Then, also, society honestly believed, and made others suffer as scapegoats the consequences of, what was stubbornly held onto as contemporary truth. Ms Sontag postulates in her book that we are doing the same thing now as our ancestors did, but this time in relationship to cancer. She says: '. . . the cancer metaphor [to evil] is particularly crass. It is invariably an encouragement to simplify what is complex and an invitation to self-righteousness, if not to fanaticism.'[6]

Dr John Higgenson, founding director of the World Health Organization's International Agency for Research on Cancer, in an interview in *Science* magazine[8], stated that: 'I don't think that some people are intentionally dishonest, but rather that they found it hard to accept that general air pollution, smoking factory chimneys, and the like are not the major cause of cancer. I mean, people would love to be able to prove that cancer is due to pollution or the general environment. It would be so easy to be able to say "let us regulate everything to zero exposure and we have no more cancer". The concept is so beautiful that it will overwhelm a mass of facts to the contrary.' As Dr Higgenson told the American Cancer Society, and as a recent study told the US Office of Technology Assessment, and as you well know, life styles — cultural, behavioural and dietary habits, particularly smoking and alcohol — rather than exposure to chemicals in the environment seem to cause most human cancers[9].

To say it plainly, we are a society that appears all too happy to encourage teenaged girls to smoke, while seeking culprits in industry under almost any pretext. There are those in our society who appear to strike out with a pride born of an anti-industry prejudice. Society, then, often directs its attention towards some vague and unproved industry health threat in the hope of finding an easy and popular scapegoat. Not learning from the history of ignorance, are we condemning ourselves to repeat our mistakes?

INDUSTRY HEALTH MANAGEMENT

With those comments as background, we turn more directly to our topic. It is important to begin with a truth essential for the business manager to comprehend and act upon. Simply stated, good pollution control, health and safety at the plant level, as well as responsible product handling . . . is good and effective management.

Attention paid to process control, to the efficiency of the process in terms of avoiding emissions and spills, results in increased control of the manufacturing process.

The health and safety of the workers, male and female, are outstanding measures of how well a plant is working.

Good safety training reflects good communications within the plant.

Proper care and use of facilities and equipment is a result of good safety training and results in quality product.

Product quality has a direct relationship, not only to product safety concerns, but also, more importantly, to productivity.

All of these aspects of management will result in improved health protection and lower business liabilities.

There is every good reason for the businessman, for his own internal management processes, to believe in and practise responsible environmental health and safety management. Management is losing a chance for competitiveness if it does not accept the environmental safety and health challenge as an opportunity.

The process of hazard management (that is, hazard identification and assessment and then control) is critical. It is easy to understand that the pollution control, health, product safety or safety professional (the environmental professional) must be schooled in his or her particular field to understand the degree of hazard (including toxicity), the degrees of exposure and the method of control. It is more difficult to understand that many business decisions which appear to be non-environmental also require an input of hazard management identification and assessment of control alternatives. This is often true of decisions to manufacture a new product, to build or expand a plant, or to market an existing product for a new use, for example. Moreover, it is also true of the everyday business and operating decisions of, say, the middle manager, or the plant superintendent or plant engineer with respect to such questions as the level of plant maintenance, or the effect of a cut in quality control or process monitoring, or even the budget for night supervision, or allocation of resources for testing, monitoring or training.

Business functions should have procedures for dealing with hazard management, including excellence in health monitoring and data management for their own long-term protection. Environmental professionals in the disciplines of pollution control, safety and loss prevention, medical services, occupational health including industrial hygiene, product safety and toxicology are able to bring specific professional knowledge to the identification of both hazards and control. Hazard identification and control should become routine[10].

INDUSTRY GUIDELINES

Turning now to industry action, I shall offer some specific guidelines. Hazard falls into one of these groups: local or acute hazard; chronic but apparent hazard; and genetic or latent hazard. Control of the hazard relative to workers (male or female) is critical.

Preventing acute hazards will usually be the same for either sex. The simplest example would be a sharp cutting edge presenting danger. Many chronic hazards, too, are applicable to either sex (say loss of hearing over a period of time due to high noise levels and absence of noise reduction programmes and hearing protection); but there are acute and chronic hazards which require special industrial attention relative to women – for example, simply dealing with individual or routine lifting hazards, which are explicitly regulated in France as to women.

Genetic or latent hazards are most in point, perhaps. The admonition in our Preface to 'guard the patient's welfare' should be controlling. Where the hazard may directly and specifically affect women or the potential offspring – such as in the case of lead dust in the battery work place, for example – women may have to be treated separately, individually or as a group in control of the hazard. The law is growing to recognise that, and so do we, as I shall discuss.

I have taken this route to the issue of protecting women in the industry work place, because protecting women as a part of the obligation to protect all workers is a paramount continuing obligation of management which it must handle routinely and with excellence if it is to remain competitive over the long term.

Again, a few obvious truths are critical:

(1) A paramount obligation of industry is to afford a safe and healthy work place for each of its workers — men and women.

(2) There are hazards which appear to affect women because of their sex, or the fetuses they may be carrying or may carry in the future.

(3) Protection of the fetus or potential fetus must be a primary concern where the danger is evident and uncorrectable under present feasible technology. Health liability concerns can not be ignored.

The issue has come to a head in Wright v. Olin Corporation[11], in which the US Court of Appeals for the Fourth Circuit ruled that: 'Employers have the burden of demonstrating that a significant risk of harm to unborn children justifies a company policy barring women from holding jobs that involve exposure to hazardous chemicals.' The court laid down the following guidelines, which are instructive even as they will be further tested for determining whether women are a special case to be protected by removal from the work place due to hazard:

(1) The burden [of proof] is upon the employer to prove that significant risks of harm to the unborn children of women workers from the exposure during pregnancy to toxic hazards in the work place make necessary the restrictions that apply only to women, and that the programme of restriction is effective for the purpose.

(2) The essential elements of the defence must be supported by the opinion evidence of qualified experts [outside the company] in the relevant scientific fields.

(3) The employer is not required to show a consensus within the scientific community; rather the employer must 'show that within the community there is so considerable a body of opinion that significant risk exists, and that it is substantially confined to women workers, that an informed employer could not responsibly fail to act on the assumption that this opinion might be the accurate one'.

(4) The women plaintiffs may rebut the defence by proof that there are other acceptable policies or practices that would better protect against the risk of harm, or lessen the differing impact between male and female workers.

When dealing with the issue of protecting women in the work place, these guidelines by the circuit court will be valuable, too, in setting a rational philosophy and programme.

Men and women workers must be provided a safe and healthy environment in which to work. Where there are special hazards to either men or women, they must be analysed and controlled. If that can not be done, the workers potentially harmed must be removed or the operation terminated.

There are many means of *control*, including:

(1) Designing, engineering out or removing the hazard – for example, by holding the hazard level below a certain dose over a certain set period of time.

(2) Personal protection – for example, by use of gloves, safety glasses or respirators.

(3) Limiting exposure – for example, by administrative measures such as job rotation.

(4) Monitoring medical factors – for example, blood lead levels – and removing the worker before he or she reaches detrimental exposure levels.

Control is the key, but where control cannot be attained realistically, then women of child-bearing potential or pregnant women may need to be removed or treated differently from men.

Dr John Inglefinger, former editor of the *New England Medical Journal*[12], wrote: 'Arrogance enters when those, reaching various decisions in the absence of adequate data, fail to recognize or to admit how empty their cupboard of information is. Superior scientists or doctors, I should like to believe, are always aware of how little they know. Doubt tempers arrogance.' Dr Inglefinger's warning about avoiding arrogance is important in terms of understanding and rationally controlling hazard.

Management should not rely fully on the fact that its operations will conform with company policies and procedures, no matter how independent its professionals, how well organised its people, how thoroughgoing the training and indoctrination. Self-doubt should suggest systems of self-checking. It should commend a system of surveillance to sample on a routine basis whether in fact the operations are complying with the laws, regulations, company policy and procedure. A regular and routine programme of plant inspections and reviews of operations will tell the management whether its operations are within the parameters of the risk assessment and control. Together with rigorous follow-up on all deficiencies found to assure that preventive measures are in place, the surveillance programme will confirm to the middle managers, supervisors and employees of the company that the company means to carry out its environmental policies and programme. That will assure that the control processes, which are the key, stay in effect.

In all cases a clear sense of purpose, resolve and authority of the decision-makers as to hazard control should be understood within the organisation. Whatever the organisation structure, it is essential that effective hazard identification and control be communicated throughout the organisation as demanded by management.

We should not delude ourselves: we are at the beginning of analytical ability and knowledge as to the existence or non-existence of many hazards. A very simple question was asked in the enlightening *New York Times* article: 'With the energy crisis, the economic crisis, and the growing fears about the environment, many people have become prophets of doom. Are they right, or is it still possible to believe in the future?'[13] Reiterating, a system of control and follow-up where there is suspected hazard must be the key for industry if we desire rational functioning of an industrial society and problem-solving instead of non-productive doom and gloom forecasting.

It would seem that the doom prophets have broken faith with society. They have abandoned the social contract, which states, basically, that one gives a little for the common good. It is interesting, as the *New York Times* article points out, that: 'Doomsayers blame what they do not like on others — scientists, militarists, industrialists, politicians, advertisers, bankers, lawyers. All enter into the script like masked figures of the vices in a mortality play.' If we are going to manage problems involving hazards in a work place by managing our efforts and resources, then we must convince our colleagues in industry, the administrators and policy-makers in government, and our peers and contemporaries who claim to advocate the protection of health and the environment that rational systems of control are the ways to make progress.

William Shakespeare wrote in *Hamlet* 400 years ago

'What a piece of work is a man. How noble in reason! how infinite in faculty! . . .'

We must as individuals, through excellence in the creation of systems of control, exercise our reason and faculties to continue to protect the health and safety of our workers — female or male.

REFERENCES

1. Eisenman, B. (1980). *What Are My Chances*, Saunders Press (Holt, Rinehart and Winston, New York, p. 3
2. Widlavsky, A. (1979). *American Scientist*, **67**, 32
3. *The New York Times*, 6 April 1982, Section C, p. 1.
4. Thurow, L. C. (1980). *The Zero Sum Society*, Basic Books, New York, p. 32
5. *The New York Times*, 20 June 1981
6. *The New York Times*, 18 May 1983
7. Sontag, Susan (1978). *Illness as Metaphor*, Farrar Straus and Giroux, New York, p. 85
8. *Science Magazine*, **205**, 1364 (1979)
9. *Science News*, **115**, 23 June (1979)

212 · *J. Plaut*

10. Gardiner, A. Ward (Ed.) (1982). *Occupational Health: 2*, Chapter 14, Wright-PSG, London
11. *Occupational Safety and Health Reporter*, reporting on Wright v. Olin Corporation (No. 81-1229), 6 January 1983, pp. 612–613, US Court of Appeals for the Fourth Circuit ruled 23 December 1982
12. Inglefinger, J. (1980). *New England Journal of Medicine*, 24 December 1509
13. Starr, R. (1979). *New York Times Magazine*, 19 August

16

Legal Considerations of Reproductive Hazards in Industry in the United Kingdom

STEVEN J. LORBER

'The Health and Safety Commission must recognise that industry's capacity to produce wealth, provide employment and compete effectively in overseas markets are priorities just as vital as the maintenance of good health and safety standards' (Confederation of British Industry evidence to House of Commons Employment Committee)[1]

'"Reasonably practicable" is a narrower term than "physically possible" and seems to me to imply that a computation must be made by the owner in which quantum of risk is placed on one scale, and the sacrifice involved in the measures necessary for averting the risk (whether in money, time or trouble) is placed in the other' (Asquith, L. J., in *Edwards* v. *National Coal Board*)[2]

The Health and Safety at Work Act 1974 (HASAWA) imposes a duty on every employer to 'ensure, so far as is reasonably practicable, the health, safety and welfare at work of all his employees'. What is reasonably practicable and the relationship between (ultimately) profit and the employees' health determine in large part the approach of the law to reproductive hazards at work.

Until the 1970s work hazards to reproduction were largely ignored by UK legislation. The Factories Acts, which had their origins in nineteenth century restrictions on the length of the working day and child labour, removed women from a limited range of processes, primarily lead-related[3] and prevented the employment of women within the 4 weeks following childbirth[4].

The old approach, the blanket removal of women from specific industries, is inadequate. As will be clear from other chapters in this book, reproductive hazards may be caused by a wide range of agents – physical, chemical or biological. The work environment may be a hazard not only to the fetus, but also to sperm, libido, potency, ovulation and other facets of reproduction[5]. The legislature is faced with a dilemma. If it were to be consistent with the policy of

213

blanket removal, both men and women would be excluded from an increasing number and variety of work places. The number of industries affected would be great. This chapter considers the law's developing approach to the dilemma.

In response to an occupational disease or hazard at work taking effect over a period, there are three approaches: (1) one can do nothing; (2) one can adopt a hazard-based approach by substituting for or reducing the hazard; (3) one can adopt a worker-restricting approach, by providing protection for the worker (e.g. special clothes), or by suspending or limiting the employment of the worker. That is schematic, but it provides a basis for considering the operation of the law. In practice, a combination of approaches is usually adopted. It is generally cheaper to adopt a worker-restricting approach, particularly where there are two groups of workers who are differentially affected, as may be the case with hazards to reproduction. Rather than reduce the hazards for both groups, exclude one.

In this chapter, I review legislative developments in the UK and the European Community (EC) and then highlight three aspects. First, I consider whether the law in practice promotes a hazard-based approach to reproductive hazards. Second, if a hazard-based approach fails, I look at who is restricted and how the criteria for restriction operate. Finally, where a worker is restricted and suspended from work, I consider the rights offered by the law to that worker.

UNITED KINGDOM AND EUROPEAN COMMUNITY LEGISLATION

It is not possible to review here all aspects of UK law bearing on reproductive hazards at work. In particular, there is no discussion of maternity rights under employment protection legislation. Since the UK's accession to the EC, much legislation has been in consequence of Community directives. The EC's approach involves not only direct control of potential hazards, but also indirect measures by providing information and education on possible risks.

In 1980 an EC Directive was approved on the protection of workers from risks related to exposure to chemical, physical and biological hazards at work[6]. This was principally concerned with direct control of hazards and established a framework for further specific directives. The first specific Directive following the framework Directive was on exposure to lead[7]. Draft proposals are being formulated on further directives which include control of asbestos[8], noise[9] and carcinogens[10].

As well as direct control of hazards, the EC has approved Directives on classification, packaging and labelling of dangerous substances and on notification to a national authority of details of new substances prior to marketing. These details include the results of tests for teratogenicity and mutagenicity[11].

In response to the EC Directives, the UK has passed regulations under HASAWA which relate to reproductive hazards: Packaging and Labelling of Dangerous Substances Regulations 1978 (as amended); Notification of New

Substances Regulations 1982; Control of Lead at Work Regulations 1980 and approved Code of Practice. Draft proposals have been made for control of ionising radiation and general control of substances hazardous to health.

Finally, the Sex Discrimination Act 1975 should be mentioned. It should be mentioned because it is, surprisingly, largely irrelevant. This contrasts with the position in the USA, where it has proved possible to attack legislation on the basis that it discriminates. The Sex Discrimination Act has no bearing on prior legislation[12]. Thus, HASAWA passed a year before cannot be challenged on the basis that it, or particular practices relating to health and safety, discriminate.

The reluctance of the courts to give the Sex Discrimination Act significance is illustrated by the case of a woman who was dismissed because she was pregnant. The court held, with rather dubious logic, that there was no discrimination, because: 'When she is pregnant a woman is no longer just a woman. She is a woman, as the *Authorised Version* accurately puts it, with child, and there is no masculine equivalent'[13]. The decision falls into the (sex-plus) trap. Its logic is that there is no sex discrimination because one is not discriminating against women generally, but against a sub-class (in this case, pregnant women). Discrimination is usually based on alleged female attributes. There is rarely discrimination against a woman purely because she is a woman. The decision has not yet been successfully challenged.

CONTROL OF HAZARDS – SO FAR AS IS REASONABLY PRACTICABLE

In theory, the law gives priority to a hazard-based approach. It assumes that it is better to prevent a hazard than to exclude the worker. Thus, the framework Directive contains a preamble which suggests a hazard-based approach: protection should 'as far as possible be ensured by measures to prevent exposure or keep it at as low a level as is reasonably practicable'[6]. Articles 4 and 5 of the Directive specify a number of control measures, including limitation of use, prevention by engineering control, hygiene and individual protection measures where exposure cannot 'reasonably be prevented by other means'[6].

The Control of Lead at Work Regulations appear to emphasise a hazard-based approach. They provide in regulation 6 that: 'Every employer shall, so far as is reasonably practicable, provide such control measures . . . as will adequately control the exposure of his employees otherwise than by the use of respiratory protective equipment or protective clothing by those employees.' The control measures are elucidated in the approved Code of Practice.

Thus, the obligations in UK legislation and EC directives are to use hazard-based measures unless they are not reasonably practicable or exposure cannot reasonably be avoided. This is in line with the general obligation upon employers under HASAWA to ensure the health and safety of employees so far as is reasonably practicable.

What is practicable may depend upon scientific or technical knowledge. 'Reasonably' qualifies 'practicable'. Its meaning is subjective and will depend on a policy decision by the courts as to the presumptions to be applied and the criteria to be used in determining reasonability. I look at this first in general and then in the specific context of lead.

'Reasonably practicable' has been considered by the courts. According to L. J. Asquith, in *Edwards* v. *National Coal Board*, it depends on a balance of quantum of risk against sacrifice to avert the risk[2]. He lists money, time and trouble. He intended employers to balance quantum of risk to employees against the cost of preventive measures. The test is inadequate. On their own, the factors considered by Asquith are incommensurable. What is measurable, and more likely to be calculated, is the risk to the business (e.g. chance of prosecution or liability for compensation) against the cost of preventing the hazard. The risk to the business is reduced because some costs are redistributed by insurance or subsidised (e.g. by the NHS). Further, the risk depends on the likelihood of enforcement or litigation in practice. As explained above, if there are two groups with different safety thresholds, there is a tendency for it to be cheaper to adopt a worker-restricting approach than to eliminate the hazard. This is likely to be the case in the context of hazards to reproduction, where the financial criteria make the test particularly unhelpful. The quotation at the beginning of this chapter from the CBI[1] treating wealth and effective competition on a par with health and safety underlines the weakness in 'reasonably practicable' as a formula.

The limitations of 'reasonably practicable' and (there being an assumption that two groups have different safety thresholds) the resulting discrimination against women are illustrated if one considers the case of lead. Paragraph 26 of the Code of Practice on lead deems hazard-based measures to be adequate where they control the exposure of the employee to the lead-in-air standard ($150 \mu g/m^3$ air). The obligation is only to achieve this so far as is reasonably practicable (see regulation 6 above). According to the Health and Safety Commission (HSC) the lead-in-air standard is likely to produce blood-lead levels of about $60 \mu g/100$ ml[14]. That is higher than the blood-lead level of $40 \mu g/100$ ml at which women of reproductive capacity are suspended. Thus, since control measures are deemed adequate at lead-in-air levels unacceptable for women of reproductive capacity and since the obligation is only to achieve those so far as is reasonably practicable, it is unlikely that an employer will expend money to reduce the lead-in-air level to one which would permit women of reproductive capacity to work. It will not be reasonably practicable.

WORKER-RESTRICTION FOLLOWING THE FAILURE OF THE HAZARD-BASED APPROACH

Background

Where a hazard-based approach is not implemented or is not sufficient, worker-restricting measures will be considered. The formula determining which workers are to be restricted is vital, particularly in the light of knowledge that hazards are not limited to the fetus, but may affect other aspects of male and female reproduction. The old approach of simply removing women from certain industries was inadequate. In 1975 the Equal Opportunities Commission (EOC) was established with statutory duties which included reviewing such discriminatory health and safety legislation[15]. Its review *Health and Safety Legislation: Should we Distinguish between Men and Women?* was published in 1979[16]. I shall consider the terms of the review and its proposals as to changes in the formula of who is to be excluded. I shall then look at objections to the proposals. Finally, I shall discuss the case of lead, which exemplifies a general reluctance to face the real nature of reproductive hazards.

EOC Report on protective legislation

The Report considered protective health and safety legislation. Such legislation adopted a worker-restricting approach, by excluding or limiting the employment of women and children. According to the EOC, its origins stemmed from a belief that 'moral and spiritual degradation' accompanied female employment. The Report identified mixed motives, not all of which were disinterested, for protective legislation: '... sympathy for woman's weakness and the fact that women reproduce; an idea of womanliness which increasingly saw women's place as in the home; and a strong feeling that women should not take work away from men ... it intensified competition.' The EOC concluded that the legislation encouraged a trend towards housewifery and tended to restrict women's employment opportunities. Men benefited[16].

Part of the EOC's Report is concerned with existing and proposed restrictions on workers exposed to lead and ionising radiation. Though specifically related to lead and ionising radiation, the EOC expected that the approach would be used for legislation on other toxic substances.

The Health and Safety Commission (HSC) advised the EOC that women were at no greater risk than men in general. The EOC concluded (reference 16, para. 431) that: 'When permissible levels of exposure to toxic substances and other harmful agents are being considered, it may be decided that the fetus needs special protection, and therefore the level of exposure for women of reproductive capacity should be lower.'

'Women of reproductive capacity'

The HSC and the EOC have different views as to who a 'woman of reproductive capacity' is.

The HSC's view is that a woman of reproductive capacity is 'any woman capable of conceiving and carrying a child'. It is she who must be restricted or prohibited from working. They mention four factors which make it impossible for a woman to conceive and carry a child. They are (1) bilateral oophorectomy; (2) bilateral salpingectomy; (3) hysterectomy; (4) congenital conditions having the same effect as (1), (2) or (3). The HSC consider that surgical sterilisation, age or contraception should not on their own exclude a woman from a restriction on work. They conclude that a woman should be assumed of reproductive capacity unless she provides a medical certificate stating that she is incapable of bearing a child (reference 16, para. 406).

The EOC were more liberal. In addition to women within the HSC category, they would include (a) women who are very unlikely to bear children, but might, and (b) women who have no intention of bearing children and, if necessary, are taking active steps to prevent pregnancy. They observe that if the HSC's view were accepted, its effect on women's employment might be great, particularly if, as they anticipated, it were applied to other legislation on toxic substances (reference 16, para. 435).

Objections to proposals

There are objections to the definitions proposed and assumptions made by both the EOC and the HSC:

(1) Both definitions concentrate on the effect to the fetus. They ignore other effects that toxic substances may have. The US National Institute of Occupational Safety and Health lists reduced fertility in men as a suspected reproductive hazard of lead. In respect of ionising radiation, it suggests that carcinogenesis, reduced fertility, spontaneous abortion, mutagenesis and teratogenesis may result[17]. As a result there is a failure to consider the question of exclusion of men where their reproductive potential is affected. No doubt, one can argue about whether a hazard to reproduction has been established and what steps to take if it is only 'suspected', but, in the context of a report which anticipates its findings being applied more widely to toxic substances, it is a surprising omission.

(2) The HSC's definition potentially includes all but a few women below their late 40s. This is far wider than their real area of concern – namely the possibility of a teratogen acting early in pregnancy and before a woman is aware of the pregnancy.

(3) In order to work, a woman would have to get a medical certificate

stating that she could no longer reproduce and submit it to her employer. This is a considerable intrusion on her privacy. Her working would, no doubt, lead to comment by other employees.

(4) The HSC assume that women should not have control of reproduction, or are not to be trusted, if there is a risk to the fetus. This is patronising. It is true that pregnancy can happen 'by accident', but accidents occur in many areas of life, not least in the work place. No one suggests that the careless party be prohibited from working.

(5) One objection raised by the HSC to the narrower EOC definition is the possibility of a successful claim for prenatal injury under the Congenital Disabilities (Civil Liability) Act 1976. The Act was passed after the thalidomide litigation. The HSC may have been unduly optimistic. The remedy provided by the legislation and common law, whether compensatory or preventive, is weak. A child would have to prove negligence or breach of statutory duty, and causation of a disability by an occurrence affecting its mother during pregnancy.

In considering whether an employer was negligent or in breach of statutory duty, a court would take into account the statutory limits laid down under the Control of Lead Regulations. The HSC were in the process of considering a formula which would be used in these, so the employer would be in a strong position[18]. Causation was examined by the Royal Commission on Civil Liability and Compensation for Personal Injury. It concluded that such were the problems of proof (in a legal sense) that: '... only a minute proportion of those who are born with congenital defects may be able to establish causation and prove it was due to negligence, and ... there is little prospect that this proportion will increase'[19].

(6) There is a contrast between the certainty of the HSC definition and the flexibility generally present in post-Robens health and safety legislation:

(a) By virtue of section 2 HASAWA, the duty owed by employers is only to ensure health and safety so far as is reasonably practicable.

(b) Robens stressed self-regulation and individual responsibility for health and safety. He believed that if employees and employers participated actively in the formulation of safe and healthy practices at work, this would reduce risks[20]. The HSC suggests that women should be denied such a role.

(c) There is a variation of views as to what are acceptable exposure limits and a general acceptance of a degree of risk.

(7) Finally, but most importantly, neither the HSC nor the EOC give sufficient consideration to the primacy of a hazard-based approach.

In effect, the EOC offers a woman a choice between her fetus and her work. The HSC offers no choice at all; it makes the apparently unquestioned assumption that the possibility of harming a fetus should take precedence over the certainty (given their definition) of unequal employment opportunity and sex discrimination. This is close to the view that a woman's real place is in the home. It is not clear how far Victorian ideas about women and work, discussed above in relation to women and protective legislation, persist. The way in which the problem of reproductive hazards is viewed and the solutions are considered suggest that those ideas may still inform the debates.

Control of Lead at Work Regulations

The terms and background of the Control of Lead Regulations suggest an unwillingness properly to confront the nature of reproductive hazards and, in particular, the formula of 'women of reproductive capacity'.

The Draft Directive on lead proposed by the European Commission on 28 December 1979 contained considerably stricter exposure limits than the final approved version. It explicitly distinguished between workers generally and workers of child-bearing capacity[21]. The Draft Directive was considered by the European Parliament and its Committee for Environment, Public Health and Consumer Protection. While welcoming the control of lead, it was concerned about sex discrimination and expressed the view that 'the limit values proposed [were] only a first step towards the equal and fullest possible protection of both men and women'[22].

The UK Control of Lead Regulations 1980 provide higher exposure levels than in the Draft Directive and do not explicitly refer to stricter standards for women of reproductive capacity. That was dealt with in an approved Code of Practice. The Regulations were passed before the EC Directive on lead. This appears to be in line with the assessment of the Chair of the HSC that: '. . . the best posture for us to adopt is to be slightly in front of the EEC but not out of sight. This would give us the advantage of being able to set the mood for the legislation which is going to come from the EEC. Any country which has already thought it through and has reached some stage of progress towards legislation is bound to be in a position where it can be the pacemaker in the EEC'[23]. While it is not clear that the Chair of the HSC had lead in mind, the EC's final approved Directive was much more in line with the Control of Lead Regulations. The Directive contained no explicit reference to higher standards for women of reproductive capacity, only to permitting the provision of greater protection for workers. The standards adopted were similar to the weaker UK levels (although the UK regulations will need to be tightened slightly)[7].

The bland formula giving workers an option of greater protection in the lead Directive, when compared with the Draft Directive, suggests an attempt to appear non-discriminatory. It does permit members of the EC to achieve equality, if they wish. At least in form, it meets the objections of the Committee for Environment, Public Health and Consumer Protection.

Surprisingly, the Code of Practice and Regulations do not define a woman of reproductive capacity. Given the disagreement concerning the meaning of reproductive capacity, and particularly the possible criminal sanctions, it is strange that the Code does not define the expression and achieve a degree of certainty.

The EOC reported in 1979 on protective legislation. Since then, the HSC has been reviewing its policy. No proposals have been forthcoming. It is not a priority in its programme for 1983–1984 and beyond. It is unfortunate that the HSC has not made a decision in principle on the matters covered in the EOC Report. There is a danger that the matter will be resolved by default.

SUSPENSION – THE EMPLOYEE'S RIGHTS

Faced with an employee who is not able to continue working in consequence of a statutory provision relating to health, an employer has three options: (1) to suspend; (2) to offer alternative work; (3) to dismiss. The framework Directive requires that workers temporarily suspended must where possible be provided with another job[6].

(1) The intention of the UK legislation as set out in section 19 of the Employment Protection (Consolidation) Act 1978 is that, where a worker must be suspended from work on medical grounds (broadly, grounds relating to lead and ionising radiation: there is no statutory protection in respect of most toxic substances), the worker will be paid for the period of suspension or up to 26 weeks. Unless the employee's contract provides otherwise, there is no obligation to pay after the end of 26 weeks. This option will cost the employer up to 26 weeks' pay and possibly remuneration for another employee to perform the job of the first. When compared with the other options, it is perhaps the least attractive to the employer.

(2) The employer can offer suitable alternative employment which, if unreasonably refused, leads to loss of the right to be paid while suspended. In practice, if an employer offers unsuitable work (with, for example, poor promotion prospects, lower status or pay) which is refused, to ensure pay during suspension the employee must apply to an industrial tribunal. The employer stands only to lose the suspension payment, which would normally have to be paid in any case. There would be considerable pressure on the employee to agree to whatever job was offered.

(3) It is when one looks at dismissal that the lack of protection for employees becomes apparent. Employees dismissed may be able to claim an award for unfair dismissal, provided that they first satisfy certain qualifying conditions. An employee does not qualify unless he or she has worked for 4 weeks and either works 16 hours or has been employed by that employer for 5 years and works more than 8 hours per week[24]. An employee having qualified, it is not automatically unfair to dismiss on medical grounds. A tribunal considers whether the reason for dismissal was fair.

In considering the operation of employment legislation, it is important to have regard to the structure of the labour market and the nature of women's employment. This is discussed in more detail elsewhere in this book by both Garcia in Chapter 21 and Oakley in Chapter 10. Women are less likely to meet the qualifying conditions than men. Women are more likely to work under 16 hours than men, particularly after a first child. They are less likely to have worked for a continuous period of 5 years[25,26].

A further significant limitation is that there is no right to claim unfair dismissal if one works under an illegal contract of employment. Such a contract is void and one is not treated as an employee[27]. The most frequent example is non-payment of tax and national insurance contributions by an employer. The employee often has no choice as to whether contributions are paid or not. If the employer will not pay contributions, the employee can accept the position or leave. In some industries[26] it is the norm to work on illegal contracts. Such workers have no rights to employment protection[25,28]. Home workers, nearly all women, are recognised as having particular health and safety problems. The HSC has issued draft regulations on the hazards of home working. The vast majority work on illegal contracts.

Although the qualifying conditions will tend to exclude women, the major limitation of a claim for unfair dismissal is the size of the potential award. In 1980 the average award was £598, considerably less than 26 weeks' pay. Tribunals can award reinstatement or re-engagement, but this is rare. In 1980 it was only awarded in 0.8 per cent of cases[29].

It is not clear that the legislation meets the requirements of Article 6 of the framework Directive[6] — namely, that a suspended worker shall, where possible, be provided with another job. The test of possibility imposes greater obligations than under the Employment Protection (Consolidation) Act 1978. An employer's failure to offer alternative employment will be considered in assessing the fairness of a dismissal, but, particularly in view of the sanction for not making an offer, it is far from a positive obligation.

CONCLUSIONS

The approach of the HSC and EOC to exclusion of women of reproductive capacity offers protection to a fetus. It ignores the effects of non-teratogenic reproductive hazards.

The definition proposed by the HSC as to which women should be excluded is inadequate because it encompasses and includes a field far greater than the HSC's real area of concern.

Neither the HSC nor the EOC sufficiently emphasise a hazard-based approach to avoid sex discrimination and unequal employment opportunity.

The statutory formula 'so far as is reasonably practicable' is inadequate to deal with the problem of reproductive hazards at work, and, in particular, the potential exclusion of women.

Where an employee is suspended, the law offers in practice insufficient protection, which can be readily circumvented. An employee should only be suspended if there are no safe, suitable alternatives, and in these circumstances should have full and effective protection of his or her position at work.

The law offers poor solutions considered on their own. It is not possible to divorce legal solutions from, for example, greater knowledge of reproductive hazards, more effective trade union involvement and the other solutions discussed in this book.

The conclusions and criticisms made in this chapter suggest certain legislative change. There are grounds for hoping that this may happen. In the light of increasing knowledge of not only the number of hazardous agents, but also the variety of effects to both men and women, the approach of the law is becoming increasingly untenable. In considering legislative change, it is always essential to distinguish formal aspects of law – what the law says – and law in practice – what really happens. In the case of health and safety law, there is a considerable gulf.

REFERENCES

1. Employment Committee (1982). Sixth Report: *The Workings of the Health and Safety Commission and Executive: Achievements since the Robens Report* (HC400), London, HMSO
2. [1949] *1 All England Law Reports*, 743 at 747
3. Section 74 Factories Act 1961
4. Section 181 Factories Act 1961
5. Barlow, S. M. and Sullivan, F. M. (1982). *Reproductive Hazards of Industrial Chemicals*, Academic Press, London, pp. 4–8
6. Directive of 27 November 1980 (80/1107/EEC). *Official Journal*, No. L327 (3 December 1982), 8
7. Directive of 28 July 1982 (82/605/EEC). *Official Journal*, No. L247 (23 August 1982), 12
8. Draft Directive. *Official Journal*, No. C262 (9 October 1980)
9. Draft Directive. *Official Journal*, No. C289 (5 November 1982)
10. Anon. (1983). EC directives, draft proposals and work in progress. *Health and Safety Information Bulletin*, No. 88 (April), 12–15
11. Sixth Amending Directive of 18 September 1976 (79/831/EEC). *Official Journal* (15 October 1979)
12. Section 51(1) Sex Discrimination Act 1975. See *Page* v. *Freight Hire (Tank Haulage) Limited* [1981]. *Industrial Relations Law Report 13*
13. *Turley* v. *Allders Department Stores Limited* [1980]. *Industrial Relations Law Report 4*
14. Submission to the Secretary of State for Employment by the HSC in respect of the Control of Lead at Work Regulations 1980 and associated Code of Practice, Para. 32
15. Section 55 Sex Discrimination Act 1975
16. EOC (1979). *Health and Safety Legislation: Should we Distinguish between Men and Women?*, pp. 98–106

17. Anon. (1979). Health hazards for women working in chemicals and pharma-ceuticals. *Health and Safety Information Bulletin*, No. 46, October, 4–5
18. *Albery-Speyer* v. *BP Oil Limited and Shell (UK) Limited*: Court of Appeal (Friday, 2 May 1980)
19. *Royal Commission on Civil Liability and Compensation for Personal Injury*. Cmnd. 7054, HMSO, London, 1978, Para. 1452
20. *Safety and Health at Work: Report of the Committee* (1970–1972). Cmnd. 5034, HMSO, London, 1972, Para. 452–459
21. Draft Directive of 10 December 1979. *Official Journal*, No. C324 (28 December, 1979), 3
22. European Parliament Working Documents 1980–1981 (1–453/80), (9 October 1980), 5
23. Anon. (1980). The European Communities explained . . . and how this affects UK health and safety legislation. *Health and Safety Information Bulletin*, No. 50 (February), 4
24. Section 64(2) and Schedule 13 Employment Protection (Consolidation) Act 1978
25. Coote, A. and Campbell, B. (1982). *Sweet Freedom*, Pan, London, 63–66
26. Crine, S. and Playford, C. (1982). *From Rags to Riches: Low Pay in the Clothing Industry*, Low Pay Unit, London
27. Section 153(1) Employment Protection (Consolidation) Act 1978
28. Hakim, C. (1980). Home working: Some new evidence. *Employment Gazette* (October), Department of Employment, HMSO, London, 1105
29. Anon. (1981). Unfair Dismissal Statistics 1980. *Employment Gazette*, Department of Employment, HMSO, London

17

Legal Considerations of Reproductive Hazards in Industry in the United States

N. A. ASHFORD

Clearly, the human risks posed by reproductive hazards in the work place are both serious and far-reaching. An effective control strategy, then, must be one that emphasises prevention while preserving employment opportunities for the worker. It is hoped that employers will recognise the need for voluntary abatement of reproductive hazards. It must be recognised, however, that employees may need to avail themselves of legal mechanisms to encourage preventive actions. In many cases the most readily available mechanisms for preventive relief will be those created by federal statute; in other instances, private actions may be required. Legislative and statutory mechanisms include standard-setting for reproductive hazards; access to exposure and medical records; the rights of workers to individually refuse hazardous work; and antidiscrimination protection. Private actions include the court injunction; collective bargaining by unions; and suits for damages suffered.

LEGISLATIVE AVENUES FOR PROTECTIVE RELIEF

There are two comprehensive federal statutes that address the problem of regulating hazards in the work place. The Occupational Safety and Health Act (OSHAct)[1] focuses on the prevention of exposure to work place hazards in general, and is designed to provide relief for the worker only, and not for his or her offspring. On the other hand, the Toxic Substances Control Act (TSCA)[2] provides a means for the regulation of the general production and use of chemical substances. Its mechanisms can be utilised on behalf of both parents and offspring.

Section 6(b)(5) of OSHAct gives the Secretary of Labor the responsibility for setting health and safety standards for the work place. The statutory delineation of this responsibility[3] clearly indicates that it was to be utilised to develop

225

standards which reduce reproductive hazards: 'The Secretary, in promulgating standards dealing with toxic materials or harmful physical agents under this subsection, shall set the standard which most adequately assures, to the extent feasible, on the basis of the best available evidence, that no employee will suffer material impairment of health or functional capacity even if such employee has regular exposure to the hazard dealt with by such standard for the period of his working life.' To the extent that they pose a danger to the health or functional capacity of the exposed worker, or perhaps to that worker's future offspring, reproductive hazards are a proper subject for standard setting under Section 6(b).

Physical injuries are certainly within the scope of this provision. The impairment of reproductive or sexual capacity by mutagens or other toxic substances, for example, clearly constitutes a 'material impairment of . . . functional capacity'. Similarly, damage to the pregnant mother as a result of exposure of the fetus to a teratogen is a material impairment of the mother's health. Further, Section 6(b) would appear to envisage the regulation of reproductive hazards for their effect on the mental or emotional health of the worker-parent, although the Occupational Safety and Health Administration's (OSHA's) regulations have not yet been extended to the prevention of other than physical damage. For while OSHAct was not designed to produce a trauma-free work place, it was intended to reduce the health risks posed by physically harmful hazards. The mental health dangers posed by a worker's physical exposure to teratogens or germ cell mutagens are no less a material impairment of health than a number of physical impairments for which regulations at present exist[4], and should be given consideration in devising appropriate control mechanisms for reproductive hazards. Finally, the United States Court of Appeals for the District of Columbia has indicated that the health of future worker offspring must be considered in the setting of OSHAct standards[5].

The Secretary's authority to regulate such hazards is quite broad. So long as he or she remains true to the goal of securing a safe and healthful work place environment, the Secretary may embrace a variety of regulatory alternatives in setting work place standards. A mechanism which may prove useful in the regulation of reproductive hazards is medical removal protection (MRP). In essence, MRP involves the removal from one work area of employees who are particularly susceptible to a hazardous exposure within that area and the reassignment of those employees, at comparable salary and seniority levels, to another work area within the plant where the hazard is not present. It may also involve a layoff with pay[6]. The District of Columbia Court of Appeals has approved an MRP programme for lead exposure as a valid exercise of the Secretary's authority under Section 6(b)[7], and this mechanism may well be appropriate for the protection of workers, who may prove to be particularly susceptible to damage from reproductive hazards. MRP programmes would appear to be sensible only where their cost is exceeded by the cost of actually removing the reproductive hazard from the work place. When properly utilised, however,

MRP programmes appear capable both of encouraging beneficial job redesign and of facilitating worker co-operation with programmes of periodic biological monitoring.

Recognising the fact that the Section 6(b) standard-setting procedure would be incapable of addressing all possible hazards in a timely fashion, Congress imposed an affirmative duty on employers to remove serious hazards from the work place even where such hazards are not the subject of a specific OSHAct standard. Section 5(a)(1)[8] mandates that each employer 'furnish to his employees employment and a place of employment which are free from recognised hazards that are causing or are likely to cause death or serious physical harm to his employees. Reproductive hazards were intended to be included within this duty. Clearly, a work place hazard which impairs the sexual or reproductive process, or which endangers the health of the mother through damage to the fetus, is an affront to the physical integrity of the affected worker.

While the general duty clause requires the employer to provide a work place free of recognised hazards likely to cause serious physical harm to his workers, the courts have not yet addressed the question of whether OSHAct permits the employer to achieve compliance with Section 5(a)(1) by excluding from the work place those employees for whom a particular condition poses a hazard. This is a particularly critical question in the context of reproductive hazard control. A number of employers have implemented policies which exclude fertile females – and, in some cases, non-sterilised males – from jobs which involve exposure to certain reproductive hazards[9]. While usually done in the name of worker protection, the benefit of such policies inures largely to the employer, who avoids the cost of removing the reproductive hazard from the work place while, at the same time, ensuring against future liability from damages to the offspring of the exposed workers. To the extent that they discriminate against employees of one sex, policies of this nature may well violate Title VII of the Federal Civil Rights Act. In addition, they may also violate OSHAct.

Thus far, reproductive hazards have been given little attention under OSHAct. Work place exposure to DBCP has been regulated primarily because of its danger as a reproductive hazard[10]. Further, while compliance with the permissible exposure level for lead will not ensure against reproductive damage[11], the lead standard does include an MRP provision intended to protect both male and female workers from reproductive effects[12]. Most reproductive toxins, however, have thus far escaped regulation under either Section 6(b) or the general duty clause.

The general duty clause has also been under-utilised with regard to reproductive hazards. One difficulty in regulating reproductive hazards under OSHAct is the frequent lack of conclusive evidence that a particular substance causes a particular reproductive injury. The precise human effects of many known or suspected mutagens and teratogens may be especially difficult to discern. A degree of uncertainty is almost always a part of the regulatory process, however, and was certainly present in the development of standards for the carcinogens and other toxins which are currently regulated under OSHAct. Persuasive animal carcinogenicity, even in the absence of confirmatory epidemiological evidence, has been deemed sufficient to regulate a substance as a potential human carcinogen[13]. Indeed, under the Occupational Safety and Health Administration's (OSHA's) generic cancer policy, suspect carcinogens are subject to regulation.

OSHAct does not require certainty. Under Section 6(b), the Secretary must show that it is more likely than not that a hazard poses a risk of material impairment before it may be subjected to regulation. Interpreting this section in the light of Section 3(8) of the Act[14], the Supreme Court has added the requirement that the probable risk be significant with regard to frequency of occurrence[15]. Section 5(a)(1) also pertains to probable risks. It does not require a determination that a substance will cause serious physical harm, but only that it is likely to cause such harm. While these evidentiary burdens cannot be taken lightly, they are far from insurmoutable.

Regulation of reproductive hazards in the work place may also be pursued through the Toxic Substances Control Act. TSCA contemplates a two-tiered approach to the control of chemical toxins. It provides a mechanism for the systematic testing of potential toxins to determine whether they present a risk of injury to human health or the environment, and further provides a means to control the production or use of those substances which present an unreasonable risk of such injury. Congress clearly intended that TSCA be used to regulate reproductive hazards. Section 4(b)(2)(A)[16] is specific in its enumeration of this coverage: 'The health and environmental effects for which standards for the development of test data may be prescribed include ... mutagenesis, teratogenesis, behavioral disorders ... and any other effect which may present an unreasonable risk of injury to health or the environment.'

TSCA requires the testing of a potentially dangerous chemical substance to be undertaken by the manufacturer of that substance. In the case of an existing chemical being put to an existing use, Section 4(a) requires testing where that chemical 'may present an unreasonable risk of injury to health or the environment', or where the chemical is produced in substantial quantities and either 'may reasonably be anticipated to enter the environment in substantial quantities' or 'there ... may be significant or substantial human exposure'[17]. Section 5 imposes similar requirements for new chemicals, and for existing chemicals put to a significant new use. Here, however, additional safeguards exist, such as production or new use may not begin until 90 days after all required testing is completed[18].

The purpose of the testing requirement is to provide the necessary data for a determination of whether regulation of a production or use is appropriate. Responsibility for the development of this regulation, and for the enforcement of the Act, rests principally with the Administrator of the Environmental Protection Agency (EPA). The Administrator may impose a temporary production or use standard, pending required testing, under Sections 5(e) and (f)[19], may file action in Federal District Court to enjoin the production or use of an imminent hazard under Section 7[20], and may impose permanent standards on the production or use under Section 6[21]. For toxic substances generally, the Administrator is required to develop a permanent standard, or take other decisive action, upon a finding that there is 'a reasonable basis to conclude' that a substance poses an 'unreasonable risk to health or the environment'[22]. In the case of carcinogens, mutagens or teratogens, the Administrator is given a more specific statutory directive.

Section 4(f) provides that whenever there is information 'which indicates to the administrator that there may be a reasonable basis to conclude that a chemical substance or mixture presents or will present a significant risk of serious or widespread harm to human beings from cancer, gene mutations, or birth defects, the administrator shall . . . initiate appropriate action under Section 5, 6, or 7, to prevent or reduce to a sufficient extent such risk or publish in the Federal Register a finding that such risk is not unreasonable'[23]. Section 9 of TSCA requires the Environmental Protection Agency (EPA) to report findings under Section 4(f) to OSHA for appropriate action, but does not preclude EPA's exercise of authority over the suspect chemical itself[24].

This section provides an excellent mechanism for the control of many serious reproductive hazards. To date, however, EPA has not invoked the provisions of Section 4(f) for any suspected teratogen or mutagen. This appears to be a failure to fulfil a direct statutory mandate. While the language of Section 4(f) arguably allows the Administrator a degree of discretion in determining whether a substance poses a significant risk, it also clearly anticipates that the Administrator will take regulatory action in the face of scientific uncertainty. Section 4(f) requires some action whenever there may be a reasonable basis to conclude that a significant risk exists. Certainly, a number of teratogens and mutagens are eligible for regulation on this basis.

Access to information regarding the identity of chemicals to which a worker may be exposed, actual exposure data and medical records is essential to ensure that the worker utilise the avenues open to him or her for protecting reproductive health. Under OSHAct, two regulations have been issued: the Hazard Communication Standard[24a] providing limited information on chemical identity and Access to Employee Exposure and Medical Records[24b]. The latest regulation provides that the workers be given access to recorded information of adverse health effects, but it does not by itself require the recording of such information. It is under Section 8(e) of TSCA that EPA (not the worker) must be informed of a substantial risk of injury to health.

In addition to general regulatory controls, federal statutes also provide workers with avenues for individual relief. In the context of reproductive hazard control, the two most valuable statutory self-help mechanisms are the right to refuse hazardous work and the right to be free of sexual discrimination in the work place.

Under both the National Labor Relations Act (NLRA) and OSHAct, employees have a limited right to leave the work place rather than submit to hazardous working conditions[25]. When properly exercised, this right protects an employee from retaliatory discharge or other discriminatory action for refusing hazardous work. The nature of this right under NLRA depends on the nature of any relevant collective bargaining agreement. Non-union employees, and union employees whose collective bargaining agreements specifically exclude health and safety from a no-strike clause, have the right to stage a safety walkout under Section 7 of the Act[26]. If they choose to stage such a walkout on a good faith belief that working conditions are unsafe, they will be protected from retaliatory action by their employer[27]. Union employees who are subject to a comprehensive collective bargaining agreement may avail themselves of the provisions of Section 502[28]. Under this section, an employee who is faced with *abnormally dangerous conditions* has an individual right to leave the job site. Such right may be exercised, however, only where the abnormally dangerous nature of the working conditions can be objectively verified[29].

Under a 1973 OSHA regulation, the right to refuse hazardous work under OSHAct extends to all employees of private employers, regardless of the existence or nature of a collective bargaining agreement. The scope of this right, however, is not yet clear. Section 11(c) of OSHAct protects an employee from discharge or other retaliatory action arising out of his or her exercise of any right afforded by the Act[30]. The Secretary of Labor has promulgated regulations under this section which define the right to refuse hazardous work in certain circumstances; where an employee reasonably believes that there is a 'real danger of death or serious injury', where there is insufficient time to eliminate that danger through normal administrative channels and where the employer has failed to comply with an employee request to correct the situation[31]. This regulation has survived challenge in the Supreme Court. The unanimous Court held that the Secretary's action was authorised by Section 11(c), and noted that the regulation 'simply permits private employees of private employers to avoid workplace dangers that they believe pose grave dangers to their own safety'[32].

Although it has not been widely used for this purpose, the right to refuse hazardous work does appear to provide a limited means of relief for employees facing reproductive hazards in the work place[33]. An employee who contemplates the exercise of one of these three statutory rights, of course, should take care to ensure that his or her work place situation meets the criteria for such exercise. Clearly, the Section 7 right is the broadest of the three, as it permits a subjective determination of work place danger. As noted, however, it applies only to certain categories of employees, and contemplates a concerted action. This usually means that more than one employee must be involved, although an individual work stoppage could qualify if it is intended to serve the interests of other workers. Exercise of the Section 502 right requires an objectively verifiable hazard, and thus does not protect against retaliatory action should the employee's subjective determination prove to have been incorrect. Under Section 11(c) of OSHAct, as noted by the Supreme Court, '... any employee who acts in reliance on the regulation runs the risk of discharge or reprimand in the event a court subsequently finds that he acted unreasonably or in bad faith'[34]. Here the standard is one of reasonableness, not correctness, of hazard perception. Proof of the violation of an applicable OSHAct standard or general-duty clause citation should provide at least a partial basis for proof of the existence of a hazard, or of the reasonableness of the perception of a hazard[35]. The employee exercising either the NLRA Section 502 or OSHAct right must determine that the danger was sufficiently 'hazardous' to warrant such exercise. Proof of an 'abnormally dangerous' condition under Section 502 may be particularly difficult in inherently dangerous jobs, as this section is usually applied only to conditions that are not a normal part of the job[36]. For this reason, reproductive hazards will probably be addressed more easily under the OSHAct right. Certainly, any reproductive hazard presents concrete risk of a serious injury. The key question will be whether that risk is of such an immediate nature as to present a real danger of injury before administrative procedures can be utilised. Hazards such as germ cell mutagens, which can cause serious and irreversible harm after only a short-term exposure, would appear to meet this criterion.

A final limitation on the right to refuse hazardous work is its uncertain applicability to injuries to a worker's future offspring. The OSHAct right appears to be applicable only to hazards which affect the health and safety of workers, and the exercise of this right would appear to be based on potential damage to the worker[37]. The applicable language of the NLRA is not limited to worker health and safety, however, but rather contains broad protections against discriminatory action and coercion, and is quite clearly designed to provide remedies for mental distress[38]. Thus, a work place teratogen may very well constitute a dangerous condition under Sections 7 and 502.

Another self-help mechanism is found in Title VII of the Civil Rights Act, which provides that '. . . women affected by pregnancy, childbirth, or related medical conditions shall be treated the same for all employment-related purposes . . . as other persons not so affected, but similar in their ability or inability to work . . .'[39].

This provision, designed to protect women from sexual discrimination in the work place, calls into question the permissibility of the fetus protection policies. An employer who excludes fertile women from a work place because they may become pregnant is discriminating against those women on the basis of their potential to become 'affected by pregnancy, childbirth, or related medical conditions'. A number of commentators have argued that such discrimination is violative of Title VII[40]. This interpretation, if followed by the courts, should provide female workers with a valuable tool for addressing work place hazards[41].

An employee who feels that her right to be free of sexual discrimination has been violated may petition for relief under the Civil Rights Act. If she is successful, she will ordinarily be entitled to recovery of attorneys' fees and costs, as well as appropriate redress for the discrimination[42]. There are two principal defences to a Title VII action. One is the bona fide occupational qualification

(BFOQ) defence, which requires the employer to demonstrate that the policy of discrimination was reasonably necessary both to the essence of its business and to the promotion of worker safety or efficiency[43]. In the case of a 'fetus protection' policy, this would require a strong showing that women of child-bearing capacity are unable to efficiently and safely perform their job. The second defence is based on business necessity, and requires the employer to demonstrate that the discriminatory policy is absolutely essential to the continuation of the business, and, upon a showing by the plaintiff that alternatives are available, that the continuation of the business cannot be protected through any reasonable alternative to the policy[44]. Both defences have been rather narrowly construed by the courts[45], and some commentators have concluded that the successful assertion of either defence will be difficult for employers seeking to justify a fetus protection policy[46]. In the past, the business necessity defence has been available only where the policy in question was not discriminatory on its face[47]. Thus, as discrimination 'on the basis of pregnancy, childbirth or related medical conditions' has been specifically designated as sex discrimination under Title VII, this defence would not appear to be available where the 'fetus protection' policy applies only to fertile women. Nonetheless, the Fourth Circuit has characterised one such policy as 'literally expressed in gender-neutral terms', and has held that business necessity, if properly established, is an appropriate defence[48]. This position conflicts with that taken by some commentators[49], as well as with the articulated position of at least one federal district court[50], and appears inconsistent with the plain language of the Civil Rights Act[51].

One commentator has argued that Title VII will permit fetal protection policies only if they are applied equally to fertile employees of both sexes[52]. Indeed, as discussed previously, there is substantial scientific evidence to oppose a policy that isolates fertile women from reproductive hazards without also isolating fertile men. A recent report of the Council on Environmental Quality summarises the available information as follows: 'The scientific basis for differential regulation is limited. Reproduction involves a wider range of processes in females than in males, and some processes in females involve critical periods of differential and development. However, it does not necessarily follow that women are more sensitive to the action of any given agent. Where extensive data have been compiled on both sexes (e.g., for anaesthetic gases and smelter emissions), evidence has been found for adverse effects resulting from exposure of both men and women, including some evidence for adverse fetal effects following exposure of males (citations omitted).'[53]

An employer's recognition of the fact that it may face liability as a result of fetal damage caused by the exposure of male employees to a reproductive hazard may well tip the balance in favour of a more healthful work environment. As noted by Wendy W. Williams of Georgetown University: 'The option of excluding workers at risk may well seem less attractive in light of such evidence than it did when the employer assumed that only women workers transmitted fetal hazards. A workplace composed exclusively of sterile men and women and post-menopausal women will be unappealing to most employers. Under these circumstances, the employer may be inspired to develop solutions short of exclusion, thus not only protecting itself from liability and advancing the health of offspring but promoting the employment interests of workers as well.'[54]

OTHER MECHANISMS FOR PROTECTIVE RELIEF

In addition to specific statutory remedies, there are more general avenues of relief which may be used to seek protection from reproductive hazards. The two most important of these are the common law injunction and the collective bargaining agreement.

The equitable right to an injunction has long been recognised as common law[55]. Through injunctive relief one can, under appropriate circumstances, obtain a court order prohibiting another from taking or continuing a particular action. Although the availability of injunctive relief varies with the particular facts of each case, the right to an injunction is generally dependent on the demonstration of three factors: the existence of a continuing or recurrent risk of irreparable harm, the existence of a legal duty to refrain from causing such harm, and the inadequacy of other available remedies in preventing that harm. As a number of reproductive hazards in the work place appear to meet these criteria, injunctive relief may be an excellent mechanism for addressing those hazards. Injunctive relief may prove especially valuable in dealing with hazards that primarily affect the offspring, rather than the parents, as most states provide rights of action for such hazards at common law.

Another useful preventive mechanism may be the collective bargaining process. Clearly, health and safety considerations are a proper subject of collective bargaining. In a recent Landmark set of three cases decided by the National Labor Relations Board, the withholding of information regarding chemical identity and health effects may be a violation of the employers' duty to bargain in good faith[56]. If workers become sufficiently cognisant of the potential effects of work place hazards on their ability to bear children, they may well seek to include abatement or reduction of reproductive hazards as a condition of employment under their collective bargaining agreement. The inclusion of this topic in labour/management negotiations, especially when coupled with the use of other mechanisms for protective or compensatory relief from reproductive hazards, might do much to improve work place safety. Any attempt to place provision of this nature into a collective bargaining agreement, however, should take care not to waive the right to utilise any of these other avenues of relief.

CONCLUSIONS

The remedies outlined above, if properly utilised, can do much to reduce occupational exposure to reproductive hazards. But the effort cannot be a piecemeal one. As these various actions will provide incentives for change at different levels of the industrial process, it is their integrated use which will bring about the most meaningful and pervasive reduction of potential damage to reproductive health.

Industrial control of reproductive hazards — whether through the reduction of exposure to hazards from existing processes or through a shift to different, less hazardous technology — will come in two principal ways. Either industry will change on its own, in response to economic constraints, or it will change in compliance with government regulation. Both OSHAct and TSCA provide attractive avenues for regulatory relief, as both articulate a comprehensive federal policy for the control of occupational toxins. Nonetheless, the limitations of the regulatory process, and the apparent unwillingness of OSHA and EPA to act aggressively against reproductive hazards, suggest the need to pursue other avenues of control. The available self-help mechanisms for both preventive and compensatory relief can provide an important complement to agency regulation. On the one hand, they can provide economic — and, in the case of injunctive relief, judicially imposed — incentives for changes in industrial behaviour. Further, by focusing attention on a particular problem, they can be an important impetus for a comprehensive regulatory response.

In utilising and refining the various regulatory and legal mechanisms discussed here, however, one cannot afford to lose sight of the underlying political context. These remedies developed, in large part, out of a strong and organised concern for work place health and safety. Without a concentrated effort to maintain that level of concern, we could see some of these avenues of relief narrowed, or even eliminated. Thus, it is perhaps the extent to which they can be used successfully as political, as well as legal, tools that will ultimately determine the extent to which these mechanisms are useful in safeguarding the reproductive health of workers and their offspring.

NOTES

1. 29 U.S.C., Section 650, *et seq*. (1970).
2. 15 U.S.C., Section 2601, *et seq*. (1970).
3. 29 U.S.C., Section 655(b) (1970).
4. The courts have long recognised the fact that mental and emotional trauma can grow out of physical injury, and have allowed recovery for damages for such trauma in both tort and worker compensation action. See Charles N. Miller, Recovery for psychic injuries under worker's compensation, *Case and Comment*, 87, No. 5, 40 (1982), for a recent discussion of this topic. There

is no reason to believe that Congress was unaware of this precedent when it passed OSHAct, and there is nothing in the language of Section 6(b) to indicate a limitation to purely *physical* consequences of work place exposures.

5. Although it is not clear whether a reproductive hazard which affects *only* future offspring, and not the workers themselves, is subject to regulation under OSHAct, the Court of Appeals for the District of Columbia Circuit has indicated that both 'workers' and 'the children they will hereafter conceive' must be given consideration in the setting of permanent and temporary standards under OSHAct. *Public Citizen v. Auchter*, No. 83-1071, United States Court of Appeals for the District of Columbia, Slip Opinion, at 6 (15 March 1983). As a practical matter, the court may well be giving tacit recognition to the *emotional* damage suffered by the worker who must face the knowledge that his or her future children may be damaged by a current work place exposure.

6. A medical removal *protection* provision should thus be distinguished from a simple medical removal provision, such as is mandated for vinyl chloride [29 CFR, Part 1910.1017(k)(5)], which does not include wage or seniority protections, and from the various employee exclusion policies instituted by many employers, without OSHA directive or authorisation, whereby fertile workers (usually women) are simply removed from their jobs. OSHA has thus far declined to develop a generic MRP policy.

7. *United Steelworkers of America v. Marshall*, 647 F.2d 1189, 1230 (D.C. Cir. 1980). Cert. Den. U.S. Supreme Court 80-1134, *Lead Industries Association Inc., et al. v. Donovan*, 29 June 1981, 49 *Law Week*, 3629.

8. 29 U.S.C., Section 654(a)(I) (1970).

9. Reportedly, employers who have implemented exclusionary policies of this nature include: Amax, American Cyanamid, Dupont, General Motors, B. F. Goodrich, Olin, Sun Oil, Gulf Oil, Bunker Hill Smelter, Union Carbide, Allied Chemical, Monsanto, TWA and Dow Chemical. The Lead Industries Association is reported to have endorsed this 'female exclusion' approach in 1974. (Joan E. Bertin, Discriminating against women of childbearing capacity, paper presented at the Hastings Center, 8 January 1982, p. 2.) For a rather reasoned discussion of some of the social issues raised by this trend, see Ronald Bayer, Women, work and reproductive hazards, *The Hastings Center Report*, October 1982, p. 14.

10. The standard for DBCP is found at 29 CFR 1910.1044. Appendix A to this regulation, at Section II.B.2, notes that: 'Prolonged or repeated exposure to DBCP has been shown to cause sterility in humans.'

11. The lead standard is found at 29 DFR 1910.1025, with a specific discussion of reproductive effects at Appendix C, Section II, 5. The inclusion of an MRP provision intended to protect, *inter alia*, against reproductive damage is a clear acknowledgement that such damage can occur under the permissible exposure levels.

12. The medical removal protection provision is found at 29 CFR 1910.1025(k). Although the automatic removal provisions (based on particular blood-lead concentrations) will not necessarily protect against reproductive damage, the general removal provisions are applicable: '... temporary medical removal may in particular cases be needed for workers desiring to parent a child in the near fugure or for particular pregnant employees. Some males may need a temporary removal so that their sperm can regain sufficient viability for fertilization ...'.

13. Three examples are: 4, 4-methylene-bis(2-chloroaniline), 29 CFR, Part

1910.1005 (since deleted); 2-acetylaminofluorene, 29 CFR, Part 1910.1014; and *N*-nitrosodimethylamine, 29 CFR, Part 1910.1016.

14. 29 U.S.C., Section 652(B).
15. *Industrial Union Department, AFL-CIO v. American Petroleum Institute*, 448 U.S. 671 (1980).
16. 15 U.S.C., Section 2603(b) (2)(A) (1976).
17. 15 U.S.C., Section 2603(a) (1976).
18. 15 U.S.C., Section 2604(a) (1976).
19. 15 U.S.C., Section 2604(e) and (f) (1976).
20. 15 U.S.C., Section 2606 (1976).
21. 15 U.S.C., Section 2605 (1976).
22. 15 U.S.C., Section 2604(f) (1976).
23. 15 U.S.C., Section 2603(f) (1976).
24. 15 U.S.C., Section 2608 (1976).
24(a). 29 CFR 1910 March 19, 1982.
24(b). 29 CFR 1910.20 May 23 1980.
24(c). 15 U.S.C.A. Section 2607(e).
25. For a detailed discussion of the right to refuse hazardous work, see: Nicholas A. Ashford and Judith I. Katz, Unsafe working conditions: employee rights under the Labour Management Relations Act and the Occupational Safety and Health Act, 52 *Notre Dame Lawyer* 802 (1977).
26. 29 U.S.C., Section 157 (1970).
27. For a more detailed discussion of this issue, see Ashford and Katz, *supra*, at note 48, pp. 803–805.
28. 29 U.S.C., Section 143 (1970).
29. For a more detailed discussion of this issue, see Ashford and Katz, *supra*, at note 48, pp. 805–818.
30. 29 U.S.C., Section 660(c) (1970).
31. 29 C.F.R., Section 1977.12 (1973).
32. *Whirlpool Corporation v. Marshall*, 445 U.S.C., 21 (1980).
33. The right to refuse hazardous work appears to have been extended to reproductive hazards in Canada. The Labour Minister has recently ruled that a pregnant employee who left her job because she felt that a hepatitis risk at the work place posed a danger to her unborn child had properly exercised her right to refuse unsafe working conditions under the Canadian Occupational Health and Safety Act. The Minister is reported to have ruled that, because 'there is no distinction between a pregnant worker and her unborn child', the fetus may be protected under the Act even though there is no specific provision of such protection. See Women can refuse if fetus in jeopardy, *At the Source*, Ontario Foundation of Labour, Occupational Health and Safety Centre, Vol. 4, No. 2 (March/April, 1983). For a discussion of the right to refuse hazardous work in Canada, see Brown, Canadian occupational health and safety legislation, 20 *Osgoode Hall Law Journal* 90, 96–102 (1982).
34. *Whirlpool, supra*, see note 32.
35. For a more detailed discussion of this issue, see Ashford and Katz, *supra*, at note 48, pp. 831–835.
36. *ibid.*, p. 806, and the cases cited therein.
37. The regulation creating the right pertains only to situations 'when an employee is confronted with a choice between not performing assigned tasks or subjecting *himself* to serious injury or death . . .', 29 C.F.R., Section 1977 12(6)(1) (1973) [emphasis added].

38. Section 7 on NLRA speaks broadly of the rights of employers to organise for their 'mutual aid or *protection*' [emphasis added], and the overall spirit of the Act is freedom from coercion, both physical and emotional.

39. 42 U.S.C., Section 2000e(k) (1978). This section, known as the 'Pregnancy Discrimination Act', was a Congressional response to *General Electric v. Gilbert*, 429 U.S. 125 (1977), where the Court held that pregnancy was not a sex-related disability. See, e.g., Mattson, The pregnancy amendment: fetal rights and the workplace, *Case and Comment*, **86**, No. 6, 33 (1981).

40. Five somewhat divergent viewpoints, all coming to this same general conclusion, are represented in the following articles and papers: Joan E. Bertin, Discrimination against women of childbearing capacity, presented at the Hastings Center, 8 January 1982; Lynn Paul Mattson, The pregnancy amendment: fetal rights and the workplace, *Case and Comment*, **86**, No. 6, 33 (1981); Gary Z. Nothstein and Jeffrey P. Ayers, Sex-based considerations of differentiation in the workplace: exploring the biomedical interface between OSHA and Title VII 26, *Villanova Law Review* 239 (1981); Wendy W. Williams, Firing the woman to protect the fetus: the reconciliation of fetal protection with employment opportunity goals under Title VII, 69 *The Georgetown Law Journal* 641 (1981); Nina Stillman, The law in conflict: accommodating equal employment and occupational health obligations, presented at the American Occupational Health Conference, Anaheim, California, 2 May 1979; and V. Bor, Exclusionary employment practices in hazardous industries: protection or discrimination?, 5 COL. JOUR. ENV. L. 97 (1978). As noted by Ronald Bayer of the Hastings Center, underlying the Title VII furore over female exclusionary policies is 'a recognition that the American economy so limits the possibilities of its woman workers that they would demand, as a sign of liberation, the right to share with men access to reproductive risks'. Bayer, *op. cit.*, p. 19, *supra*, at note 9.

41. The only circuit court decision that construes the 1978 amendment in the context of a fetal protection policy is *Wright v. Olin Corp.*, 697 F. 22 1172 (4th Cir. 1982). Under Olin's 'fetal vulnerability' policy, all women up to age 63 are assumed to be fertile, and are excluded from certain jobs which may require exposure to teratogenic or abortifacient agents unless Olin's doctors determine that they cannot bear children. In addition, most pregnant women are excluded from certain other jobs which involve more limited exposure to these substances, and non-pregnant women may work in such jobs only after signing acknowledgement of risk. In reversing the district court [*EEOC and Olin Corp.*, 24 FEP Cases 1646 (W.D.N.C. 1980)], the Fourth Circuit held that, 'the existence and operation of the fetal vulnerability program established as a matter of law a *prima facie* case of Title VII violation' (697 F22 at 1187). The court remanded the case to the district court to allow Olin an opportunity to attempt to demonstrate that the policy was justified by business necessity. See note 48, *infra*. In *Hayes v. Shelby Memorial Hospital*, 2d FEP 1173 (N.D. Al a, 1982), federal district court in Alabama invalidated a 'fetus protection' policy under Title VII; the case is at present on appeal to the Eleventh Circuit (No. 82-7296). A Title VII challenge to the American Cyanamid 'fetus protection' policy is at present pending before the U.S. District Court for the Northern District of West Virginia (*Christman v. American Cyanamid*, Cause No. 80-0024). Two pre-amendment cases involving a General Motors policy were apparently settled in the U.S. District Court for the Southern District of Indiana (*EEOC v. General Motors*, Cause No. 76-53B-E, and *Toomer v.*

General Motors, Cause No. 76-101-0), but more recently the EEOC appears
to have taken a less activist stance in challenging policies that exclude pregnant or fertile women from the work place.

42. U.S.C., Section 2000e-5(k) (as amended, 1972).

43. The defence arises from statutory language. See 42 U.S.C., Section 2000e-
2(e) (1976). Principal cases defining the defence are: *Arrit v. Grisell*, 567
F.2d 1267, 1271 (4th Cir. 1977); *Usury v. Tamiami: Trail Tours*, 531 F.2d
224, 236 (5th Cir. 1976); and *Hodgson v. Greyhound Lines, Inc.*, 499 F.2d
859 (7th Cir. 1974). Mattson, *supra*, at note 61, p. 34 (see note 40, *supra*),
argues that the defence will not be successful in 'fetus protection' cases
'unless it can be shown that there is a definite nexus between pregnancy
risks and job performance, as opposed to a potential risk to the fetus'.

44. The business necessity defence was judicially created. See *Griggs v. Duke
Power Co.*, 401 U.S. 424, 431 (1971).

45. The Supreme Court has characterised the BFOQ defence as an 'extremely
narrow exception' to the prohibition against sex discrimination: *Dothard v.
Rawlinson*, 433 U.S. 321, 334 (1977). In *Griggs v. Duke Power Co.*, 401
U.S. 424, 431 (1971), the Court characterised the business necessity test as
requiring a 'manifest relation to the employment in question'; in *Albermarle
Paper Co. v. Moody*, 422 U.S. 405, 425 (1975), the Court indicated that the
availability of an alternative policy which would meet the same business
necessity 'would be evidence that the employer was using [the challenged
policy] merely as a "pretext" for discrimination'. See also *Robinson v.
Lorillard Corp.* 444 F20 791 (4th Cir.), *cert. denied*, 404 U.S. 1006 (1971).

46. Again, though they do not always agree on particulars, this is the general
conclusion reached by the commentators cited *supra* at note 83.

47. The defence was developed by the Supreme Court in conjunction with the
court's recognition that an employment practice that was neutral *on its
face* could still violate Title VII if it was discriminatory *in its effect: Griggs
v. Duke Power Co.*, 401 U.S. 424, 431 (1971). The court has not extended
the defence to racially discriminatory policies.

48. *Wright v. Olin Corp., supra*, 697 F.2d 1172. In describing Olin's 'fetus
vulnerability' policy as 'gender-neutral', the court appears to have rejected
the argument that discrimination on the basis of childbearing capacity was
sex discrimination *on its face*, and thus to have found the policy discriminatory only *in its effect*. As noted, application of the business necessity
defence would be consistent with such a determination of racial neutrality.
The court indicated that protection of the fetus was an appropriate business
purpose under that defence: '. . . we believe the safety of unborn children is . . .
appropriately analogized to the safety of personal service customers of the
business . . . we cannot believe that Congress meant by Title VII absolutely
to deprive employers of the right to provide any protection for licensees and
invitees legitimately and necessarily upon their premises by any policy
having a disparate impact upon certain workers.' 697 F.2d at 1189. In
setting forth guidelines for cases of this nature, the court indicated that the
burden of establishing the defence is on the employer, that it must be
established by independent, objective evidence, and that it must be supported by the opinion evidence of qualified scientific experts. The court
further indicated that the employer need not show a scientific consensus,
but must show that there is so considerable a body of opinion that (1)
significant risk to unborn children exists and (2) such risk is *confined to
the exposure of women workers*, that an informed employer could not

responsibly fail to act. Finally, the court indicated that the defence, if established, may be rebutted by proof of acceptable alternative policies or practices.

49. See Nothstein and Ayers, *supra*, note 40, at 306–312; and Williams, *supra*, note 40, at 667–678.

50. The Western District of Michigan has offered the following statement of the law: '. . . in evaluating employment practices subsequent to [the Pregnancy Discrimination Act], policies which create distinctions or discriminate on the basis of pregnancy are in violation absent a showing of a bona fide occupational qualification' (*Thompson v. Board of Education of Romeo Community Schools*, 526 F. Supp. 1035, 1039 [W. D. Mich. 1081]).

51. Although the rather direct language of the Pregnancy Discrimination Act would appear to be central to any analysis of the treatment of 'fetus protection' policies under Title VII, the court does not address this language in any detail. The apparent inconsistency between it and the court's position may well be reconcilable, but the rationale for such a reconciliation does not appear to be found in the decision. Rather, the court simply notes that if it were to limit the employer to the BFOQ defence, it would 'prevent the employer from asserting a justification defense which under developed Title VII doctrine it is entitled to present' (697 F.22 at 1185, note 21).

52. Wendy Williams, *supra*, note 61 (see note 40, *supra*).

53. Clement Associates, Inc., *Chemical Hazards to Human Reproduction*, prepared for the Council on Environmental Quality (January, 1981), pp. VII–4. See also Judith S. Bollin, Genes and gender in the workplace, *Occupational Health and Safety*, 16 (January 1982).

54. Williams, *supra*, note 61, pp. 703–704.

55. A general discussion of the availability of injunctive relief to abate work place hazards can be found in Alfred W. Blumrose *et al.*, Injunctions against occupational hazards: the right to work under safe conditions, 64 *California Law Review* 702 (1976), 1 *Industrial Relations Law Journal* 25 (1976).

56. See Michelle C. Mentzer, *Industrial Relations Law Journal*, 5(2), 247–282 (1983).

18

What Can be Done in Antenatal Care?

ANN FOSTER

In this chapter are described some of the existing schemes and initiatives concerned with facilities and formal policies directed towards pregnant women at work, and the response of those involved in these schemes, and the early development of very recent work initiated in one region of the Health and Safety Executive is outlined.

The report of the House of Commons Social Services Committee on *Perinatal and Neonatal Mortality* (the Short Report)[1] considered evidence given by representatives of the health care professions, Members of Parliament, trade union and employers' organisations and many others concerned with the, then, lack of significant success in reducing perinatal and neonatal mortality rates. Evidence was also given on behalf of two companies from the private sector of British industry who had prepared formal policies directed towards pregnant employees. The companies concerned were Strathleven Bonded Warehouses Ltd, Scotland, and Park Cakes Ltd, Oldham. For the purpose of this chapter, discussion will concentrate upon the work done in the Oldham company. This is in no way meant to negate the work done in Scotland but is merely because of the personal experience of the author at Park Cakes.

Oldham is one of the traditionally working class cotton spinning towns of the North-west of England. It is situated at the foot of the Pennines dividing Lancashire from Yorkshire and, hence, the cotton trade from the woollen trade.

At the turn of this century, the traditional work in this area was mostly cotton spinning and heavy textile engineering. The decline of the cotton industry left its legacy of empty mills and the health problems prevalent in social classes IV and V, highlighted in the Black Report[2]. Changes in industry have run parallel with the changes in the population profile. Light manufacturing units have replaced many of the mills. The influx of Asian immigrants in the 1960s and 1970s has contributed to the formation of a multiracial community which exists in mutual tolerance and harmony.

Park Cakes Ltd is a large employer within this community. It is the bakery

241

division of the Northern Food group of companies, employing around 2000 people of mixed ethnic origin. Bakery work is unskilled work, traditionally performed by women, some 80 per cent of the work force. It is arduous, repetitive work, is labour-intensive and involves long periods, invariably standing, at a conveyor belt. It is hot work, especially during summer. Under these conditions (of employment) pregnancy may not be the most pleasant of conditions. The minor problems assume quite a high priority. Frequency of micturition can be very inconvenient when maintaining production levels at a conveyor belt. Varicosities can be uncomfortable if most of one's working day is spent standing. While one sponge cake can smell quite nice during cooking, the smell of a thousand can deliver a full-blown assault on the olfactory senses; at 8.0 A.M. on a warm summer day in a hot bakery these minor problems require extreme sensitivity in being overcome.

The socio-economic factors prevalent in this work force indicate that these may be just the women who are likely to be unsure of their dates, smoke heavily, lack adequate nutrition, have high underlying morbidity rates and have inadequate natal care, because of either lack of uptake or deficiencies within the system. In 1978 the perinatal mortality rate for Oldham was 21.2 per 1000 total births, as opposed to a national figure of 15.5 per thousand[3].

Part of the work of any Occupational Health Department (OHD) is to monitor the health of vulnerable groups of employees — either vulnerable because of hazardous working processes or at risk because of personal health or social factors. To these aims, an information monitoring service had been offered to pregnant women at Park Cakes for some time; however, in 1980 it was decided to develop a formal policy regarding provision for pregnant employees. This policy followed a lengthy period of planning involving the local Health Education Department.

The aims were defined as:

(1) To increase the awareness of the need for early and regular antenatal care.

(2) To offer a programme of formal health education to pregnant employees.

(3) To study the ergonomics between pregnancy and work, exclusive to Park Cakes.

This scheme was to contribute to the overall regional objective of reducing the neonatal and perinatal morbidity and mortality rates. The work began in early 1980, and is essentially a practical exercise in health education, public relations, improved communication and ergonomics.

The contribution of the OHD is primarily in co-ordinating the health education sessions which are held during production time. The health educators are midwives, health visitors, dieticians, health education officers, dental hygienists and the company safety officer, occupational health nurses and a member of the personnel department, who gives specific advice regarding maternity grants, benefits and allowances. The health educators explain why antenatal care is important, give advice regarding nutrition, the dangers of smoking and alcohol consumption and the indiscriminate use of non-prescribed drugs, and provide a translation service for midwifery and obstetrical jargon. The health educators from outside the company meet the women on their own ground. The consumers of this education contribute freely and a frank and interesting exchange of ideas and views often occurs. The atmosphere is often lively and conducive to a mutually beneficial experience.

The OHD closely studied the individual personal ergonomics between work and pregnancy. There are three main ergonomic problems of pregnancy in a bakery: backache, balance, bulk.

Backache will be exacerbated by long periods of standing at a conveyor belt. The OHD were aware that the availability of seating for pregnant employees would have implications for the work force in general. Backache may also be exacerbated by the posture adopted during working, and this requires individual investigation and advice.

Slipping is a common hazard in a bakery whether the female employee is pregnant or not; obviously, when pregnant, balance is even more precarious. The pregnancy scheme focused attention on this problem and provided renewed impetus for a solution.

The pros and cons of schemes such as this one described are not peculiar to Park Cakes. Other schemes, such as the one initiated by the Cleveland Area Health Authority[4] in the North-east of England, which has a similar social profile to that of Oldham, were focused upon the provision of information to smaller companies in the area who do not have established OHDs. There are initiatives in areas in Scotland[5] and England where local obstetricians have taken part of their antenatal clinics into the community health centres or onto industrial estate sites. There are many different examples of reaching the consumer[6] of antenatal care. There is no blueprint of what is the right way to do this and what is the wrong way. Each group must identify its own needs and ways of meeting these needs. However, there are considerations of overall strategy which are common to these schemes.

(1) The need for adequate preparation, consultation and communication.

(2) The need for flexibility to reassess in the light of information evolving from group discussion with a women involved.

(3) The need to recognise and reconcile areas of potential conflict[7] in the woman, who may be sole wage earner, mother of other children, daughter of an ill mother or mother-in-law, etc., and who also just happens to be pregnant. This is especially important when considering the extended family unit, which can bring additional burdens, especially in the Asian culture.

Employers also have needs when considering the pros and cons of such schemes. Alistair Robertson, Director of Personnel, Strathleven Bonded Warehouse Ltd, has spoken of the need to audit such schemes, to monitor the use and its effect and future needs[8]. Evaluation of such schemes must include whether or not the needs of all those involved are being met.

From January 1980 to January 1983, a total of 113 pregnancies were recorded among the employees of Park Cakes (table 18.1). Twenty-six pregnancies were with non-Caucasian mothers.

Table 18.1   Pregnancies 1980–1983 among employees at Park Cakes

Age of mother	Jan.–Dec. 1980	Jan.–Dec. 1981	Jan.–Dec. 1982	Totals
16–19	3	5	8	16
20–29	28	20	23	71
30–39	14	4	5	23
40–49	2	1	–	3
> 50	–	–	–	–
Totals	47	30	36	113

There was one uncharacteristic exception to the uptake of this, obviously voluntary, scheme. The provision of time off for visits to GPs or the local antenatal clinic for antenatal care has been costed at around £1500 per year for the whole scheme.

An analysis by the Health Education Officer (HEO) in Oldham has revealed that the scheme users are those who prove to be traditionally more difficult to reach with hospital-based services and those who reflect a lower uptake rate of preventive services and may be, consequently, at risk. An evaluation recently prepared by Dominic Harrison[9] (HEO) states: 'In some senses the high uptake [by the employees] and the continuance and expansion of the scheme are the most articulate advocates of its success.'

Undoubtedly, the tremendous response of the pregnant women at Park Cakes is a challenge to all health educators who contribute to the scheme. Consumer participation is plentiful; reticence is almost unknown, even among the women whose background has not encouraged the demand of knowledge. This is now *their scheme*. The OHD may have created the framework or established the opportunity, but it is now the women who define their needs and provoke reaction from the health care professionals. The women are eager to contribute to their own care and the care of their babies. They have spoken on regional radio programmes about the scheme: these are the same women who 3 years ago felt silly about asking a very simple question at a visit to the antenatal clinic.

The challenge extended to the health care professionals has not been ignored. Midwives have examined their attitudes and approaches to the provision of their services in an attempt to meet the needs of the consumer[10,11]. Working parties have been convened by midwives, and jointly with others, to consider pregnancy at work[12]. Two years ago, the wrath of obstetricians was incurred at a one-day conference at the Royal College of Physicians, entitled 'Pregnant at Work', by a complaint that the response of obstetricians did not run parallel with that of other professions in identifying and contributing to the solution of the problems of pregnant women at work. It is hoped that this would not happen today, for obstetricians do contribute to the scheme at Park Cakes, obstetricians are examining different ways of selling antenatal care to the consumer and obstetricians are participating in conferences such as that at the Royal Society of Medicine.

Health care professionals have begun to identify the general problems of the additional burden at work on pregnancy and to co-ordinate some solutions. It is logical that the identification of occupational exposure to hazards which may affect reproduction follows.

We now need to identify the role of occupational health practitioners in answering the questions that are asked by both male and female workers and fellow health care professionals.

A survey, currently at the pilot stage, is being carried out in the North London Region of the Employment Medical Advisory Service of the Health and Safety Executive in collaboration with the National Health Service staff and other disciplines within the Health and Safety Executive. A visitor's perception of London sometimes belies the underlying community of varied manufacturing activity, hospitals and universities. It is a community of overwhelming interest and unconventional charm. It is also a community beset by the problems of the inner city, which are not unique to London but are common to many cities in the USA. This survey involves two Employment Nursing Advisers (ENAs) attending the booking clinic in two large hospitals in London in order to collate information with regard to:

medical and obstetrical history
pregnancy and neonatal history
occupational history
current occupational profile and level of exposure to:
  noise
  vibration
  high temperature
  low temperature
  dust
  fume
  lifting
  standing

        ionising radiation
        non-ionising radiation
        other hazards
   domestic work burden
   occupational exposure of husband (father of child)
   infertility
   pregnancy outcome

The survey aims to assess the size of the problem, and at this pilot stage we have set ourselves three questions to answer:

(1) What proportion of pregnant women are exposed to possible occupational hazards?
(2) What sort of hazards are they?
(3) What can we do to modify the working environment?

The current work place can be visited and recommendations and reassurance given as necessary. Further investigations — for example, the taking of biological or environmental samples — can be arranged and follow-up visits made as indicated.

Information regarding potentially reproductive hazards in the work place will be incomplete if we do not include information from both male and female employees. That information will be more speedily and efficiently obtained if we moderate our attitudes and expand our lines of communication. Men and women have the right to conceive a child free from the worry of the effects of their work on that child. There is diversity in the backgrounds and disciplines of the contributors to this volume; we are not mutually exclusive in providing some solutions to the problems of pregnant women at work.

REFERENCES

1. House of Commons Social Services Committee (1979–80). Report: *Perinatal and Neonatal Mortality* (Short Report), HMSO, London
2. Black, D. (Chairman) (1980). Report of Research Working Group: *Inequalities in Health*, DHSS
3. Office of Population and Census Surveys. HMSO, London
4. Wright, L. (1981). Forging links between the Health Service and local employees. Paper presented at *Pregnant at Work* Conference, April 1981
5. Reid, M. E. and McIlwain, G. M. (1980). Consumer opinion of hospital antenatal clinic. *Soc. Sci. Med.*, **14A**, 363–368
6. Dowling, S. (1984). The workplace as a focus for antenatal health education and the promotion of antenatal care. In *Health for a Change*, Child Poverty Action Group and National Extension College, Cambridge
7. Graham, H. and Oakley, A. (1981). Competing ideologies of reproduction; medical and maternal perspectives on pregnancy. In Roberts, H. (Ed.), *Women, Health and Reproduction*, Routledge and Kegan Paul, London

8. Robertson, A. (1981). The role of management. Paper presented at *Pregnant at Work* Conference, April 1981
9. Harrison, D. P. (n.d.). An evaluation of the Park Cakes Educating Programme (unpublished)
10. Flint, C. (1982). Antenatal clinics. 1. Where have we gone wrong? *Nursing Mirror*, 155, 24 November, 26–28
11. Flint, C. (1982). Antenatal clinics. 2. Get off the conveyor belt. *Nursing Mirror*, 155, 1 December, 37–38
12. Rodmell, G. and Smart, L. (1982). Pregnant at work (Joint OU/Kensington, Chelsea and Westminster ANA Research project). *Midwives Chron.*, 95(1), November, 408–409

19

The Contribution of the Occupational Health Services

FRANCES J.T. BAKER

Evidence seems to demonstrate quite conclusively that women who receive continuous antenatal care throughout pregnancy have a better chance of a safe delivery and a healthy baby than those who do not. The traditional antenatal care team comprises doctor, midwife, health visitor and a variety of associated paramedical workers. To this group I would add occupational health personnel, and for the purpose of this chapter emphasise the role of the nurse.

More women now go out to work and, in consequence, are likely to be at work while pregnant. The amount of medical care they receive will depend on the extent of managerial support to avail themselves of statutory provisions, or their individual energy or interest to pursue what is possible.

The feasibility of managerial support for antenatal care in the work place immediately raises several issues:

Should management be expected to have a role in what appears to be essentially a personal matter?
How costly would such an endeavour be?
What benefits could the organisation expect?

It is only fair that such issues be considered, for it is too easy to see the care of the pregnant woman at work as yet another burden to be placed on management, a sort of medical VAT. Rather should the topic be considered for what it more appropriately is – a concern for the whole society.

Historical experience has shown that actions frequently follow events. When the Boer War demonstrated how unhealthy the average working man was and how many recruits had to be rejected, the need for social legislation was apparent; measures were taken and provisions such as the School Health Service commenced[1].

The need today is less dramatically obvious, but is it too fanciful to equate the lack of energy which so many adults show with a latent result in inadequate

249

antenatal care, social factors which so often surround this and the subsequent life-long effects? Lest some readers see such statements as a plea for more cash as the solution to our problems, we hasten to add that cash subsidies do not automatically equate with healthy babies, although additional financial provision may well be part of the solution. Rather, the way ahead lies in a greater vision of what is reasonably possible within the existing limitations while striving continuously for a better future.

Table 19.1 shows a short questionnaire put before a number of occupational health nursing students in 1979.

Table 19.1   Questionnaire answered by occupational health nursing students

(1) Are you automatically notified about women in the organisation who become pregnant?

(2) Do you have another method whereby you discover the information?

(3) Could there be pregnant women at work without your knowledge?

(4) What particular care are you able to give pregnant women at work – for example, rest, diet or blood pressure?

(5) What are your views on antenatal clinics at work run by community midwives and occupational health nurses?

(6) The perinatal mortality rate in the UK is not good, particularly in industrial areas and in social classes IV and V. What contribution do you think that the occupational health nurses can offer?

The responses were interesting. The first question was almost uniformly answered in the negative. The follow-up questions 2 and 3 showed that such knowledge came in a variety of ways: women presenting at the Medical Centre feeling sick and requiring treatment, information from the Personnel Department, casually from the woman herself attending for reasons unconnected with the pregnancy, and information acquired in the course of visits to the work place (an important aspect of the function of an occupational health nurse).

The care which could be given in answer to question 4 included direct care such as weight checks, blood pressure, nutrition advice and guidance about provisions. There was also the special care needed for groups such as diabetics and those known to have a degree of hypertension.

In response to question 5 regarding clinics, it was felt that, unless the work force was largely female, this was an unrealistic approach. There was felt to be no reason, however, why there should not be closer contact between midwives and occupational health nurses, and, indeed, in my own area midwives on the Health Education Certificate course are expected to teach a session to the occupational health nursing students with this view in mind. Midwives who were based in districts where there was a poor usage of antenatal clinics were particularly interested in such liaison. For women in these areas, activities such as clinic visits were equated with time lost from work (which could mean reduced wages), reduced shopping time, the complications of caring for other children and the additional effort of going out in the evening after a day at work. In this situation care at work can look very attractive and may well be providing for the woman most at risk.

Certainly, however, if they were organised, the most important feature would have to be the co-operation and liaison between the occupational health nurse and the community midwife. Obviously, management could not easily be convinced of the value of clinics in work-time, but lunch breaks and immediately after work are possible alternatives (particularly if husbands could be encouraged to attend as well).

The role of the occupational health nurse, however, extends much further than organising and sharing in antenatal clinics[2]. There are many aspects of work which have a considerable bearing on the health of a pregnant woman. Obviously, no such woman should be in contact with known toxic substances, and legislation gives clear guidance on this matter. However, legislation is only as useful as the means which exist for its implementation. A trained occupational health nurse would be in a good position to see that such provisions were strongly adhered to.

There are other work processes, however, which, while not seriously affecting health, do produce unpleasant effects, resulting in nausea and vomiting. Equally, the work operation in which the mother is involved could well benefit from ergonomic-type considerations. Machines are certainly not designed with pregnant women in mind, nor are they likely to be, but this need not remove the obligation to notice when her altered shape no longer fits the process on which she is involved. Such gross difficulties are less likely to be the norm; more commonly the factor will be quite simple — can the job be done sitting when it has been usual to stand? Minor adaptations may provide a solution, or in an extreme situation a different job might be indicated. Whatever the action, the situation would greatly benefit from supervision by an occupational health nurse who has the training to assess the problem from a physiological and industrial perspective.

If one considers the management of pregnancy chronologically, one of the first events is likely to be its confirmation and subsequent hospital booking, after which antenatal care commences. It is also the stage at which delays occur which are not sufficiently recognised. An unpublished study relating to attendance at the antenatal clinic of a Manchester hospital has demonstrated that the first visit, on average, takes place considerably later than one might assume — at 16 weeks. By this date early pregnancy problems could easily be established and, perhaps more seriously, wrong health patterns adopted.

In 1980 Laurence *et al*. wrote in the *British Medical Journal* describing the increased risk of pregnancies complicated by fetal neural tube defects in mothers receiving poor diets, and the possible benefit of dietary counselling[2]. While admitting that in any prospective study it is difficult to obtain a sample size large enough to show important clinical differences when the incidence of the disease is low, the researchers nevertheless concluded by suggesting that 'improving the quality of the diet, especially during the first trimester of pregnancy in women at risk . . . may improve some environmental factors acting on the fetus'. They further added that 'all the recurrences and nearly all the miscarriages occurred following pregnancies in women receiving a poor diet or severely unbalanced diet'.

During the important first trimester a pregnant woman will almost certainly be at work, and, as the Manchester statistics indicated, will be unlikely to have made a first appearance at hospital. In such a situation the role of the occupational health services becomes one almost of crisis management rather than the probably desirable one which we have envisaged. The health education role here is more properly one for the schools, for a good nutritional programme cannot be either acquired or expected to produce maximum results overnight. How ready the school system will be to incorporate this approach is questionable. A colleague, involved in education, recently approached three schools in the North-west of England with a request to be allowed to introduce a *nutrition for pregnancy* module into the Home Economics Course. In each case her request was met with refusal. Such a situation is probably a fairly accurate reflection of the attitudes which prevail both inside and outside the Health Service towards preventive medicine. Repeatedly problems are treated when they arise with expert intervention backed by high technology. On the whole, the message of medical history, that controlling the environment is the best approach, goes unheeded.

It is worth giving consideration to both the food the woman eats at work and where it is consumed. It is hoped that the surroundings are at least minimally appropriate, being away from the work operation, although, despite legislation, even this cannot in every case be assumed. The canteen, or its equivalent, may be cramped, noisy and smoke-filled, none of which features are helpful to the pregnant woman. The canteen food is more likely to err towards fried and filling stodge than the fresh fruit or lightly cooked vegetables which we know to be more appropriate. Yet these simple aspects may be among the most crucial for the woman's health. Unfortunately, by their very simplicity they may be ignored as insignificant.

Many factories and other commercial concerns are constantly busy raising money for sophisticated medical machinery whose worth has not yet been properly evaluated and the cost of which, both initial and for the subsequent operations, is astronomical. There is certainly the will among ordinary people to improve health standards, but the direction is sometimes inappropriate. Much of the blame for this must lie with the professionals and the media, whose aims and objectives are not always either clearly defined or appreciated by the relevant consumers.

Some aspects of the care of a pregnant woman may well be appropriately complex, but many will not. A good number of years ago, pupil midwives were frequently admonished with the words: 'Childbirth is a natural event; you are merely there to assist nature should the need arise.' Surely, it is natural that we provide a proper environment for the pregnant woman at work. As already indicated, this proper environment will exclude her from contact with known toxic substances and will consider the ergometric implications of her manner of working. Her diet will be in accord with what she had learned at school as being advisable for an expectant mother, and will have been observed for at least as long as the decision to commence a family. She will have no problem in following the pattern at work, because such an approach will be the norm. With so much support, extra rest during the day will not be necessary at this stage, but, should the need arise, then the Occupational Health Centre ought to have the facilities to cope. To advice and help regarding rest could be added topics such as exercise, dental care, the taking of drugs and, of course, attitudes to smoking.

The trained occupational health nurse is able to look at the environment. Just as it would be wrong to overestimate the number of nurses in industry as a whole (Radwanski, lately of EMAS, suggests 9000 or 3 per cent of nurses), so, too, would it be erroneous to envisage them all having specialised skills. A great many have no additional training for this very different kind of nursing, and although many may desire it, there is no compulsion for an employer to give the necessary permission and support for training time.

The occupational health nurse can be a source of considerable support, both directly in the ways suggested and as an information resource. A trained occupational health nurse will be aware of the various rights and benefits available to the pregnant woman, but the knowledge she possesses is useful not so much for advising the woman about the financial and other provisions to which she is entitled – others can more appropriately deal with such matters – but because in her role as a counsellor such knowledge is crucial. Counselling is a non-directive approach and part of the training of such a nurse. It is a useful skill in many situations, not least in the present context, for not all pregnancies are either planned or desired, as we all know. The nurse at work ought to be someone to whom the woman, possibly with her mind in turmoil, can turn, knowing that objectivity will be combined with a caring approach to the problem. Some time ago, at a British Institute of Management Conference on 'Stress at Work', a consultant psychiatrist replied to the question, 'What can I practically do to reduce stress in my organisation?' with the words, 'Get yourself a trained occupational health nurse . . .'.

There are clearly many areas where the occupational health services have a potential role to play in the care of the pregnant woman at work.

Whether or not this happens will depend on a number of factors, most obvious among which will be whether in the first place such a service exists. Until such time as there is a statutory requirement, provision is likely to be uneven and inequalities of care will continue. The simple reason for the imbalance could be identified as financial, but until there is an acceptance of the importance of health care at work the situation is unlikely to change. Since the National Health Service itself, with certain notable exceptions, has been somewhat tardy in introducing occupational health for its own employees, it is difficult to imagine the demand gathering momentum.

Second, where there is such a service, the extent to which its members have specialised training will be significant. As already indicated, there is at present no legal requirement for such training, although the recent document from the Health and Safety Executive, *First Aid at Work*, which recognises for the first time the existence of a qualified occupational health nurse, has pointed the way ahead[3]. However, some major national firms might try to twist the letter of the law and use the document as evidence that a nurse can be dispensed with.

It may be that the last thing the pregnant woman wants is for her pregnancy to be an aspect of what happens at work, and this right of privacy obviously must be observed while making sure that she is aware of all the facilities which exist.

Where an occupational health service exists and where its various team members are trained, the potential is considerable. During 1981 and 1982 we carried out a survey of 20 work places in order to demonstrate the potential of occupational health nurses for health education[4]. The study was connected with nutritional standards and indirectly with smoking behaviour, aiming to show that the occupational health nurse has a significant role in health promotion, in contrast to her readily understood treatment role. At the same time we must bear in mind that industry and commerce exist primarily to make a profit, not to promote health education, although benefits for them in doing the latter can be identified.

The population for the study was drawn from 20 industrial and service organisations, all but one within a 15 mile radius of Stoke-on-Trent, in North Staffordshire. The sample was to be representative of all those workers attending the medical centre during a particular week, not necessarily a true sample of the whole work force, which would have required a more sophisticated procedure and would not necessarily have been more appropriate. The study aimed to give nurses an opportunity for assessment and health education with a sample of their client group. Any workers attending the medical centre fulfilled this criterion.

On the whole, the nurses taking part had no experience of survey methods. In consequence, the approach adopted was made as straightforward as possible. The overall aim was to demonstrate and give opportunity for health education; this took precedence, although certain safeguards were built into the study in order to minimise possible bias. For example:

(1) An outline numerical plan was described for determining who should be included.

(2) The participants identified over a period of 4 days included, where appropriate, shift and night workers.

(3) Where possible the sample included all social classes and was representative of the various working groups. Similarly, a health profile was included to ensure that the sample did not contain an inordinate number of people with significant health problems.

Questions were also asked about visits to GP or hospital, about medication and self-health assessment. It should be remembered, however, that occupational health departments are likely to be used with much less premeditation than takes place when patients visit their GP or other statutory services.

The study took place over a period of 6 months, including an initial stage and a follow-up. The 20 organisations taking part gave a possible study total of 660 persons. The actual number who completed the initial stage was 509 (77 per cent of the population); 40 per cent of this total were smokers. Of these, 81 per cent were considered to have a potentially inadequate diet, compared with 43 per cent of the non-smokers. Health education information concerning nutrition and smoking was then given to all participants.

Five months later a follow-up took place; 74 per cent of those who had completed the initial survey completed this second stage. Twenty-eight per cent originally considered potentially at risk had improved their diet; 18 per cent who had been smokers 6 months earlier had now ceased smoking. Both of these behaviour changes were found to be statistically significant. In addition, the follow-up response rate was found to be significant for social classes IV and V.

Health education ideally aims to make contact with populations before problems arise. The work place is largely comprised of healthy people and would seem an important focus for primary prevention using the likely co-operation of the resident health professionals. The future of any nation clearly lies with its young. That the mother-to-be in the last decades of the twentieth century is likely to be at work is a fact of life. For social classes IV and V this will be particularly the case, and among these groups working conditions likely to be poorest and morbidity statistics most significant. There are already health services in many industries which could be utilised more effectively to deal with the problem.

There needs, too, to be more honesty among health professionals concerning the appropriate approach to certain types of health problems and with this a greater practical will to apportion available resources. We already have much of the necessary knowledge to solve the problems raised in this book. What is needed is an adjustment in the balance of interest and provision.

The realisation may well take time to come to fruition. In the meantime we must give thanks for the pioneers at Park Cakes, Oldham, and Strathleven Bonded Warehouses, Dumbarton, who have already had the courage and energy to act. I enjoyed teaching my students about the notables in occupational health history, from Ramazinni, through Thackrah to Legge, Philippa Flowerday, Hunter and Marion West. It is heartening to know that the tradition continues.

REFERENCES

1. Charley, I. H. (1960). *The Birth of Industrial Nursing*, Baillière, Tindall and Cox, London
2. Laurence, K. M. *et al.* (1980). Increased risk of pregnancies complicated by

foetal neural tube defects in mothers receiving poor diets and possible benefit of dietary counselling. *British Medical Journal*, **281**, 1592–1594
3. *First Aid at Work* (1981). Health and Safety Series Booklet HS(R)11
4. Baker, F. J. T. (1982). *Working for Health*, unpublished MSc thesis, Faculty of Medicine, Manchester University
5. Slaney, B. (1980). *Occupational Health Nursing*, Croom Helm, London

20

Educating Workers, Management and the General Public

J. McEWEN

The title of this chapter may give two false impressions: the first is that the three groups are completely separate and that there are three educational tasks; the second is that these groups will be the passive recipients of a series of lectures. With the type of problems we are considering and the groups of people involved, those with responsibility for health need to come together and learn together, seeking to solve their common dilemmas and uncertainties. A variety of different people with special skills and resources can be used in this problem-solving approach.

Currently there is a chance to make use of public interest and the motivation of people concerned about health and prevention, to build on existing groups and social networks and to make use of the facilities and expertise available in industry, unions, the health services and the community. The ideal may not always be attainable, and therefore every opportunity must be utilised by those in responsible positions – management, unions, health professionals, pressure groups and community groups – to initiate appropriate health education and to respond to requests for help and advice.

I shall begin by discussing the basis of health education and then examine the needs of the community. Health education has made limited advances in the work place, but it is necessary to consider some of the problems before looking ahead to the opportunities.

INFORMATION AND SKILLS – A NECESSARY PARTNERSHIP

In the field of health education, we have been bedevilled by problems of terminology.

What do we mean by health education?
What do others understand it to be?

257

Recently, there has been an explosion of new terms, perhaps indicating the uncertainty, yet the real interest, that exists. The terms include: 'preventive medicine', 'health promotion', 'health maintenance', 'health protection', 'anticipatory care', 'education for life styles' and 'health education'. Although the varying terminology may relate in part to a casual view of health education, more frequently it reflects a real division between the medical and educational approaches. The differing philosophical bases of medicine and education are compounded by separate professional training and inherited professional prejudices. For health education to be effective and realistic, there needs to be a combination of the epidemiological, social, psychological and anthropological sciences with the science and skills of education (figure 20.1). Perhaps some of

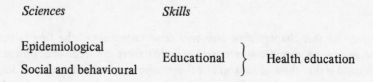

Sciences   *Skills*

Epidemiological
                              Educational } Health education
Social and behavioural

Figure 20.1   A necessary partnership

the failures of health education in the past would have been avoided if there had been multidisciplinary research leading on to multidisciplinary practice. The WHO definition of health education[1] provides a useful beginning: 'The focus of health education is on people and actions. In general, its aims are to persuade people to adopt and sustain healthful life practices, to use judiciously and wisely the health services available to them and to take their own decisions, both individually and collectively, to improve their health status environment.'

Health education in the widest sense is a continuous process which begins in early infancy and continues throughout life. Educationists recognise the importance of formal health education in the early years of schooling (one aspect being to prepare young people for the world of work)[2], but this is a small part of a much wider process involving family, friends, peer groups, professionals and the media. The field of health education is, therefore, justified in examining and developing other settings that offer opportunities for health education, including the health education of adults in the work place. After school children, pregnant women have been accorded high priority for health education. The Education and Preparation for Parenthood Programme is one of the major programmes of the Health Education Council. It is an integrated longitudinal programme, which begins with preconception care and seeks to co-ordinate all activities related to this important area, through publications, mass media, and education and training initiatives.

Although in this volume we are considering *Pregnant Women at Work*, it is unreasonable to expect individuals to be concerned with, or assume responsibility for, an isolated aspect of health – or indeed to see health as isolated from other areas of life such as housing, education and the environment. This chapter will attempt to provide an overview and indicate some ways in which the practice may be improved. Equally, the health of a pregnant woman relates to attitudes and behaviour which are long-standing and to an environment which involves both work and community in all aspects – social, psychological and physical. Accordingly, it is necessary to consider both specific programmes for pregnant women and long-term programmes of education for all employees, management and the public.

It is also useful to mention the changing emphasis in health education as has been described by Kickbusch[3] from the European Region of the World Health Organization. She outlines four conceptual re-orientations that are taking place: (1) from health prescription to health promotion; (2) from individualistic behaviour modification to a systematic public health approach; (3) from medical orientation to recognition of lay competence; (4) from authoritarian health education to supportive health education. She believes that the more imaginative forms of health education and information that the above strategy requires can be developed along three main lines: (1) raising individual competence and knowledge about health and illness, about the body and its functions, about prevention and coping; (2) raising competence and knowledge to use the health care system and to understand its functioning; (3) raising awareness about social, political and environmental factors that influence health.

NEEDS – THE CHALLENGE OF INEQUALITY

Much has been written about the inequalities in health, so comprehensively summarised by the Black Report[4]. The importance of antenatal care and the health of mothers was particularly noted. The failure of health education, the limited use of preventive health services and the adverse effects of the working environment were among the factors that were considered to contribute to inequality in health. However, it is recognised that the social, economic, educational and environmental aspects of our communities are the major determinants of health, and, although we may not be in a position to affect them directly, we should ensure that health services do seek to promote health and prevent illness and that we are prepared to pursue the social policy implications on a wider level.

In the work place there are particular risks and problems associated with specific jobs and environments. Those with knowledge and status within the management structure have a responsibility to identify such hazards and to ensure that the risks are minimised. Special precautions and educational initiatives should be undertaken. As already indicated, many health concerns cross the work–non-work barrier. The spectrum of chronic disease extends from the serious disabling diseases to the less well-defined conditions which nevertheless produce much suffering and handicap and reduce the quality of life.

Terris[5] has claimed that we are in the period of the second epidemiological revolution (the first having been the effective attack on communicable disease) and that we now have the weapons for the conquest of the leading non-infectious diseases through preventive measures: control of the environment; screening; health education. Health education, he suggests, should include: educating the public to understand the scientific basis for the new public health programmes; educating individuals to change their behaviour in the interests of disease prevention; education to counter the opposition of vested private interests.

Although in the past we have concentrated our efforts on high-risk groups (and this must continue), Rose[6] argues that we must now seek to bring about a smaller alteration in risk factors in a large majority of the population who are at lower risk. 'The mass approach to prevention is the only way to prevent mass disease.' For this, a mass approach with an emphasis on education is the only way. In such an approach the safety of the intervention must be high and this is likely to be so if there is: restoration of biological normality; removal of an undesirable influence; addition of a safe and positive influence.

Such activities are the prime concern of those seeking to promote occupational health and safety, and apply directly to the special group of pregnant women. While the facts of inequality in health indicate a failure, they also point to the exciting possibility of reducing mortality and morbidity and of the gains in both quantity and quality of life that might be achieved if the gap were to be abolished or narrowed.

HEALTH EDUCATION: FAILURES, BARRIERS AND UNCERTAINTY

One of the complaints often levelled at health education is that its most visible component, the mass media campaign, has been ineffective. Perhaps this has been based on a failure to understand not only the wider aspects of health education, but also what can reasonably be expected from mass media campaigns. Budd and McCron[7] have indicated the value of mass media in setting the agenda in health education, but the public recognise the key role of health professionals as sources of advice and information. Health professionals are deemed to be the first source of advice, but the public are frequently disappointed with the quality of advice given. Studies from general practice and occupational health indicate that individuals have considerable contact with health professionals and confirm the potential for health education[8]. While the separation of prevention and care may have been appropriate in the nineteenth century, the complex nature of current health concerns renders the continuing separation illogical at both the theoretical and practical levels.

In Britain prevention and health education are clearly a responsibility of the National Health Service, but they are not the prerogative of any single part of the Service. However, many regard health education as an optional extra or irrelevant in their busy professional practice. Clearly, specialists in community medicine and health education officers have a responsibility for overall policy, support, advice and encouragement to all those who are directly involved in providing care, whether or not they are working in the National Health Service.

The Royal College of General Practitioners[9] has emphasised the importance of prevention and health education in primary care and has indicated the implications for practice.

Many other organisations have a responsibility for education, but there is often misunderstanding, conflicting advice or apathy.

The Health and Safety Commission[10] have a defined responsibility for prevention and for providing information and advice: to identify health hazards; to advise on environmental control; to advise and inform workers and employers of risks; to advise on medical aspects of employment. As their remit is to professionals, employers, employees, unions and the public, they have a most extensive responsibility and are recognised as a source of specialised expertise.

Unions, who are responsible for the welfare of their members, have indicated their involvement in health and safety matters by the development of training programmes for safety representatives, through the publication of booklets and pamphlets and, at the central level, by participation in policy decisions.

Local authorities have a responsibility for environmental health which includes a preventive and health education component in all their routine activities, and, in addition, have certain responsibilities imposed on them by the Health and Safety at Work Act related to work places.

With regard to occupational health services, since there is no legal requirement to have one, there is obviously no legal commitment to any particular activity. The functions of occupational health services are determined by the staff, the management and the particular problems of individual work places. Where there are no occupational health services, there must by law (dependent on the size of the establishment) be the appropriate number of first aiders, but they do not usually have a preventive role.

The responsibility for health and safety as laid down by the Health and Safety at Work Act is well known: in summary, it is a joint responsibility by employer and employee, the employer to provide and the employee to avail himself of what is provided. In industry it is generally accepted that responsibility is associated with status and a person's position in the structure of the organisation[11]. It is accepted that individuals as well as the organisation are liable to allegations of negligence if they do not exert the responsibility that is commensurate with their position — ignorance or failure to prepare themselves for responsibility is no defence.

Is there or should there be a separation between general and specifically occupational prevention and health education? The failure to answer this question has been a key factor in the failure to have effective initiatives in the work place. The ambiguity is based on artificial professional boundaries, lack of certainty about the function of services, professional dog in the manger attitudes

262   *J. McEwen*

and a general lack of training in skills necessary for prevention and health education. We need to base our activities on two aspects of epidemiology – general and specific occupational and combining these to seek to prevent illness and promote health. This can be put into practice by means of two approaches, the first a long-term broad-based health education programme, with accompanying specific programmes for special groups – in this case, educational programmes for pregnant women at work, combining general health and specific occupational problems and hazards.

Finally, there is the necessity of evaluation. Much criticism has been levelled at health education for the failure to demonstrate effectiveness. There are enormous problems in the evaluation of such long-term programmes as health education, but new tools are being developed which may provide an additional dimension to traditional measures of outcome. One is the Nottingham Health Profile (Hunt and McEwen[11a] and Backett *et al.*[11b]). Figures 20.2 and 20.3 show the scores on the Profile, which is a measure of perceived health in a pilot study of women with normal pregnancies.

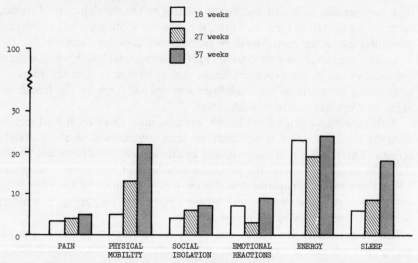

Figure 20.2 Median scores on part I of the Profile at 18, 27 and 37 weeks' pregnancy

PRESENT STATE OF PREVENTION AND HEALTH EDUCATION IN THE WORK PLACE

The Employment Medical Advisory Service Study[12] carried out in 1976 is the only recent national study of occupational health services. It indicated clearly that the most commonly practised activity within occupational health services is the treatment of acute emergencies, minor illness and injury. This study was

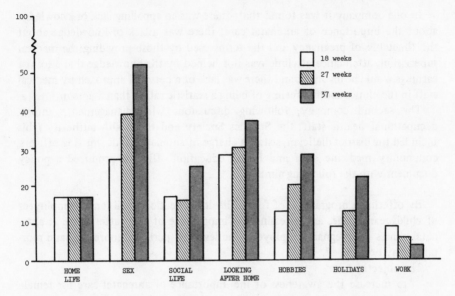

100
50
40
30
20
10
0

□ 18 weeks
▨ 27 weeks
▨ 37 weeks

HOME LIFE   SEX   SOCIAL LIFE   LOOKING AFTER HOME   HOBBIES   HOLIDAYS   WORK

Figure 20.3   Percentage of women reporting problems in each of the seven areas of daily life, at 18, 27 and 37 weeks' gestation

on reported and not recorded activities. Preventive activities and health education did not rank very highly — health education being fifteenth out of eighteen items. A survey based on a questionnaire to occupational health nurses and health education officers is now being analysed. The Health Education Council will publish these results as a follow up to the discussion document on *Health Education in the Work Place*[16]. It is hoped that by reporting these activities, it will encourage others to examine their current practice and develop new programmes.

Probably most prevention and health education at present is opportunistic (apart from routine health examinations) and is related to individual contact through consultation, and therefore is similar to primary care[13]. Here the ease of access to occupational health services provides a continuing and acceptable source of advice and support for the pregnant woman.

Several large companies have long-established screening programmes — usually well women or executives — and, although popular, their value has been challenged. Possibly the greatest value may be the chance to discuss personal and environmental aspects of work and life. Specially designed programmes for groups such as pregnant women have been arranged. Two British companies employing large numbers of women have investigated the problems of pregnant women at the work place and have developed similar practical programmes to meet the perceived needs.

In one company it was found that: there was an appalling lack of knowledge about the importance of antenatal care; there was a lack of knowledge about the timetable of pregnancy and the terms used by those providing the medical supervision; attendance at clinic was not helped by the knowledge that a loss of earnings would be involved; and there was lack of a personal approach by medical staff in the clinics and the feeling of being a statistic rather than a person.

The second company, following discussions with management, unions, occupational health staff, the Spastics Society and the health authority (this included the district dietician, sister in charge of antenatal clinic, nursing officers, community medicine staff and health education officers), produced a policy document with the following aim:

By offering a programme of formal health education to all female employees of child-bearing age, and stressing the importance of early attendance at antenatal clinics for pregnant employees, the levels of perinatal morbidity and mortality may be reduced.

The objectives are:

> to increase the awareness of the importance of antenatal care for female staff;
> to increase rubella vaccination uptake prior to pregnancy;
> to encourage earlier antenatal attendance and to lessen defaulting at antenatal clinics;
> to improve nutrition during pregnancy;
> to increase infant birth weight;
> to reduce smoking during pregnancy;
> to reduce excessive alcohol intake during pregnancy;
> to improve prescribed drug compliance during pregnancy;
> to decrease non-prescribed, non-approved drug taking during pregnancy;
> to increase knowledge of rights — for example, maternity grants, benefits and allowances;
> to support and advise occupational health staff.

A detailed educational programme was devised and a number of incentives were offered to pregnant employees.

An alternative approach has been a planned long-term programme of health education, such as a topic a month, with displays, materials, films, articles in company newspapers, agony columns and referrals to specialist agencies. In some places there has been a renewed interest in sports and exercise, with the emphasis on personal fitness and enjoyment rather than inter-company matches. The LAY (Look After Yourself)[13a] scheme supported by the Health Education Council, which consists of health information, practical exercises and relaxation, is now being developed for greater use in the work place. This approach to positive health would assist in ensuring good general health prior to pregnancy.

Recently the occupational importance of excessive alcohol intake has become a matter of great concern, with companies realising that any policy on problem drinking requires a preventive and educational component. A pilot study in a large national organization, supported by the Health Education Council, will explore the development of educational materials and staff training on alcohol education. The controversial aspects of alcohol intake and pregnancy could be discussed with informed occupational health staff.

Several European countries regard the work place as one target for a wide-ranging and integrated prevention and education programme. This is usually based on a strong national preventive medical approach, and anti-smoking or the related problem of heart disease has often served as a focus. By integrating a series of related programmes aimed at different audiences, it is hoped to achieve maximum impact. It has, for instance, been suggested that it is possible to aim to abolish smoking in one generation. Specific programmes for workers are part of the wider national project. Discussions are taking place between the Health Education Council and the Trades Union Congress over a combined approach to smoking education in the work place.

Health education programmes have been developed more extensively in the USA than in other countries, and this may reflect the high costs to industry of illness and the differences between Britain and the USA in national health care. These programmes are usually broad-based and comprehensive, covering both general health issues and specific occupational problems. Active participation by all concerned in the planning of courses is encouraged. An example of a participatory approach is found in an American study[14] which 'was designed to inform and educate rank and file and low level union leadership' and encourage workers to inform their fellows about the nature of the problem at work. The components of the programme included:

training workers to identify specific occupational hazards and to use legal resources in having these corrected;

developing contact between workers and occupational health specialists;

stimulating understanding of and interest in job health by helping workers write leaflets and hazard information sheets;

setting up accident and health hazards reporting systems;

facilitating links among unions and worker groups facing similar problems.

A reversal of site is found when safety representatives[15] bring their skills to the general practitioners' waiting rooms. There they do the following:

find out what jobs the patients are doing or have done and what conditions were/are like;

supply them with information on hazards at work;

organise meetings around particular issues (e.g. work-related deafness and asthma);

give advice on claiming state benefits and compensation;

point out to the doctors in their practices the role of work in their patient's ill-health.

Health education has made great advances in the schools – through influencing teacher training and through the preparation of well-planned and appropriate curricula. A new generation of young people will be entering the work place with differing attitudes to health, participation and health service provision. They will insist on a great openness to the personal and collective issues of health and the interrelationship between the influences of family, home, work, leisure and unemployment on health.

AN INTEGRATED APPROACH AT THREE LEVELS

Currently, although there are some outstanding examples of new health education programmes, the general picture is one of confusion, misunderstanding, apathy and inactivity. If there are to be any widespread developments, an integrated and co-ordinated approach would seem to be essential. This will require to bring together the three groups mentioned in the title of this chapter and to co-ordinate what is being done within an organisation, with community programmes and at a national level.

Within an organisation

Individuals or sections within an organisation need to be identified to assume responsibility for co-ordination, but even more important is the recognition by management that health should be seen as a policy matter. Health concerns should figure in all major decisions and health issues such as pregnant women should be the subject of specific policies. In small organisations individuals who already have some responsibility for health and safety (e.g. managers, safety representatives or first aiders) should be encouraged to co-ordinate health education.

Local community

The most appropriate way to achieve an integrated and effective approach to health education is to base the responsibility for co-ordination and support at the district health level in the UK. There is a need to co-ordinate activities within an organisation and to relate these to initiatives in the community. Unless we are to postulate substantial increase in funding, additional experienced staff and massive public support, any new development in health education must:

utilise existing resources;
make use of existing health professionals;
be acceptable to public and professionals;
be firmly related to our existing services;
be capable of local adaptation;
not be isolated from health and education;
be related to continuing professional education.

The many opportunities for health education can only be accepted if all health professionals recognise the educational component in their everyday tasks. Not all health professionals have the necessary educational skills, and district health authorities, through their specialists in epidemiology and their health education officers, can provide the appropriate support and help. They can seek to bring about an integrated approach at the primary care level. It is important to integrate activities at the occupational level to community activities — perhaps involving local media and community groups — and to national mass media, publications and debates. Co-operation with health professionals involved in primary care will encourage a common message, and may avoid conflict and discover gaps in advice and support.

One useful way may be to encourage the client group approach, which in the case of pregnant women should bring together prevention and care in an integrated manner for all the relevant health professionals in hospital, community, general practice and the work place.

National

It looks as though the Health Education Council may be able to assume a co-ordinating role. During the past few years it has arranged conferences, seminars and workshops with the aim of bringing diverse people together to lay a foundation for future activities and to stimulate interest. Papers have been prepared and some research has been supported. Perhaps the major role can be in supporting training in health education. Certificate courses in health education exist in centres throughout the UK, and attempts are being made to promote health education in the appropriate basic, undergraduate and professional training.

Continuing professional education may provide a focus and by learning together it may be easier to work together. The proposal for a Primary Health Care Unit for Continuing Education at the Open University for the entire primary care team would seem to be a most significant step in this direction.

The national bodies involved with policy, such as the Health and Safety Commission, the Department of Health and the Health Education Council, already co-operate and should be encouraged to tackle the subjects of common concern. Unlike some other countries, Britain does not have defined health policies or national objectives for health. Such policies, involving differing aspects of government, industry, commerce and service organisations, might do much to stimulate those working at local level.

THE POTENTIAL OF THE WORK PLACE

The potential of the work place can be appreciated if it is considered along-side the settings which offer opportunities for the health education of adults.

The work place has direct contact with a large number of adults of different ages, sex, social class and ethnic group. A significant proportion of this audience, including higher-risk groups, may not be reached effectively in so-called community or patient health education settings. ('Community' refers here to those activities that are organised outside school, clinical or occupational settings. 'Patient' refers to those activities that are organised in clinics, hospitals or general practice surgeries.) Many community health education activities, for example, are criticised because they frequently involve only voluntary or highly motivated people – that is, preaching to the converted. Patient health education activities, by definition, most frequently involve people who are already symptomatic and therefore, typically, are concerned with secondary or tertiary prevention (restoration of health).

The continuity of contact that exists between most adults and their place of work is also valuable: it offers opportunities for reinforcement methods to be built into health education programmes. The work place can offer opportunities for a great variety of health education methods to be applied: one-to-one education or counselling; small group work; talks to larger groups; and use of communication media, such as leaflets, posters, displays or work newspapers.

Occupational health, where it exists, has several advantages which would enable it to act as a focus for new initiatives in prevention and health education. It is clearly established as a discipline involved in preventing ill-health and accidents, and through education and training encouraging health and safety. It is accepted by the adult population as relevant to their needs. In practice it combines prevention and care. Staff are recognised as having a multiplicity of roles. Perhaps the occupational health nurse is one of the best examples of the extended role of the nurse – encompassing care, prevention, education, counselling, administration, environmental monitoring, training and participation in many aspects of the day-to-day functions of the organisation.

Rather than seeing the work force as a captive population who can be subjected to unplanned and irrelevant health education or meaningless routine medical examinations, the challenge is to devise a programme that relates to defined needs, making use of existing staff skills and facilities. It has been traditional for professionals committed to prevention and health education to define the problems as they see them, rather than adopt a participatory approach to planning.

The work place provides an easy route to a better educational strategy of starting where people are and, as in other concerns in the work place, a joint approach to health issues – which may involve education, screening, environmental monitoring, patient education, etc., and the production of policies on shiftwork, smoking, alcohol or canteen meals. There can be an easy interchange between the different health communities of primary care and the work place. As Kickbusch[3] has pointed out: 'People are not just consumers of health care, they provide it themselves.'

CONCLUSIONS

This chapter has addressed itself primarily to health professionals and indicated the task for all of us. This should not be taken to imply that the task is theirs alone. The role of unions, health and safety groups, pressure groups, self-help groups, community groups and individuals must be recognised. The role of different professionals and lay people should ideally be a partnership – providing differing expertise and experience, defining issues and facilitating learning together. Sometimes conflict will be inevitable, as aims and objectives may differ and at times lay expertise may be seen as a threat by the ill-informed professional who is reluctant to participate.

To some the fight for the realisation of health is very much at the centre of the conflict between capital and labour which takes place at the work place and heightens in moments of crisis. Others see the work place as one where people can co-operate to promote health, prevent accidents and improve the quality of life.

There is a strong imperative on us all to participate fully in educational activities related to health and safety – using our existing knowledge and skills and adding to them as necessary. There is no evidence that an effective and planned education approach to health and safety can be other than helpful.

REFERENCES

1. WHO (1969). *Planning and Evaluation of Health Education Services*, Technical Report Series No. 409, WHO, Geneva
2. Department of Education and Science (1977). *Health Education in Schools*, HMSO, London
3. Kickbusch, I. (1981). Involvement in health: a social concept of health education. *International Journal of Health Education*, 24, 3–15
4. DHSS (1980). *Inequalities in Health* (Report of a Research Working Group), DHSS, London
5. Terris, M. (1981). The primacy of prevention. *Preventive Medicine*, 10, 689–699

6.   Rose, G. (1981). Strategy of prevention: lessons from cardiovascular disease. *British Medical Journal*, **282**, 1847–1851

7.   Budd, J. and McCron, R. (1982). *The Role of the Mass Media in Health Education* (Report Prepared for The Health Education Council), Centre for Mass Communication Research, Leicester

8.   McEwen, J., Pearson, J. C. G. and Langham, A. (1982). Procedures, treatments and staff roles in occupational health. *Journal of the Society of Occupational Medicine*, **32**, 101–111

9.   Royal College of General Practitioners (1981). *Health and Prevention in Primary Care* (Report from General Practice 18). RCGP, London

10. Department of Employment (1975). *Employment Medical Advisory Service: A Report of the Work of the Service for 1973 and 1974*, HMSO, London

11. Farmer, D. (1978). Personal responsibilities. *Health and Safety at Work*, **1**, 34–35

11a. Hunt, S. M. and McEwen, J. (1980). The development of a subjective health indicator. *Sociology of Health and Illness*, **2**, 231–246

11b. Backett, E. M., McEwen, J. and Hunt, S. M. (1981). *Health and Quality of Life*. Report to the Social Science Research Council, London

12. Phillips, M. and McEwen, J. (1979). *Private Occupational Health Services in Britain. The EMAS Survey 1976*. Report produced for the Health and Safety Executive, Nottingham Department of Community Health

13. Stott, N. C. H. and Davis, R. H. (1979). The exceptional potential in the primary care consultation. *Journal of the Royal College of General Practitioners*, **29**, 201–205

13a. LAY (Look After Yourself) is a mixture of advertising, posters, publications and training schemes designed to encourage people to look after themselves, with special reference to diet, exercise, smoking, etc.

14. Wegman, D. H., Boden, L. and Levenstein, C. (1975). Health hazard surveillance by industrial workers. *American Journal of Public Health*, **65**, 26–30

15. BSSRS (1982). Example of safety representatives in a doctor's waiting room in Sheffield. *Hazards Bulletin*, August, 12

16. Randell, J., Wear, G. and McEwen, J. (1984). *Health Education in the Workplace*, Health Education Council, London

Part 4
Conclusions

21

Future Research on Work in Pregnancy

JO GARCIA and DIANA ELBOURNE

In this chapter we shall review studies which deal with the association between paid employment and pregnancy outcome and end by proposing lines for further research. Although we do not deal with specific work place hazards, we shall mention particular aspects of work which seem to be associated with pregnancy outcomes.

PAID EMPLOYMENT

In 1981 married women accounted for about a quarter of the economically active population in Great Britain[1]. Their pattern of activity by age is compared with that of men in table 21.1.

Of those married women who are employees (as opposed to unemployed or self-employed), more than half work part-time[1]. Whether or not they have dependent children not surprisingly influences their participation in paid work, as indicated in table 21.2. Whether married or unmarried, women tend to be

Table 21.1 Economic activity rates (%) by age for men and for married women, Great Britain, 1981[1]

Age (years)	Men (%)	Married women (%)
16–19	68.6	47.8
20–24	90.3	55.6
25–34	97.2	51.3
35–49	96.9	67.5
50–59	92.4	57.7
60–64	69.6	23.2
65 and over	10.5	4.7

273

Table 21.2 Percentage of women aged 16–59 working, by presence of dependent children in household, Great Britain, 1980[4]

	No dependent children in household		All with dependent children in household	Youngest child 0–4
	Non-married	Married		
Working full-time	60	42	17	7
Working part-time	7	26	36	23
Not working	33	31	46	70
No. in sample (= 100%)	2172	2441	4175	1485

concentrated in certain sectors of the economy (distribution and services, as opposed to industry) and to work in certain jobs within those sectors (particularly clerical jobs). Their earnings, while substantially lower than men's (women's median earnings just prior to a pregnancy were about 60 per cent of their husband's in a study carried out in 1979[2]), play an important part in maintaining household income[3]. Although a smaller proportion of married women are classified formally as unemployed compared with men and non-married women, there is evidence that married women are far more likely to be seeking work but not registered as unemployed[4]. A proportion of them are also interested in employment but do not seek work because of child-care difficulties. In general, women with young children are liable to work part-time in a succession of poorly paid jobs with little or no career progression[5]. The majority of men with dependent children are in full-time employment and, incidentally, are likely to spend more hours a week at work than men without children[5].

UNPAID WORK

Housework and the care of children and other adults takes up an important part of the time and energy of most women. Results from surveys and time-budget studies suggest that neither the increase in mechanical and technical aids for housework nor the larger proportion of women in paid employment has much reduced the time spent by women on housework, or increased the amount of housework done by men[6]. Housework is often physically taxing, especially for those who care for children or elderly people. The burden of such work may be increased for those who are less well off and who lack private transport or live in substandard housing. Even for the better off, housework is often lonely and isolated work. Women's participation in paid work may be relatively easy to measure but gives an incomplete picture of the demands made upon women's time and energy.

Douglas[7,8], in his analysis of the data derived for a national sample of births in 1946, was particularly concerned to take into account all aspects of the circumstances of child-bearing women. He found that help with household tasks in late pregnancy was least available to those who needed it most. Mothers with more children and those married to men in manual occupations were less likely to receive help and more likely to start full household duties sooner than other mothers. The help available to mothers married to men in manual and in professional occupations is illustrated in figure 21.1. Douglas also found that help in the home from relatives and friends in the last 3 months of pregnancy was associated with a lower proportion of babies of low birth weight among primiparae and

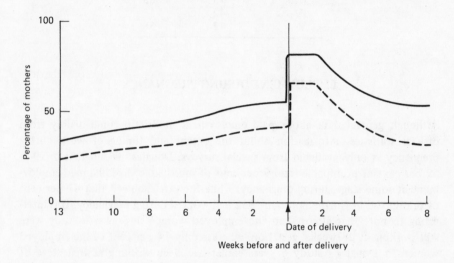

Figure 21.1 Help in the home before and after birth. Professional and manual worker groups compared, Great Britain 1946. Solid line, professional and salaried workers' wives receiving help; dashed line, manual workers' wives receiving help. (From reference 7)

mothers with a confinement within the preceding 2 years. He concluded[8]: 'Only a small proportion of women are able, or can afford, to engage domestic help during pregnancy, and assistance, often for inadequate periods, is mainly supplied by relatives or friends; even so, less than half had been helped. Every effort should be made to remedy this situation by the provision of a domestic help service for women during the last weeks of pregnancy as well as during the lying-in period.' Daniel's study[2] of a national sample of 2400 recent British mothers carried out in 1979 showed that women married to men in social classes IV and V were less likely than other women to have help in the home during the first month after the birth (table 21.3). It is unlikely that the need for help with domestic tasks perceived by Douglas has disappeared, and research into effective and acceptable forms of such help is desirable, though, sadly, unlikely to be given priority.

Table 21.3 Extent to which mothers had some help in the first month after the birth[2]

Social class of father	Some help (%)	No help (%)
I	59	41
II	54	46
IIIN	51	49
IIIM	45	55
IV	42	58
V	42	58

EMPLOYMENT DURING PREGNANCY

Although general data about paid employment in Britain come mainly from official statistics, information about the extent and timing of work during pregnancy is only available from special surveys. Douglas[7] found that in 1946 58 per cent of primiparae (and 9 per cent of multiparae) had had paid employment at some stage during pregnancy, while Stewart[9] showed that 41 per cent of primiparae in Northampton in 1952 had worked during pregnancy. It is interesting to note that almost half the employed women in Stewart's study were still working at 28 weeks' gestation, whereas only 14 per cent of the employed women in Douglas's study 6 years earlier had been working at that stage of pregnancy. Stewart's sample may not have been representative of the picture in the country as a whole.

Data from two recent surveys provide more up to date information about employment in pregnancy, and are presented in table 21.4. Daniel[2] found that 48 per cent of the 2400 recent mothers in his sample had been in paid employment during pregnancy and that two-thirds of these were still working 12 weeks before delivery. Boyd and Sellars' survey of 6000 British women who volunteered in response to a television programme (carried out in 1981)[10] found that 45 per cent of all women were in paid employment during pregnancy. The duration of work is not presented in a way comparable to that of Daniel's survey. Sixty-one per cent were still working at gestations of 29 weeks and over.

It is obvious, but nonetheless important, that pregnant women in paid employment differ from those without such employment. Some differences will be unsurprising and relatively easy to measure — for example, parity or educational level. Others, such as health or access to a social network that provides jobs, may be more subtle but are nevertheless important in interpreting any observed differences in pregnancy outcome.

Parity emerged as a crucial influence in Daniel's study. Eighty-five per cent of first-time mothers and less than a third of other mothers had been in paid work

Table 21.4 Employment during pregnancy at different gestations in recent British studies

Time of ceasing work in weeks before delivery[a]	% of employed mothers[a]
≤ 11	57
≤ 12	72
13–20	9
17–25	11
≥ 26	6
Time of ceasing work in weeks' gestation[b]	**% of employed mothers[b]**
≤ 12	6
13–20	7
21–28	26
29–36	57
37–40	4

[a] Reference 2.
[b] Reference 10.

12 months before the birth of their baby. Although a small number of respondents gave up work just before becoming pregnant, these figures give a reasonable guide to the characteristics of those employed in pregnancy. Most first-time mothers worked full-time compared with only about a tenth of those with children. It is interesting to note that single women and those married to unemployed men were less likely than other women to be working during their first pregnancy. By contrast, when expecting a second or subsequent baby, single and separated women were more likely to be working.

Studies from other countries, which will be described in more detail below, show differences between employed and non-employed women in terms of parity, age, marital status, educational level, ethnic origin, region of residence and other characteristics. Some of these differences are illustrated in the French data[11] given in tables 21.5–21.7, which also show that employed women attend antenatal care earlier and more regularly (table 21.8) and are more likely to be seen antenatally by an obstetrician or in the hospital where they plan to give birth.

Observational studies which relate employment to pregnancy outcomes are difficult to interpret because of the range of documented and undocumented differences which we have discussed. This is just one reason why the subject is one where the potential for fruitful collaboration between researchers with medical and social or economic backgrounds is particularly great.

Table 21.5 Characteristics of employed and non-employed pregnant women, France, 1976[11]

	Employed (%)	Non-employed (%)
Age		
19 or less	6.1	10.3
20–24	41.2	34.1
25–29	38.7	34.2
30–34	10.4	13.9
35 or more	3.6	7.4
No. of women	1942	1251

Table 21.6 Characteristics of employed and non-employed pregnant women, France, 1976[11]

	Employed (%)	Non-employed (%)
Parity		
0	57.8	26.8
1	33.6	37.5
2 or more	8.6	35.7
No. of women	1947	1262

Table 21.7 Characteristics of employed and non-employed pregnant women, France, 1976[11]

	Employed (%)	Non-employed (%)
Profession of child's father:		
agricultural	4.0	3.4
small businesses	4.9	5.7
higher professional	10.5	10.1
middle professional	17.0	9.7
employees (n.m.)	15.1	11.4
skilled workers	25.1	24.7
other workers	23.5	35.0
No. of women	1811	1152

Table 21.8 Antenatal care of employed and non-employed pregnant women, France 1976[11]

	Employed (%)	Non-employed (%)
No. of consultations:		
less than legal minimum	4.4	10.1
legal minimum	24.9	34.8
more than legal minimum	70.7	55.2
No. of women	1935	1251
First consultation after 3 months' gestation	5.7	7.4
No. of women	1724	1049
Antenatal preparation (for primiparae)	49.7	29.8
No. of women	1102	336

INFLUENCE OF EMPLOYMENT ON PREGNANCY OUTCOME

The main question posed by researchers is whether women's paid employment itself is associated with particular adverse pregnancy outcomes. Additional questions relate to the impact of work at different gestations, the risks and benefits of particular kinds of employment and the effects of other aspects of work such as fatigue, duration and posture. Because few studies have sufficiently large populations, the adverse outcomes examined have only rarely included mortality and have tended to focus on birth weight, gestational age and sometimes on measures of pregnancy illness. An Appendix gives a description of the main studies considered here, and summarises the results of each study.

Of the three British studies carried out in the late 1940s and early 1950s[7,9,12], two[7,9] found evidence of an association between employment in the later months of pregnancy and reduced birth weight in primiparous women.

In Stewart's study this association persisted after taking into account differences between employed and non-employed women in respect of the social class of their husbands, and their civil status at the time of conception. No association of birth weight with employment was observed in the study by Illsley and his colleagues[12]. Douglas was surprised to note that women who worked in the early part of pregnancy had a smaller proportion of babies of low birth weight than those who did not work at all. He suggests that this might be due to the higher proportion of the former who had some domestic help in the last 3 months of pregnancy.

Although most of the other available studies have been carried out since 1970, data from the 1959–1966 US Collaborative Perinatal Project have recently been published[13]. This study shows an association between reduced mean birth weight in full-term infants of women working in the last trimester of pregnancy, as compared with women not in paid work, and women who gave up work at earlier gestations. Those with low pre-pregnancy weight, a small pregnancy weight gain and hypertension have lower average birth weights. These data are difficult to interpret because the process of selection of the women studied is not indicated. Numbers of women in the various categories of the analysis are not given and the impact of withdrawing pre-term deliveries is not explored. The authors conclude that standing work is associated with reduced mean birth weight, but the data presented on standing and sitting work are difficult to assess. The adoption of the mean birth weight of those women not working outside the home as a standard is also problematic. The paper does, however, indicate that women working late in pregnancy (15 per cent of white women and 10 per cent of black women were employed at 33 weeks' gestation in their sample, which may not be representative of pregnant women in the US at that time) may be at risk of having babies of reduced birth weight in certain circumstances, especially if other adverse factors are present.

McDowell *et al.*[14] have used longitudinally linked data from the 1971 census and vital registration to examine the mortality of children born to mothers whose employment status was recorded at the census. Despite the small numbers, they discerned an increase in infant deaths among pregnant mothers who were employed at the time of the census. Nevertheless, almost all the observed differences might have been expected, because women having pre-term births would be more likely to be working at the census date than women whose pregnancies lasted longer.

In 1972 the first French national birth survey[15,16] showed a positive association between paid work and low birth weight for gestational age, but negative association with curtailed gestation and stillbirth (table 21.9). In 1976 a second national survey[11,17] showed no significant association between paid employment and either mean birth weight, birth weight less than 2500 g or low birth weight for gestational age (table 21.10). There were higher rates of all these outcomes for those without paid employment but these associations could all be ascribed to chance. Pre-term delivery, however, was significantly associated with

Table 21.9 Pregnancy outcomes according to the employment status of the mother, France, 1972[11,15]

	Employed	Non-employed
Stillbirth rate	6.7 per 1000	13.7 per 1000
Curtailed gestation ($<$ 37 weeks)	7.4%	9.3%
Low birth weight for gestational age	6.1%	3.9%

(All statistically significant at 0.001 level)

Table 21.10 Birth weight and gestational age according to occupational status of mother during pregnancy, France, 1976[17]

Indicator	Work in pregnancy	
	Yes	No
Mean birth weight (g)	3282	3310
	(1951)	*(1259)*
Birth weight < 2500 g (%)	5.4	6.1
	(1951)	*(1259)*
Gestation ≤ 36 completed weeks (%)	5.1[b]	7.5[b]
	(1866)	*(1171)*
Intrauterine growth retardation (%)[a]	5.0	5.8
	(1795)	(1114)

Figures in italic type show numbers of women.
[a] Birth weight lower than the 5th percentile of birth weight distribution according to gestational age.
[b] $P < 0.01$.

lack of paid employment. Gofin[18], in his study of women in West Jerusalem in 1970–1972, found a statistically significant association between low birth weight and lack of paid employment, but no association with duration of gestation.

The most recent French findings, taken together with Gofin's study, suggest a clear advantage for women in paid employment, although the authors stress the differences between those with and without paid employment, both in social and demographic characteristics and in terms of their access to antenatal care. These studies also draw attention to certain categories of working women who do not seem to share in the advantage associated with paid work. In Gofin's study these are women married to men in lower social classes and those born in North Africa or Asia (as opposed to Europe, America or Israel). In both these groups women's own work during pregnancy was more likely to be classified as involving moderately heavy or heavy physical activity, as opposed to light.

The first French national birth survey shows quite marked differences in the proportion of pre-term deliveries between women in different occupations, with manual, shop and service workers having higher rates. The 1976 figures show similar differences which do not reach statistical significance. Two other French studies show high rates of pre-term delivery among women in medical work[19,20].

Aspects of the work itself have been linked to pre-term delivery in several French studies[11,19,20]. In the 1976 survey higher rates of prematurity were associated with standing work, a working week of over 42 hours, and a long journey to work (for those women working 42 hours a week). Mamelle and co-workers[20], in a study in Lyon, showed a positive association between pre-term delivery and an index of fatigue which comprised measures of posture, machine work, physical effort, repetitive gestures and other physical aspects of the work.

Overall, the varied and sometimes conflicting findings of these studies should not surprise us. For one woman paid work may entail a long working week, poor surroundings, long bus rides and physical and emotional stresses. For another, paid work may mean companionship, regular breaks and a good working environment. For both women the potential importance of earnings to their own well-being and that of their families should not be underestimated. Not only do women differ in the kinds of paid work that they do, but also the characteristics of those who are in paid work vary widely between and within countries. In some places child-bearing women may go out to work only where compelled to by poverty. In other settings those who stay at home are the least favoured in financial or educational terms.

Although the studies reviewed here provide little basis for fearing adverse effects of paid employment for the majority of women, they offer rather limited guidance to an individual woman. How can a woman weigh up, for example, suggestions that the kind of job she does or the hours that she works may be associated with a small increase in the chance of a baby of low birth weight? She may be the family's sole breadwinner. She may have ample help at home.

Clinicians also face problems in trying to advise individual women about employment (and, incidentally, many other activities in pregnancy). Mamelle's findings of an association between pre-term labour and a cumulative index of fatigue could provide occupational health staff and other care-givers with an opportunity to support a woman's request for a change of work during pregnancy.

SOME DIRECTIONS FOR RESEARCH

It is probably not useful or interesting to go on asking whether employment *per se* is a good or a bad thing in pregnancy. Women, policy-makers, trade unionists and clinicians are looking for information about aspects of employment, housework and other activities which can be taken into account in the often limited space for making decisions.

On the basis of existing findings, such as those of Mamelle, researchers could usefully analyse existing data sets for further information about particular aspects of employment. It may, however, be necessary to mount special prospective observational studies in order to collect detailed data on aspects of employment not routinely available. Large numbers are needed for successful analyses. Mamelle's findings raise the question of particular aspects of housework that may be identified in the same way as she has found associations between features of paid employment and an adverse pregnancy outcome. Quantification of household tasks is certainly not easy, but is an important next step.

At a rather basic level, women's often limited choices about paid employment in pregnancy can be extended by a knowledge of the existing financial and employment measures. These measures, such as paid leave or paid time off to attend antenatal care, are often very difficult to understand and to benefit from. Very few studies have looked at women's own perceptions of work of all kinds during pregnancy, or have explored the decisions that families are making. An exception was a study of 30 women in London who had worked during pregnancy[21], which, among other findings, gave some useful insights into the way that employment protection legislation works in practice. Daniel[2] provided information which was unavailable from routinely collected statistics, about the workings of the British employment protection legislation and the practical consequences of child-bearing for women's employment. Policy-makers in most Western countries have already taken the view that both prohibitive and protective measures should be introduced to regulate the employment of pregnant women. Paid maternity leave has the dual function of encouraging women to stop work and providing income maintenance.

Information derived from observational studies is used in debates about legislative changes[8,22]. The interaction of protective legislation with fiscal policies, employment trends and child-care provisions has led to a complex situation where, at least within the present political context, measures likely to benefit particular categories of workers are not always easy to discern[23,24]. For example, legislation which protects women from particular kinds of employment may have adverse consequences for some women in terms of income. An important first requirement is often documentation of the impact of new policies. Do women make use of paid time off for antenatal care or take advantage of their rights to maternity leave?[2] Second, if we introduce a policy with the aim of securing an improvement in health or well-being, however defined, can we provide any evidence that such an improvement occurs and is linked to the policy change? In many instances it is impossible to draw such a conclusion. Observational studies may suggest policy changes (political and moral values enter and influence the changes we want), but the adequate evaluation of such changes often demands experimental studies.

This is a field where some experimental studies are clearly ruled out for practical or political reasons. The possibilities of allocating pregnant women at random to different kinds of employment or of manipulating statutory rights are limited. There is room, however, for some useful and imaginative experimental studies in this field. One study, which seeks to evaluate the impact of a family worker on the outcome of pregnancy in women who may be at risk of giving birth to a baby of low birth weight is already under way in Manchester[25]. Another, which puts more emphasis on social support and the consequences of stress in pregnancy, has been proposed[26]. Both studies employ a randomised design.

Work place studies could, for example, allow a comparison between fixed and flexible rest breaks for pregnant women. A French policy document[22] suggested that the extent of sick leave taken during pregnancy might indicate the need for an extension of paid maternity leave. A case could be made out for a comparison of extra leave taken at any point in pregnancy with a fixed period added to that already given. Allowing women greater scope for changes in the type of work that they do during pregnancy could also be assessed with a randomised design. In all these cases care is needed both in the preliminary exploration of the situation and in seeking appropriate outcome measures. Unintended consequences are very likely when interventions are made in an already complex situation.

We need to embark on research which takes seriously the whole context of women's paid and unpaid work and which can examine the impact of minor or major changes in their social or economic circumstances or the health care that they receive.

ACKNOWLEDGEMENTS

We should like to thank our colleagues at the National Perinatal Epidemiology Unit for their comments on this chapter and the Department of Health and Social Security for their support of the Unit.

REFERENCES

1. Office of Population Censuses and Surveys (1982). *Labour Force Survey 1981*, HMSO, London
2. Daniel, W. W. (1980). *Maternity Rights: The Experience of Women*, report No. 588, Policy Studies Institute, London
3. Hamill, L. (1978). *Wives as Sole and Joint Breadwinners*, Government Economic Service Working Papers, No. 13, HMSO, London
4. Office of Population Censuses and Surveys (1982). *General Household Survey, 1980*, HMSO, London
5. Moss, P. and Fonda, N. (Eds.) (1980). *Work and the Family*, Temple Smith, London
6. Oakley, A. (1981). *Subject Women*, Martin Robertson, Oxford
7. Douglas, J. W. B. (1948). *Maternity in Great Britain*, Oxford University Press, London
8. Douglas, J. W. B. (1950). Some factors associated with prematurity: the results of a national study. *J. Obstet. Gynaecol. Br. Emp.*, 57, 143–170
9. Stewart, A. (1955). A note on the obstetric effects of work during pregnancy. *Br. J. Prev. Soc. Med.*, 9, 159–161
10. Boyd, C. and Sellars, L. (1982). *The British Way of Birth*, Pan, London
11. Saurel-Cubizolles, M. J. (1982). Activité processionnelle des femmes enceintes: comportement medical et issue de grossesse: approche socio-historique et epidémiologique. Thesis, University of Paris I
12. Illsley, R., Billewicz, W. Z. and Thompson, A. M. (1954). Prematurity and paid work during pregnancy. *Br. J. Prev. Soc. Med.*, 8, 153–156

13. Naeye, R. L. and Peters, E. C. (1982). Working during pregnancy; effects on the fetus. *Pediatrics*, **69**, 724–727

14. McDowell, M., Goldblatt, P. and Fox, J. (1981). Employment during pregnancy and infant mortality. *Pop. Trends*, **26**, 12–15

15. Rumeau-Rouquette, C. and Unit 149 (1979) *Naitre en France*, INSERM, Paris

16. Saurel-Cubizolles, M. J. (1979). Influence de l'activité professionnelle de la femme enceinte sur la déroulement et l'issue de la grossesse. *Mémoire de Maîtrise en Sociologie, Université René Descartes, Paris*

17. Saurel, M. J. and Kaminski, M. (1983). Pregnant women at work. *Lancet*, 475 (letter)

18. Gofin, J. (1979). The effect on birth weight of employment during pregnancy. *J. Biosoc. Sci.*, **11**, 259–267

19. Estryn, M., Kaminski, M., Franc, M., Fermand, S. and Gerstle, F. (1979). Grossesse et conditions de travail en milieu hospitalier. *Rev. Fr. Gynec.*, **73**, 625–631

20. Mamelle, N., Munoz, F., Colin, D., Charvet, F. and Lazar, P. (1981). Fatigue professionnelle et prematurité. *Arch. Mal. Profess.*, **42**, 211–216

21. Rodmell, S. and Smart, L. (1982). *Pregnant at Work: The Experiences of Women*, The Open University

22. Inspection Generales des Affaires Sociales. (1980). *Protection Sociale et Mutations Socio-economiques*, Rapport annuel, Paris

23. Equal Opportunities Commission (1979). *Health and Safety Legislation: Should We Distinguish Between Men and Women?* HMSO, London

24. Coyle, A. (1980). The protection racket? *Fem. Rev.*, **4**, 1–12

25. Spencer, B. (n.d.) Personal communication

26. Oakley, A. (n.d.) Social factors and pregnancy outcome. Unpublished research proposal

27. Figa'-Talamanca, I. (1980). A study of environmental and behavioural factors affecting pregnancy outcome in an Italian community. *Pop. Environ.*, **3**, 107–124

28. Marguet, G., Michel-Briand, C., Quichon, R. and Schirrer, J. (1977). Influence de la situation professionnelle de la femme sur l'enfant à naître. *Arch. Mal. Profess.*, **38**, 329–346

29. Hemminki, K., Niemi, M.-L., Saloniemi, I., Vainio, H. and Hemminki, E. (1980). Spontaneous abortions by occupation and social class in Finland. *Int. J. Epidemiol.*, **9**, 149–153

APPENDIX OF PUBLISHED STUDIES

Study Population

Findings

1944 working class primiparae drawn from mothers of 13 257 singleton births in one week in 1946 (Great Britain)[7,8].

Positive association between low birth weight (LBW) and later gestation at leaving work.

Positive association between LBW and no help in the home in last 3 months of pregnancy. Both associations persist when maternal age is controlled for.

206 legitimate, singleton births in 1952 and 1953 to Aberdeen primiparae matched for women's age, height, main occupation, pre- or post-marital conception and husband's social class[12].

No association between LBW and later gestation at leaving work.

1318 singleton births to Northampton primiparae, matched for maternal age, pre- or post-marital conception and social class[9].

Positive association between LBW and later gestation at leaving work.

7722 singleton births to USA mothers between 1959 and 1966. Analysed by maternal age, race, socio-economic status, education, smoking, parity, pre-pregnancy weight, net weight gain, hypertension[13].

Reduced mean birth weight in full-term births associated with employment at later gestations in some sub-samples.

161 women who had had an infant death, 92 who had had a stillbirth and 239 controls from Perugia (1970–1975)[27].

Association between type of occupation and stillbirth and infant death.

4574 births to British women in April–December 1971. Mothers' employment status recorded at the census. Gestation at census and birth not available[14].

Positive association between employment in week before census and infant mortality, which persists when maternal age, parity, housing tenure and socio-economic status taken into account.

708 singleton live births to mothers in West Jerusalem between 1970 and 1972. Multivariate analysis including parity, certain pregnancy complications, smoking, social class and country of origin[18].

No association between employment and pregnancy complications or length of gestation. Employment is associated with a lower proportion of LBW but does not emerge as a significant factor in a multivariate analysis.

French national stratified sample of 11 254 births in 1972[15,16].

Positive association between employment in pregnancy and LBW for gestational age. Negative association between employment in pregnancy and curtailed gestation. Association between certain

Study Population	Findings
	types of employment and curtailed gestation, with non-employed women having a higher proportion of pregnancies of curtailed gestation than all employed women taken together but a lower proportion than women in particular jobs.
299 women resident in one *département* who delivered in a hospital in Besançon in a specified period in 1974[28].	No association between employment in pregnancy and LBW for gestational age or curtailed gestation. Employed mothers had more antenatal visits, were more likely to breast-feed and more likely to smoke during pregnancy.
Records of all hospital in-patient admissions for spontaneous abortion between 1973 and 1975 (18 733 women) in Finland[29].	Positive association between hospitalisation for spontaneous abortion and employment in industrial and construction sector as compared with other sectors; and in unskilled workers as opposed to other occupational grades.
2100 births to women in two maternity hospitals in France between 1977 and 1979[20].	Negative association between employment in pregnancy and curtailed gestation. Positive linear association between hours worked a week and curtailed gestation. Positive linear association between a cumulative index of fatigue and curtailed gestation. No association between self-assessed household duties and curtailed gestation.
French national stratified sample of 4685 women in 1976. Analysis of employment data carried out for 3218 women[11,17].	Negative association between employment in pregnancy and curtailed gestation. No association between employment in pregnancy and birth weight, LBW for gestational age and LBW. Positive association between curtailed gestation and: standing work, long working week.

22

Adverse Influences of the Working Environment

G. CHAMBERLAIN

This volume is based upon a meeting held at the Royal Society of Medicine in 1983; the contributors to the chapters were the major speakers but much discussion was generated by the other hundred participants to the conference, and some of this forms the basis of this concluding chapter.

The problems of the pregnant woman at work is within one band of the whole spectrum of reproductive function in the modern working environment. Both male and female workers are exposed to a series of known, guessed at and potential physical and chemical factors which might affect reproductive function. They may act at many levels; there may be an effect on spermatogenesis or ovum release; potency or capacity for sexual intercourse might be affected; there may be a noxious influence causing very early abortions so that women do not even know they are pregnant; the rate of known abortions may be increased; there might be an increased incidence of congenital abnormalities affecting the unborn child. All these effects could be important in assessing total reproductive function, but this conference purposely confined itself to looking at those who got past the early pregnancy stages and actually knew they were pregnant. After childbirth there are all the influences of the working environment on lactation, infant feeding and the rearing of the child. Indeed, some would go further and suggest that reproductive success was also shown in the capacity of the offspring of the woman to reproduce also. These factors, too, while important, were outside the scope of this conference at the Royal Society of Medicine.

It was stressed many times that women work in more ways than just paid employment. Every woman has a home in which she works, often harder than outside. She is doing housework, preparing meals, clearing the house and looking after the needs of other members of the family. This is the baseline on top of which must be added the stresses of travel to and from employment, and only then can we consider the problems that occur in the work place itself.

At the place of paid work there are obviously specific hazards of a physical or a chemical nature. These are stressed in several chapters, and include solvents,

289

cleaning fluids and X-rays. Some of them we know about and can avoid, while others need more research. With some 2000 new chemicals a year being brought onto the market, the adequate testing of these for safety would present enormous logistic problems. Further, there is a ten-times backlog of chemicals already in use which have never been subjected to rigorous testing. Because of this excess of substances for testing some organisations, such as the Committee of Safety Medicine in the United Kingdom, have made a policy to test the drugs this excess of substances for testing, some organisations, such as the Committee

As well as the specific hazards, there are the general problems of pregnant women in the work place. Some jobs are demanding, and we should consider the fatigue of work, and the problems of standing at a production line or of working in unusual postures. As well as the physical loads, there is a variable amount of mental stress in certain jobs. We are bad at measuring the effects of physical agents but worse at examining the mental ones. To these can be added tiredness and the stress induced by getting to and from work.

One of the major problems in this field was the setting up of standards. We need to know more about potential feto-toxic agents. The levels of safety would need vigorous definition – a preliminary standard might be that the risk to those in any work place should not be greater than that in the general population. A good example is the current concern over use by pregnant operators of the visual display units (VDU) common in industry and business. Apparent causal associations have been fabricated with pregnancy mishap but there is little acceptably scientific evidence at the moment that shows this to be true. This might be because there is no true association or because it has not been properly assessed. Studies which present evidence of an apparently contradictory nature do not lead to easy public interpretation. More information is needed and this can come only through many disciplines. Epidemiologists in observational surveys can provide clues but often these assess a single factor after a long time has passed; it may be the best that we can do and then we have to move to interventional studies which may be required to confirm these. Perhaps the work on *Hydra* described in Chapter 11 may shorten the time period of intervention work, but trans-species extrapolations have always been suspect and are capable of misinterpretation. Physiologists can work on other species or on isolated organ systems as well as on intact humans, and they can present results which need interpretation for the whole human. Teratologists can correlate data from a wide variety of sources; allowing for species differences, they attempt to make informed hypotheses. In all, medical monitoring of reproductive endpoints can only answer specific issues at specific and laid-down points in the process.

When this information is known, the next stage will be the education of all who work or look after workers. The employees themselves, male and female, should be better informed about what we really know of hazards to the pregnant woman. Just as important, they should be informed when evidence is substantiated that a given factor is not a real hazard; thus, true judgements can be made and many women helped to take their proper place in society rather than be offered the protective attitude as an overall blanket implying that all work must be wrong because our Victorian forebears thought so.

It seems that the fetus cannot really be protected by law even in the USA. When we know more, we may be able to set up certain advisory standards, but even so it will rest upon the right of a worker to choose eventually. Further, we can only offer protection against those features we know about and it is doubtful whether we shall ever become omnipotent in this field. We can try to push back the barriers a little further each year but it is difficult to introduce preventive means with any great confidence. Those who want to hold back point first at the costs of preventive measures, and then doubt the credibility of the studies which support the implications of tighter controls in the work place.

This conference raised more questions than it provided answers, often the sign of good discussion. It showed that even with some of the best workers and interpreters of the subject in the Western World being available, there are large areas in which we are relatively uninformed. It is hoped that the meeting will act as a stimulus to more research on the subject of 'Pregnant Women and Work' so that we can build on the days spent at the Royal Society of Medicine in the summer of 1983.

Index